Individual Psychotherapy
and the Science
of Psychodynamics

D1388777

Individual Psychotherapy and the Science of Psychodynamics

Second edition

David H Malan, DM, FRCPsych
Tavistock Clinic

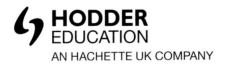

HODDER
EDUCATION
AN HACHETTE UK COMPANY

First published in Great Britain in 1995 by Butterworth Heinemann.

This impression reprinted in 2010 by
Hodder Arnold, an imprint of Hodder Education,
an Hachette UK Company
338 Euston Road, London NW1 3BH

www.hoddereducation.com

Whilst the advice and information in this book is believed to be true and
accurate at the date of going to press, neither the authors nor the publisher
can accept any legal responsibility or liability for any errors or omissions
that may be made. In particular (but without limiting the generality of the
preceding disclaimer) every effort has been made to check drug dosages;
however, it is still possible that errors have been missed. Furthermore,
dosage schedules are constantly being revised and new side-effects
recognized. For these reasons the reader is strongly urged to consult the
drug companies' printed instructions before administering any of the drugs
recommended in this book.

British Library Cataloguing in Publication Data
A catalogue record for this book is available from the British Library

Library of Congress Cataloging in Publication Data
A catalog record for this book is available from the Library of Congress

ISBN 978 0 7506 2387 2

12 13 14

Printed and bound by CPI Group (UK) Ltd, Croydon, CR0 4YY

What do you think about this book? Or any other Hodder Arnold title?
Please send your comments to www.hoddereducation.com

Contents

Preface to the Second Edition

In this second edition the approach that I have used is absolutely unchanged, consisting of illustrating the observations of psychodynamics and the technique of psychotherapy with actual case histories; but I have aimed to consider certain subjects more fully than were covered in the first edition. The most important of these are: the relation with the mother in the male Oedipus complex, disturbances in the relation with siblings, and the two obscure phenomena of masochism and the 'compulsion to repeat'. I have thought out more clearly the Law of Increased Disturbance, realizing that whether or not patients break down in psychotherapy depends to a large extent on the balance between the disturbing nature of the technique used, on the one hand, and the amount of support provided on the other.

I have also been able to add further follow-up information on many of the patients described in the first edition; and I am glad to say that most of them retained their original gains and matured further.

Several of the additional case histories are summarized from much fuller accounts given in *Psychodynamics, training and outcome in brief psychotherapy* (Malan and Osimo, 1992), also published by Butterworth-Heinemann.

I hope the result will be a more complete textbook of dynamic psychotherapy, and further strong support for the scientific status of psychodynamics.

D.H.M.

A note on how this book may be used

In this book the principles of dynamic psychotherapy, from the most elementary to some of the most profound, are presented in logical order, but almost entirely in connection with illustrative true stories which are told as they happened. Such stories are practically never simple, and hence most of them illustrate several different principles and ideas at the same time. This means that if the reader wishes to learn about such a concept as 'transference' or 'acting out', he will find it discussed and illustrated in various different places in the book in connection with a number of different stories, often with cross-references one to the other.

I hope this book is entertaining enough to be read in sequence like a novel. But it can also be used for reference. For this purpose all the reader has to do is to look up any particular concept in the index or the table of contents, and turn to the appropriate passages. In the first of these the concept will usually be defined, and in any subsequent passages it will be further illustrated and elaborated.

Throughout this book I have often used 'he', 'his' etc. as a substitute for the cumbersome 'he or she', 'his or her' etc. This is purely in the interests of brevity, and no sexist implications are intended.

D.H.M.

Acknowledgements

First of all I should like to express my deep gratitude to all those patients who have given permission for their material to be published. If any patient whose permission I have not asked recognizes himself or herself, may I both apologize and say that in most cases the material has been carefully disguised; that it is published with sympathy and respect; and that the ultimate aim is for psychotherapy to be more understood and generally accepted, and hence for more people to be helped by it.

I am greatly indebted to the following colleagues for clinical material: Enid Balint, John Boreham, Roy Butler, Austin Case, Cecilia Clementel, Beverly Cohen, Barbara Cottman, Philip Crockatt, Paddy Daniel, Nicole Desjarlais, Benjamin Esrock, Harwant Gill, Sadie Gillespie, William Grant, Dennis Heath, Peter Hildebrand, Joseph Jacobs, Wallace Joffe, Anne Kilcoyne, Jill Leonard, Agnes Main, Tom Main, Gabriel Manasse, Michael Michalacopoulos, Richard Mackie, Marilyn Miller-Pietroni, Ellen Noonan, Pippa Norris, Samuel Packer, Malcolm Pines, Eric Rayner, Andrew Samuels, Gustav Schulman, Rafael Springmann, Judith Stephens, Jane Temperley, Pierre Turquet, John Wilson.

Finally I should like to thank Virginia Law and Kathleen Sargent for typing the fair copy from my much corrected manuscript; Jocelyn Gamble, my secretary for 10 years at the Tavistock Clinic, for her constant help, support, and dedication; and my wife, Jennie, for much encouragement and constructive criticism.

1

Psychotherapy in everyday life

The economics student

An economics student in her early twenties travelled to Spain with a young man, who talked intimately to her on the train journey about his life and troubles. On arrival at the villa they were joined by a girl-friend of hers. Some days later the student began to have a depressive attack accompanied by a feeling of self-hatred, which she described as 'like descending into a pit'. After some hours there began to emerge in her mind her intense jealousy of her girl-friend, to whom the young man had been paying more attention than to her, and she went to her room and broke down into an uncontrollable fit of weeping. The other two heard her and came in, and she was able to pour out her feelings to them. The depressive attack disappeared, and from then on not only in the short term did the holiday go well, but in the long term she found herself able to relate to groups of people in a new way – no longer as an outsider, but as a participant.

In many ways this is a very ordinary and everyday story, but in many ways also it bears very close examination.

First of all, it needs no very deep insight into human nature to suggest that the basic situation on this holiday, a young man and two girls, was loaded with potential trouble. One of the girls was likely to feel jealous and left out, in this case the student, and subsequent events would depend on how well she coped with this. Many possibilities can be envisaged, one of which might have been to have redoubled her efforts to make herself attractive and then to have won the young man back again; or, failing this, to have angrily taxed him with his faithlessness and lack of consideration, and then to have put herself in a situation where she could snap her fingers at him and find someone else. In this latter way she could have got her anger off her chest and consoled herself by getting what she wanted elsewhere. Instead she developed *symptoms*, which illustrates at once the contrast between what may be called 'adaptive' and 'maladaptive' behaviour. However, once this had happened she was in fact able to express her feelings and to resolve the situation satisfactorily. So in the end her behaviour was adaptive after all.

Yet, in using this story as an illustration of general principles – here the difference between adaptive and maladaptive behaviour – we have only just begun. What about the development of depressive symptoms? Surely it is hardly possible to doubt that, in this case, the symptoms were the result of unexpressed

1

feelings – certainly they disappeared when the feelings were expressed. These feelings started by being *out of her awareness*, and they could not have been expressed unless she had come to *know what they were*, and thus it is important to note that their expression was preceded by *insight* – the knowledge that one of their main components was jealousy. But why should the feelings have been out of her awareness? Well, jealousy is a painful emotion. But this does not really seem to be an adequate explanation – we all of us have to face jealousy at one time or another, and most of us manage without getting symptoms. There must presumably be some special quality for her about the emotion of jealousy. If we examine the story for clues more closely, we may come upon the self-hatred that was prominent in her depressive attack. It is of course possible to say that self-reproaches are often a feature of depressive illness and to look no further. But a little thought will show that this gets one nowhere, and indeed it is utterly unscientific simply to dismiss phenomena by saying that they often appear. Why should self-reproaches occur in depressive illness? Could it be that part of the explanation is that depression often has something to do with *guilt*; and that in this girl's case she found jealousy difficult to face because she felt guilty about it? If this is so some of the therapeutic effect could well have followed not merely from the discharge of unexpressed emotion (though this almost certainly was a factor), but from a form of emotional discovery: that it was possible to face jealous feelings and to express them in such a way that they could be accepted by the people towards whom they were directed, and so far from making the situation worse, could actually resolve it. Another observation now falls into place: having discovered that jealousy is not such a terrible emotion after all, from then on this girl was able to participate in group situations – an unending source of potential jealousy – in a way that had never been possible for her before.

Let us now examine the fact that the two other young people heard her crying and came in to see what was the matter. Of course she described the crying as 'uncontrollable' and no doubt this was true. But is it not also possible that she did not *wish* to control her crying, or to cry silently, because – without being fully aware of it – she wanted to be heard? This would serve the purpose of getting the other two to come in, and thus providing her with a situation in which she could not help expressing the feelings to them which she had had such difficulty in facing.

Yet it seems the questions will never end. Why should this girl have been especially sensitive to jealousy and guilty about it? Of course it is possible to suggest that perhaps she had a constitutional weakness – after all, depressive illness is known to contain a hereditary factor. Once again, however, this would be an easy way out and quite unscientific – if *nature* is to be called on as an explanation, then *nurture* needs to be considered as well. One must ask, were there perhaps situations in her earlier history that could have left her with unexpressed feelings and have sensitized her to jealousy? The answer is that indeed there were such situations, but this whole question will be postponed till a later chapter.

I have chosen this true story from everyday life as an opening because it can be used to illustrate so much that is important to the kind of psychotherapy with which this book is concerned.

First of all, it illustrates the extraordinary complexity into which one is led in trying to understand even a simple incident involving human relationships;

while at the same time it illustrates that, whatever the complexities, much of what happens is intelligible in terms of the kind of insight that all of us possess. This leads at once to one of the most important qualities that psychotherapists should possess, which is a *knowledge of people*, much of which may come not from any formal training or reading but simply from personal experience. Which of us has not experienced, in ourselves or those close to us, the potential dangers of apparently innocent triangular situations; or the use of tears not merely as emotional release but an appeal for help; or the beneficial consequences of getting our feelings off our chest at once in the situation that has caused them, and the disastrous consequences of not doing so? Let us suppose that this girl had not in fact been able to do this, but had come to you, the reader, as a friend, saying that she had come back from her holiday in a state of depression. As long as you were not intimidated by the fact that she was presenting a psychiatric condition, it would be nothing more than human common sense to ask her to cast her mind back to when it started, and to make her retell the story in such a way that the issue became clear to both of you. How many patients present themselves at GPs' surgeries, or psychiatric out-patient departments, and are given a diagnosis of 'depression' (for which the treatment is anti-depressants) or 'anxiety' (for which the treatment is tranquillizers), when the true diagnosis is *unexpressed painful feeling*, for which the treatment is to express it, which in turn can be brought about with no more skill than is possessed by any thoughtful human being?

Of course it would be absurd to give the impression that psychotherapy is usually as easy as this – I wish only to show that the principles are not difficult to understand. In most cases the patient does not reach the insight spontaneously but needs to be helped by the fact that the therapist can see into the situation more deeply. In order to do this, the therapist first needs to be able to reach the insight himself, for which purpose he must examine the patient's story in a search for clues.

If this patient had failed to deal with the situation as she did and had presented herself, not to a friend, but to any professional person with the complaint of depression, then how should the latter have proceeded? The answer is, obviously, that the first thing to do is to *take a history*. Here, this particular story illustrates two fundamental principles: first that where the onset of symptoms can be dated, it is essential to find out what was happening in the patient's life at the time; and second that the content of the symptoms may give a clue to the nature of the hidden feelings involved.

The fact that the symptoms arose within a triangular situation, with all its known problems, and the clue given by the self-reproaches, could have enabled the potential therapist to say something like, 'I think the trouble was that you couldn't face your jealousy of the other two', and to wait and see how the patient responded. This is what is meant by the giving of insight through *interpretation*, which is one of the therapist's most essential tools. In turn the aim of giving this insight is to enable the patient to face what she (or he) really feels, to realize that it is not as painful or as dangerous as she fears, to work it through in a relationship, and finally to be able to make use of her real feelings within relationships in a constructive way, thus changing maladaptive into adaptive behaviour. Moreover, the aim is also that the effects of this emotional learning should be permanent – i.e. that the patient should not only be able to deal with the immediate situation, but with similar situations in the future, in a new and adaptive way. All the aims of psychotherapy are thus illustrated by this simple example.

There are of course other principles that this example does not illustrate, especially the use of the 'transference', that is the relationship with the therapist, which will be considered in later chapters. For the time being, however, I hope that enough has been illustrated to give an indication of what this book will be about. It will be concerned with a particular type of approach to human beings, which we may call 'psychodynamic', and a method of psychotherapy based on this, which we may call 'dynamic psychotherapy'. The method of course is derived from psychoanalysis, and the original insights are all due to Freud; but one of the difficulties of psychoanalysis is the lack of properly documented evidence for many of its tenets. Nothing will be presented here without clear evidence to support it.

It is important to emphasize that there are many forms of psychotherapy which this book is not about, though several of these will be mentioned when the question of the choice of therapy is being considered. It is not, for instance, about any of the psychoanalytically-based therapies that are not therapies of the individual – such as the therapy of couples, or families, or groups. Nor is it about behaviour therapy, the most important new form of therapy to emerge in the last few decades, which is quite clearly the treatment of choice in certain types of case. Nor is it about such methods as gestalt therapy or psychodrama. It is about the giving of insight and the use of this insight in relationships – which includes that with the therapist – in a one-to-one setting. There are many patients also for whom this is the treatment of choice.

2

Inner mechanisms in everyday life

More stories

While the previous chapter opened with a story, the present chapter opens with nine stories. Two are from Aesop's Fables (taken from the Penguin edition, Handford, 1954). With one exception the rest are true stories taken from modern everyday life, and although most were told in the consulting room, all happened outside it. The exception is also a true story, but is taken from mediaeval history.

The aim is to illustrate the ways in which human beings try to avoid mental pain; how they try to control unacceptable behaviour or feelings; how sometimes what is unacceptable creeps in by the back door; and finally the kinds of consequence that may ensue from all these processes. The stories will be told in the first place with no elucidation, and it might be a good exercise for the reader to analyse them for himself, using no more than self-knowledge and intuition. It is worth saying, however, that most of them are a good deal more complex than they probably at first appear.

The Spoilt Son

A young solicitor, an only child, who in recent years had begun to make his unhappiness clear for everyone to see, told how his mother was always saying that his father had spoilt him. The truth seemed to be rather that she herself had always been suffocatingly possessive and over-protective; and the father, who was effective enough at work but under his wife's thumb at home, had gone along with her in his ineffective and passive way.

The Anthropologist and the Cat

A young woman with a degree in anthropology was going through yet another crisis with her man-friend, Dick, whose pattern of letting her down seemed chronic and compulsive. She was visiting the house of a woman friend, where Dick had promised to phone her, but of course he didn't. She was sitting with her friend's cat in her lap, and her friend said to her, 'Of course you know Dick was never any good for you'. She hurled the cat across the room (who,

5

in the way of cats, fell on his feet uninjured), and walked out of the house. When she later returned, her friend was naturally furious, and could not leave the incident alone for a long time.

Upsetting the Sugar

One evening a mother came into her little girl's bedroom, to find the walls smeared with faeces. Though revolted, she did not scold her daughter and simply cleaned it all up. The next day the girl accidentally upset the sugar, and the mother completely lost control and hit her.

The Franciscans in the Middle Ages

This religious Order was founded by St Francis of Assisi in the early part of the 13th century. One of the basic principles laid down by the founder was the vow of poverty, according to which the order renounced possessions of any kind. This even applied to the *ownership* of churches and friaries, but it did not apply to their *occupation*.

In the latter part of the century the order found itself in competition with the parish clergy not only for churches, but also for such religious duties as burials and the hearing of confessions. The members of the order also set up their own teaching at universities and found themselves in competition with the ordinary dons, both for pupils and for teaching appointments. There was also competition for *holiness*, since their vow of poverty gave them a certain 'holier than thou' attitude towards the other clergy. Moreover their hearing of deathbed confessions often resulted in substantial legacies which they would use for building finer churches and friaries, and also for such items as books necessary for their status as a learned order. Thus they gave the appearance of a considerable degree of prosperity, and all these factors together brought down upon them a great deal of envy and hostility. A way out of the weaknesses in their position was then found when they induced the Papacy to take upon itself the ownership of all their possessions. The crisis occurred, however, when Pope John XXII withdrew his ownership. ...

Sour Grapes

'A hungry fox tried to reach some clusters of grapes which he saw hanging from a vine trained on a tree, but they were too high. So he went off, ... saying "They weren't ripe anyhow" '.

Roberta in Hospital

A physicist was in hospital for an operation. In the next ward was a little girl of four, Roberta, who was in for a tonsillectomy, and with whom he made friends. The day after her operation her mother visited her, but Roberta refused to respond. The physicist witnessed the incident and afterwards saw Roberta lying frozen, almost as if she was paralysed, staring at the ceiling, with the mother in another part of the ward ignoring her and talking to some other parents. He went up to Roberta's bed and said very gently, twice, stroking her hair, 'Yes it's awful being in hospital without your mother'. She let out a heart-rending sob, and the mother came over angrily, saying, 'Now look what you've done, she'll have a sore throat for days'. He said to her, through his teeth, 'I had thirty years of stammering because of an episode like this', and walked away. And what was the result? First, Roberta sobbing in her mother's arms; then walking with her up and down the corridor for twenty minutes; and then holding her mother's hand in the ward, the two of them looking happy. Needless to say the physicist received no thanks for what he had done.

The Social Worker and her Father

The father of a social worker, who had left the home when she was eleven but had kept in touch with her, phoned her one evening to say that he was in London. At the time she was needing comfort very badly and she asked him if he would come and see her there and then, but he said he couldn't and asked if instead she could come and see him the next day. In reply she was very rude, saying 'What do you think I do with my time?', but in the end she agreed. When they met he tried to put his arms round her, but she utterly rejected him and moved to the other side of the room. When she later told this story she said she had realized she didn't love him at all, she disliked him.

The Anatomy Viva

A medical student arrived in the dissecting room to find that his two companions were suggesting that the three of them should be examined on the upper part of the leg that afternoon. He did not feel that he knew enough to be ready to be examined, and protested, but the others insisted. 'All right,' he said, 'Let's have the viva this morning.'

The Snake and the Wasp

'A wasp settled on a snake's head and tormented it by continually stinging. The snake, maddened with the pain and not knowing how else to be revenged on its tormentor, put its head under the wheel of a waggon, so they both perished together.'

Discussion

Throughout its history dynamic psychotherapy has aroused a great deal of scepticism and hostility. These particular stories have been chosen because the mechanisms involved in them are easily accessible to introspection, and I would say largely undeniable; and yet they contain many of the essential principles of the theoretical basis of dynamic psychotherapy, a subject which we may call psychodynamics. If even this chapter arouses scepticism in the reader, then

I would suggest he should read no further – whatever else his accomplishments, he is not likely to be able to number psychotherapy among them, nor, for that matter, much of human interaction.

As mentioned above, and as always when human reactions are being considered, careful examination reveals that most of these stories are more complex than they seem. Moreover, they lead rapidly by association into profound and often painful truths about human beings.

Expressive and defensive mechanisms

The best starting point is the story of the Spoilt Son. Here the mechanism is relatively straightforward: the son, by implication, had begun to blame his parents for his unhappiness; and the mother then started to accuse the father of spoiling him, when the truth seemed to be that it was she who was largely responsible for the spoiling. The mechanism that she was using was described by the son in words that cannot be bettered: 'I think she's afraid of being found out, and is trying to put the blame on my father'. According to this, she was both *expressing* something, namely blaming the father, and also *defending* herself against her son's implied accusations, by deflecting them onto the father. In other words she was using the mechanism of *displacement*. Yet even this is not entirely simple, as she was surely defending herself both against her *son's blame* and against *self-blame*, because somewhere within her she must have known about her own guilt in the situation. But this was hardly likely to be something that she would readily acknowledge.

Perhaps most similar to this, though far more complicated, is the story of the Anthropologist and the Cat. Here also displacement is at work – after all, the cat had done her no harm, and the anger was with her friend. In this case, therefore, the main mechanism is largely *expressive* and involves the displacement of an *impulse* from her friend onto the cat. Yet this is only the beginning. First, the displacement was also *defensive* in the sense that, by directing her anger at the cat, she was clearly trying to avoid an angry assault on her friend; but this was only partially successful, since to hurt the cat was to hurt the friend, as was shown by her friend's reaction to the incident. Thus her action was a fusion of *defence* and *impulse*.

Next we need to ask the question, why was her anger of such intensity? Well, her friend had said something disparaging about the man with whom she was involved, which naturally would anger her. But surely this is the lesser of two determinants. The real trouble was that her friend's remark was not merely disparaging but – painfully and unforgivably – true, which she had been trying for a long time not to acknowledge to herself. Therefore there was probably yet another *defensive* function of her reaction, namely to divert her attention from acknowledging this truth. It is the attempt to escape from painful truth that makes the main link with the story of the Spoilt Son.

A third kind of displacement is at work in the story entitled Upsetting the Sugar. Here the original situation was the little girl smearing faeces over her bedroom, which the mother dealt with in the most enlightened fashion by controlling her impulse of anger and simply cleaning it all up. To all outward appearances, the incident was then forgotten. But undischarged impulses seek expression, and what then happened was almost certainly that when the mother was faced with another situation in which her daughter made a mess, her defences were completely taken by surprise, and the original anger immediately overcame her. The displacement here is thus from one *situation* onto another, the *person* towards whom the feelings were directed remaining the same in both cases. It is also an example of what Freud called the *return of the repressed*, since the original impulse suddenly erupted in a disguised form. Further, it is an example of *symbolization*, or something very like it, in the sense that in the second incident the sugar very clearly 'stood for' faeces – and this in turn reveals that symbolization is simply one particular form of displacement.

The return of the repressed

Another example of the *return of the repressed* – which is highly entertaining as long as we temper our feelings with some degree of compassion and fellow-feeling – is provided by the story of the Franciscans. Here the attempt was to control man's basic impulses of acquisitiveness and competitiveness by the vow of poverty, which meant the renunciation of property or possessions of any kind. This sounds very like an example of the mechanism of *over-compensation*, or 'trying to be better than you really are' – which puts a burden on human beings that may be more than they can bear (compare the Drama Student, p. 34). Anyhow, such was the result in this particular case: first, the acquisitiveness and competitiveness returned in all sorts of disguised forms – the acquisition of, and hence competition for, churches, for religious duties, for pupils, for teaching appointments, and finally for holiness itself. And then, since the proper discharge of their religious function depended in part on material articles such as books, they needed to acquire these; and the distinction from actual material possessions became a very fine one indeed. They then found it necessary to escape from the position into which they had got themselves by what can only be described as a piece of sophistry (dishonesty?): that all these possessions were really the property of the Pope. And so it went on. If anyone had offered them the comment that they really were highly acquisitive and competitive people, I doubt if he would have received a ready acknowledgment of the truth of what he was saying.

Let us enjoy our amusement at this piece of human frailty, at the same time remembering that, whatever political party we may support, we have almost certainly become involved at one time or another in similar mechanisms ourselves.

Guilt and concern

In passing we may perhaps make some remarks about the forces operating in human beings to hold in check their basic, primitive, and selfish impulses. Without question these controlling forces can be of immense power, as the story of the Franciscans shows. If we are religious we may refer to concepts like the Christian ideal, and say that this has been provided for us by our Maker: if we are biologists we may speak of the altruistic forces of *guilt* and *concern*, and say that they have survival value for the species and have been developed by evolution; and of course the two mechanisms are not mutually exclusive. But in my view we should thank our Maker or evolution (or both) for *concern*, but I do not feel inclined to offer any thanks for *guilt*, which is a force too powerful, too lasting, too destructive, and in the end often ineffective, as we discover time and again in psychotherapy.

Preliminary summary

But this is threatening to take us too far afield. What needs to be pointed out is that in these four stories we have illustrated a number of observations, and concepts derived from them, which are necessary to the understanding of almost all neurotic reactions, and hence which play a part every day in the processes of psychotherapy. These are as follows: (1) the concept of *defence mechanisms*, whose function is the attempt to avoid pain or conflict; (2) the observation that, as a result of the defence mechanisms, the painful or conflicting feelings are at least to some degree *kept out of conscious awareness*; (3) the *return of the repressed*, i.e. the observation that the end-product of the defence mechanism often involves in addition the disguised *expression* of the feelings that the person has been trying to avoid; and therefore (4) that the end-product as observed usually does not have a simple explanation, but contains more than one determinant, a phenomenon which is known as *condensation* or *over-determination*.

The application of these concepts to symptoms

In all these examples the end-product of the mental mechanisms consisted of a *piece of behaviour*. Now when patients present themselves for psychotherapy it may often not be unwanted behaviour for which they are asking help, but more often it is *symptoms* – e.g. anxiety, obsessions, or depression. In this case the connection between the end-product and inner mechanisms is usually not immediately obvious and not accessible to introspection. Nevertheless, exactly the same concepts may have very great explanatory power.

The Economics Student in Chapter 1 can be considered from this point of view. She suffered from an attack of *depression*. It is clear that she was trying to *defend herself* against the *painful* and *guilt-laden* feeling of jealousy. Both the jealousy and the guilt were at first *kept out of conscious awareness*. The *return of the repressed* then occurred in two ways: the guilt appeared in the form of *self-hatred*; and the *jealousy* was effectively expressed by the fit of crying, which forced the other two people to pay attention to her rather than to each other. She was then able to become aware of the hidden feelings and to express them openly, and the depression disappeared.

Depreciation or rejection of what is desired

Let us now turn to the best known of all these stories, the Fox and the Sour Grapes. No apology will be offered for using this entirely mythical example, since the type of human situation that it is meant to illustrate is obvious and presumably has existed almost as long as humanity itself.

The basic situation is that of being faced with something *desirable* that is also *unattainable*. The natural reaction to this is the pain of frustration and disappointment. However the pain is then eased by a piece of self-deception (or dishonesty): whatever it was that was desirable is made out to have been undesirable – the grapes weren't ripe – so that there is now no longer any cause for disappointment. In other words the function of this mechanism, once more, is to *avoid pain*.

Of course this formulation is correct as far as it goes, and indeed this is clearly what Aesop was intending, since the last sentence as actually written contains the words '*he comforted himself by saying* "They weren't ripe anyhow"'. But in most real-life situations, the reaction is likely to be not only the pain of disappointment, but also the *anger of frustration*; and this will be doubly true if it is *a person* who has made himself unattainable, since then the anger is the result of *being rejected*. Careful thought then indicates that the mechanism involves not only the avoidance of pain but the expression of anger, as is made clearer when one sees that the grapes in the story are being *disparaged* or *depreciated*. Of course it doesn't hurt the grapes to be called sour, so that in this situation the expression of anger is purely internal; but if the depreciation can be expressed *to* the person who has done the rejecting, then it is likely to be painful to *him*, and the anger is expressed externally and directly and is effective because it hurts. Taken to the limit, the other person becomes rejected in his turn, 'now you can know what it feels like', and the punishment fits the crime.

The two stories that illustrate this kind of mechanism are those of Roberta in Hospital, and the Social Worker and her Father. Of these the former is probably the simpler. We owe particularly to John Bowlby (e.g. 1953, 1973) and James Robertson (e.g. 1953) the realization of the devastating consequences of separating young children from their mothers for any length of time, without an adequate substitute, and an understanding of the mechanisms involved. As Bowlby has described, the first stage is that of *protest*. Driven by extremely painful and intense feelings, the child (without fully knowing what she is doing) does all in her power to create a situation in which her mother will feel forced by her own maternal instincts either not to leave her or else to return; and when this fails, she sinks into a state of *despair*. Both these stages are relatively direct and straightforward, and do not in themselves contain any pathogenic potential.

The two first stages of adult grief are essentially the same; and when all goes well they are followed by what may be called a stage of 'working through', in which the agonies of loss are faced one by one and over and over again, to a point at which they are sufficiently weakened to lose their effect. An alternative outcome, however, when the individual is not strong enough to face the feelings involved – which seems to be the usual situation when the person concerned is a small child – is that they are not weakened, but that they are buried and kept away from consciousness. The end-product is Bowlby's third stage, in which the child uses the defence mechanism of *denial* or *detachment*, which is utterly deceptive because to outward appearances she seems to have returned to normal.

If now the lost mother returns, the naive expectation is that the child will be, quite simply and straightforwardly, overjoyed to see her again. Indeed, this is what happens when a master returns to his dog; but with human beings, as the story of Roberta illustrates, the result is often very different. What in fact may happen is that the mother is rejected. The message to the mother is very like that conveyed in the sour grapes reaction – 'I don't want you any more' – and the mechanism almost certainly serves the same twin functions, which as always are not as simple as they may at first sight appear: (1) The first function is the *avoidance of pain* – as long as the child keeps up the pretence of not wanting her mother; (a) she saves herself the agonizing recovery of the buried feelings of grief (demonstrated so clearly in Roberta after the physicist had spoken to her); and (b) she forearms herself against having to go through the same stages of useless protest and hopeless agony if the mother should leave again. (2) The second function is almost certainly the *expression of anger* – there is a great deal of direct evidence for anger in young children as a response to loss (see Bowlby, 1973, pp. 146ff.) though it may not be obviously detectable in the initial rejection of the mother, and may be utterly obscured by the overwhelming grief that is later uncovered. It also would be far too sophisticated to suggest that under these circumstances young children are trying to make the mother suffer what they have been suffering themselves. This is only likely to enter at a much later stage.

The story of Roberta, therefore, illustrates much more clearly the defensive or protective function of rejecting the mother who returns. The story of the Social Worker and her Father illustrates the anger quite clearly, and the sour grapes reaction is absolutely clear in her statement that she didn't love him, she disliked him. In this story, too, the element of hurting the other person, and making him suffer what she had suffered herself, is very clear. It is also worth noting the language used, as the word 'disliked' carries with it the defensive manoeuvre of the sour grapes reaction, implying that she never wanted him anyhow, whereas the word 'hated' would have implied an involvement that she obviously did not want to acknowledge at the time.

Unconscious mechanisms and feelings

This story leads to one of the crucial points of the present chapter. So far I have described situations in which feelings were *kept out of conscious awareness* but I have deliberately avoided using the word 'unconscious'. The stories can probably be arranged in a series according to the degree to which the true feelings were or were not accessible. Thus, at one end, the Anthropologist, and the mother of the little girl who upset the sugar, both of whom were insightful and sophisticated people, would have readily acknowledged the inner mechanisms at work; in the middle, the mother of the Spoilt Son, and the Franciscans, would probably have had the greatest difficulty in acknowledging their hidden feelings, though they must really have been aware of them; and at the other end, the Economics Student was quite unaware of her jealousy until it finally forced itself on her attention.

We may now ask, at what point are we justified in introducing the word 'unconscious'? This seems to be largely a matter of choice, and surely it must be true that there is really a continuum from being *unwilling to acknowledge* at one end to being *totally unaware* at the other.

Yet, because in the case of the Economics Student the feelings were in the end relatively easily accessible, there may be reluctance to use the word 'unconscious' even here.

This is the importance of the story of the Social Worker. During many years of psychotherapy she had always regarded her father as the perfection of what a man should be. Side by side with this had gone an intense – even compulsive – awareness of the faults of *other men in her life*, to the point at which she used to say that she could never get married because she would destroy any man whom she got close to. Where on earth could such intense hatred of men have originated? She had suffered nothing at the hands of men to justify such a feeling.

Yet of course she had – she had been abandoned by her father at the age of eleven. The whole picture now becomes comprehensible if we postulate that she is using three related defence mechanisms to protect herself against the intolerable pain of hating someone whom she also loved so much: first *idealization*, which is obvious; then *splitting*, which means avoiding conflict by keeping the two kinds of incompatible feelings entirely separate; and finally, when faced with the *return of the repressed*, she is using *displacement* – displacing her anger against her father onto other men. Of course all this is only a hypothesis – and indeed, however many times she was confronted with it in her psychotherapy, she simply denied it and remained totally unaware that it had any validity whatsoever. The importance of incidents like that described in the above story was that at last the hidden anger with her father emerged, and the hypothesis was confirmed by direct evidence. Now the long process of rescuing her from her hatred of men could finally begin. It remains absolutely incontrovertible that until this point in her life the hidden feelings and mechanisms had been, in the full sense of the word, unconscious.

Self-defeating and self-destructive mechanisms

Further consideration of these two stories may be approached through a diversion introducing the last two stories, the Anatomy Viva and the Snake and the Wasp.

A quick glance at the first of these may raise a naive question: if the medical student was so unprepared that he felt unable to undergo his viva that *afternoon*, why on earth did he suddenly turn round and advocate having the viva that *morning*? A likely consequence would be that all three of them would fail together. The answer is of course very simple, namely that in doing so he hoped to turn the tables on his two fellow students, making them in their turn face the viva with insufficient preparation. The fact that this made the prospect of the viva even worse for him was ignored *because it was worth it*. This is a mild example of the situation illustrated by the fable of the Snake and the Wasp – 'not knowing how else to be revenged on its tormentor, it put its head under the wheel of a waggon, so that they both perished together'.

The point illustrated here is that the forces driving some of these mental mechanisms are often so powerful that the devastatingly self-destructive consequences that may ensue offer no deterrence whatsoever. This is one of the gloomy truths about human beings that face all of us when we undertake psychotherapy; and it results in one of our primary tasks, namely to rescue our patients from the self-destructive consequences of what they are doing, by tracing these mechanisms to their origin and uncovering the feelings that are being expressed indirectly or are being avoided.

This leads us back at once to what the physicist did for Roberta. Her rejection of her mother, if hardened into a pattern, could have set up ripples that extended, for her, to the ends of time. A single sentence, repeated once, aborted them – on this occasion anyhow. This sentence is of course an example of an *interpretation*, i.e. a communication to the suffering person designed to bring out the hidden mechanisms involved and thus to have therapeutic effects.

The triangle of conflict

Here we may introduce a concept that is absolutely fundamental to dynamic psychotherapy. The physicist's words, 'Yes, it's awful being in hospital without your mother', were in effect a direct interpretation to the little girl of the *hidden feelings* that she was *defending herself* against. It was quite unnecessary to point out to her either the *mechanism of defence* or the *reason for* the defence. It would obviously have been absurd to have said something like: 'You are pushing your mother away [defence], in order to avoid your grief and anger about having been abandoned by her [hidden feelings], because you are afraid of being overwhelmed by them [anxiety].' Yet this would have been the complete interpretation, which often *is* appropriate in psychotherapy, spelling out for the patient the three aspects of the mechanism going on inside her – *defence, anxiety*, and *hidden feeling* – the *triangle of conflict*, one or more aspects of which can be used to describe almost every interpretation that is made in dynamic psychotherapy (for further discussion see Chapter 10, pp. 90ff.).

There is also an important note on the *hidden feeling* that needs to be introduced here. In Roberta we have postulated that the hidden feeling contains two elements, grief and anger. Of these, anger may be described as an *impulse*, though grief cannot. Similarly, in the stories of the Anthropologist and the Cat, Upsetting the Sugar, and the Social Worker and her Father, the hidden feelings consisted of angry impulses; and in the story of the Franciscans the impulses were acquisitive and competitive. Moreover, as will appear later (see e.g. further discussion of the Economics Student in Chapter 7), the hidden feelings often consist of unacceptable sexual impulses. Thus, when appropriate, the word 'impulse' will often be substituted for 'hidden feeling', especially as it is more succinct. In fact the triangle of conflict is often taught as consisting of 'defence, anxiety and impulse', but this is not always correct, as the story of Roberta illustrates.

The effect on the environment; vicious circles; conjoint therapy

This story also leads to the final point of the present chapter. So far we have been entirely concerned with mechanisms *within a single person*, and have not considered either their effect on people outside, or the effect of this in turn on the person in whom the mechanisms are operating. The incident between the social worker and her father is not a good illustration, because her father was quite mature and insightful enough to know what was going on, and to cope with it by patient understanding and forbearance. But Roberta's mother was an entirely different matter, as is shown by the situation that faced the physicist, with Roberta frozen in bed and her mother ignoring her at the other end of the ward. The mother may be forgiven for a feeling of bewildered resentment when she arrives full of anticipation at seeing her little girl again and finds herself rejected; and Roberta in turn may of course be forgiven if she begins to think her mother indifferent because she pays attention to the other parents instead of sitting by her bed; but the result may well be a vicious circle of resentment based on mutual and total misunderstanding of the situation, which is of course – on both sides – one of wounded love. I do not wish to suggest that this single incident in itself would have necessarily had any permanent effect – provided the relation between mother and daughter was good enough in the first place. But if the relation was already threatened in other ways, then the consequences might well be permanent, as the physicist himself had cause to know.

All this leads to the crucial point: as it happened, it was possible to undo the situation by an intervention aimed at one half of the vicious circle only. Yet at that moment *both* figures in the drama needed help; and this would certainly have been so if the vicious circle had been allowed to establish itself for any length of time. When a patient presents with a complaint of difficulty in relation to the marriage partner, this is almost always true; and then, although it may be possible and appropriate to help by treating one partner only, it may be far better to treat both; so that the treatment of choice may well not be individual therapy but some form of conjoint marital therapy. In turn, in more complex situations, it may be best to treat the entire family. In the present book, which is specifically about individual psychotherapy, this point will not be considered further, but it is essential that everyone concerned with psychotherapy should be aware of it.

Summary

A consideration of these apparently simple and everyday stories has thus spread to covering a large part of the field of psychodynamics, and it is as well to end with a summary of the features that have been illustrated. These are as follows:

(1) Human beings adopt various defensive mechanisms in order to avoid mental pain or conflict, or to control unacceptable impulses.
(2) These mechanisms vary from being almost wholly conscious, in which case they can be undone by a few words, to being so totally unconscious that they are only revealed by years of psychotherapy.
(3) The end-product of these mechanisms is often a form of maladaptive behaviour or a neurotic symptom.
(4) The behaviour or symptom often has an expressive as well as a defensive function, containing the avoided feelings or impulses in a disguised form.
(5) The behaviour or symptom often has damaging consequences for everyone, not least for the individual in whom the mechanisms are occurring.
(6) Although some individuals may be well aware of the self-destructive consequences of what is occurring, the forces involved are so strong that they are usually powerless to control them.
(7) One of the ways in which damaging consequences occur is through the

setting up of a vicious circle between individuals and the people in their environment.

(8) One of the main tasks of the psychotherapist is therefore to analyse in his or her own mind, and then to *interpret* to the patient, the end-product of these mechanisms, in terms of (a) the devices adopted for avoiding mental pain, conflict, or unacceptable feelings (the *defence*); (b) the feared consequences of expressing these hidden feelings (the *anxiety*); and (c) the nature of the *hidden feelings* themselves. This is the *triangle of conflict*, which will be repeatedly encountered in the following pages.

3

Unconscious communication

This subject, crucial to psychotherapy, is best introduced via the subject of *association*, which in turn may be illustrated once more by a true story.

An example of association

A young research chemist, working on a military device during the War, was washing out a small clear plastic ampoule containing iodine. As he put the ampoule under the tap and the brown solution spilled over into the sink, there flashed into his mind a memory from his childhood in India, in which, at the age of seven, he and his father and mother had driven away for the day and had picnicked by a waterfall.

Puzzled by this sudden and apparently irrelevant association, he started to try and analyse it. It then came to him, first, that the water gushing from the tap and cascading from the ampoule could well have led his associations to a waterfall; then, that the brown colour of the solution reminded him of the fact that this particular mountain stream had been said to be polluted; and finally he remembered that as he and his father had walked beside the stream, they had seen on a leaf the skin shed by an insect, which had the same brown and translucent appearance as the ampoule stained by iodine. Thus three entirely independent associations led from the immediate situation to the memory of so many years ago.

If this story had been told to any of the earlier philosophers and psychologists who had studied the phenomenon of association – earlier, that is, than Freud and Jung, from Aristotle through Galton to Wundt – then they would no doubt have regarded the explanation as complete. It seems only too likely that the coincidence of these three similarities would have led uniquely to this particular association, and by the principle of economy of hypothesis no further explanation need be sought. Yet the fascinating thing is that the phenomenon of *condensation* or *over-determination*, mentioned in Chapter 2, often means that in mental phenomena the principle of economy of hypothesis does not apply; and that even when an explanation that is apparently quite sufficient has been found, it may be appropriate to seek a further explanation that applies not as an alternative, but in addition.

Association and emotional significance

This was something that the chemist only realized after his psychotherapy many years later. The picnic that appeared in his associations was not long before his father's sudden death, an event which – until he was rescued by psychotherapy – had gone a long way towards destroying his emotional life altogether; and the picnic in fact represented not only a rare moment of closeness to his often absent father, but also one of the last times that he had experienced a united family in an exceedingly secure and happy childhood, much of it spent among some of the beauty spots of the world. Thus it is quite clear that this particular association held a significance for him that not only was *profound*, but of which at the time he was *largely unaware*. In other words, even when there were three separate similarities leading towards a particular association, there was a powerful additional force at work leading towards the same end product, namely *emotional significance*, which in this case was also *largely unconscious*.

Unconscious and preconscious

We can now continue the discussion of the word 'unconscious', begun in Chapter 2. The word was used here in the strict sense introduced by Freud, namely that the *significance* of the memory (though not the memory itself) was kept out of conscious awareness by 'repressing' forces whose function was to avoid pain. This was made clear by the fact that a major feature of the chemist's psychotherapy consisted of the recovery of overwhelming grief about his childhood, which had remained out of his awareness for over twenty years.

Freud used another term, *preconscious*, for mental phenomena that are not conscious at any given moment but are readily accessible to consciousness. It seems clear that preconscious and unconscious are not sharply distinguishable but represent a continuum. The significance of the above memory was clearly unconscious. The three similarities which led to the chemist's association lay much nearer to the preconscious end of the spectrum; but they were still not fully preconscious in the sense that, say, his middle name was preconscious, since they were only recovered after considerable thought.

Free association in psychotherapy

It was of course considerations similar to these that led Freud to use 'free association' as one of the cornerstones of his technique, since he realized that whatever the more superficial reasons for the appearance of a particular association in consciousness – whether these be similarity to a previous association, or contiguity of place or time, or any other of the recognized laws of association – these would be in a sense *used* by deeper forces pressing for expression. Thus if the patient was simply required to 'say everything that came into his mind', sooner or later his associations would be sufficiently influenced by his inner conflicts for these to be first inferred by the therapist, and then brought into consciousness by questioning or by interpretations based on these inferences. If the example given above had occurred during psychotherapy, the therapist might quite naturally have asked the patient simply to think about the significance to him of this particular memory, and if the therapist had taken a proper history, he might easily have been able to infer its significance himself, and then to lead the patient towards his repressed feelings. This is one of the essential processes of psychotherapy.

There are now two further important considerations. The first is that when the underlying feelings are at least partly unconscious, then the association that appears represents a *compromise between the repressed and the repressing forces*. In the example used above the compromise consisted of the fact that the memory appeared but without any of the accompanying feelings of grief. This phenomenon is exactly similar to the twin *defensive* and *expressive* functions of certain forms of behaviour discussed in Chapter 2.

Association and communication

The second consideration is as follows: in this example the chemist was alone, and the association was a purely internal matter. When there is a second person present and thoughts are spoken aloud – whether this be in an everyday conversation or in the more one-sided situation of psychotherapy – a given association becomes a *communication*, and there may be contained in it an unconscious message. Once more there will then be a compromise between the repressed and repressing forces, the wish to conceal and the wish to reveal, so that the message may appear in disguise. This disguise often takes the form of speaking about an event or situation that has obvious parallels to a current situation about which the message is being unconsciously conveyed. Patients who readily communicate in this way are among the best subjects for psychotherapy; and it is an essential quality in a psychotherapist that he should be able to sense when this is happening, to detect the underlying message, and to know whether, and if so to what degree and in what language, to translate the disguise. All such communications should be noted, and if appropriate should be acted on, but not all such communications should be translated – particularly when they occur in everyday life – as the following example will show.

Unconscious communication in everyday life – Sandra and the Puppies

A university student in biology at last overcame his intense shyness to the point of being able to ask a girl to come out with him. It was summer, and after dining out together they went for a walk in the country. During the course of the evening the tension of shyness between them had gradually eased, and as they walked through a field he was able to turn to her and risk saying 'It's nice here'. She replied warmly 'Yes it is', and there was a short silence. Suddenly, apparently apropos of nothing, she said 'We've got a dog called Sandra, and one day she ran off for a long time, and a few weeks later we discovered that she was going to have puppies', and the conversation continued, naturally and easily, on the subject of what the puppies were like, and the kinds of home that had been found for them.

The point of this story is, obviously, the girl's sudden and abrupt change of subject to her dog Sandra and the puppies. The reader is left to decode the message, which was both of the utmost warmth and generosity, and of an acutely embarrassing nature, and far more than she would have wished anyone to know at the time – it would hardly have been appropriate to decode it for her.

Now I cannot prove that this was in fact the coded message that the girl was conveying (whatever it may be that you are thinking!), and you would be quite justified in remaining sceptical that she was speaking about anything other than her dog and the puppies. In therapeutic situations, on the other hand, it may often be the correct procedure to *give an interpretation* which decodes the message there and then, and indeed this may be what the patient is unconsciously asking for. Subsequent events then provide powerful evidence about whether or not the interpretation was correct – an example of an experimental situation in the science of psychodynamics. The following example is particularly striking.

The Neurological Patient

A man in his late forties was admitted to a neurological ward for investigation of headaches, which turned out to be almost certainly psychogenic. During the course of his stay in hospital the (male) student assigned to him encouraged him to talk about his life and the current difficulties that probably lay at the root of his symptom, which he managed to put into words with considerable relief. On the day before his discharge – no physical cause having been found – he was again talking to the student, and he suddenly began to speak as follows: 'A few months ago my wife and I went out to a meal in a restaurant. We had a most enjoyable evening, and as we were about to go I called the waitress over and asked her how I could thank her for the wonderful service she had given us. She just said that if I wanted to thank her, perhaps I could speak about it to the manager.'

We may now ask, why should the patient be talking about that particular incident? It would be easy to answer simply that it was a pleasant memory and clearly had an emotional significance for him, thus fulfilling one of the laws of association mentioned above. Whereas this is undoubtedly true, it would clearly be even better if one could explain why that incident had come into his mind *at that particular moment*. Here one might say that there is no information about the conversation that came immediately before, so how is it possible to answer?

Yet in fact there is sufficient information to make an answer possible. This subject of conversation has all the hallmarks of an *unconscious communication:* an apparently irrelevant incident that shows an obvious parallel to another situation which is highly relevant, and of which the patient might well be wanting to speak, without being aware of it. The next question is whether it is appropriate to decode the message for the patient by interpretation. The answer emerges very clearly from what actually happened.

The student simply said, 'I think you're trying to thank me for giving you good service'; at which the patient, with tears in his eyes, turned to him and said, 'Yes, I will never forget what the hospital has done for me', and the final parting was on a note of great warmth.

Rapport and its use in psychotherapy

We may use this example to introduce two concepts that are fundamental to the practice of psychotherapy. The first is *rapport*, which can be defined as the degree of emotional contact between patient and therapist. The reader may sense in the account of the conversation between this patient and his student a sudden transition following on the student's remark: a change from an apparently very ordinary and emotionally composed account of a previous incident, to an intense and heartfelt declaration of feeling about the whole of his recent experience in hospital – something that was clearly uppermost in his mind at that particular moment, just as he was about to leave the hospital and go home. In fact the patient became in touch with a feeling of great significance to him, and was not only able to express it, but to express it directly to one of the people principally involved in the feeling itself. In other words there was a dramatic *deepening of rapport*. This, together with the direct confirmation contained in what the patient said, is as near as one can ever get to scientific proof that the student's interpretation was correct.

It is one of the most important characteristics of a therapist that he should be able to sense the degree of rapport existing at any given moment in a therapeutic session. Anyone who has this capacity can set it up as a kind of thermometer between him and the patient, and can use the moment-to-moment fluctuations in the level of rapport in order to gauge the appropriateness of what he has just said. It is of course going a bit far to say that then he *cannot go wrong*, but as a way of conveying an important principle the exaggeration is worth it. (The subject is illustrated in detail with an actual example in Chapter 10 – see pp. 85ff.).

The here-and-now; transference

The second fundamental concept is that of the *here-and-now*. Whenever a patient speaks (and not only a patient, as the story of Sandra and the Puppies illustrates) he may unwittingly be making a communication about his *relation to the person he is with, i.e. the therapist, or his feelings about the therapeutic situation*. It is therefore a second most important characteristic of a therapist that he should be able to recognize when this is happening – something that it is often most difficult for a beginner to face, particularly if the feelings are uncomplimentary, and also, of course if they are embarrassingly positive.

This leads towards the concept of *transference*. Anyone who enters the field of dynamic psychotherapy will very quickly observe that his patients tend to develop intense feelings about him. Very frequently, though *not always*, such feelings really belong to someone in the patient's past, from whom they have been *transferred* – hence the word transference. This word has gradually become more loosely used for *any* feelings that the patient may have about the therapist. The whole subject will be discussed more fully in Chapter 9.

There follow some more examples in which the parallel between the patient's communication and the here-and-now situation was so clear that the therapist would have had to be particularly blind, or particularly frightened, to miss it.

The Interior Decorator

A young man of 26, recently married, came to therapy because he had been unable to consummate his marriage. He had clearly suffered for a long time from problems of self-confidence as a man, which in the past had led to over-compensation and boasting, and which of course had not been reassured by his recent sexual failure. In the second interview the therapist set him a time limit of *16 sessions* at once a week, and invited him to speak about whatever came to him. Half way through the session the patient began to speak of one of the few times when he felt he had really achieved something, when he had been in the Forces and had done a *'16-week course in navigation'*. He had really felt this was a challenge, and he had been determined to do as well as possible at it. Here the coincidence between the two numbers made it virtually impossible to miss the here-and-now communication; and when the patient was given the *interpretation* that he regarded his therapy in the same way, as a challenge in which he was determined to do as well as possible, there was a clear *deepening of rapport*, and he was able to voice some of his *mixed feelings about entering therapy* and to speak of his *difficulty in trusting people* (for further details see pp. 85ff.).

The Girl Afraid of Breakdown

Another example can be described by quotations from the interviewer's written report of the third exploratory interview with a girl of 25:

'I then told her that we could offer her group treatment, but it would mean being on a waiting list, and I couldn't guarantee when she would get a vacancy. She obviously wasn't very keen on the idea, but when I put it to her that she might have preferred individual treatment, she said she didn't really know, and a group might be good for her. It would all depend on what the other people were like.

'I deliberately allowed a silence to fall in order to get a more spontaneous communication, which in fact she gave. She asked me apropos of nothing in particular whether she had told me that her flatmate had had a breakdown recently. It turned out that the flatmate had attended a therapeutic group. Apparently all the introspection had disturbed her. This was particularly upsetting as the flatmate had seemed to the patient when she first met her to be an especially normal and stable person.'

With the two previous examples in mind, it is worth while for the reader to consider (1) the nature of the unconscious communication, and (2) what he would say to the patient at this point.

What happened in fact is continued in the interviewer's words:

'It wasn't very difficult to offer the interpretation that she was afraid she would be made worse by the group treatment here. This startled her because in fact she had not consciously seen the connection at all. She acknowledged that it was probably so, but didn't produce any further elaboration.'

Although this girl had given some evidence of psychotic manifestations both in her interviews and projection tests, she was finally felt to have enough strength to face psychotherapy and was put on the waiting list for a group in spite of her own obvious misgivings. Three months later, and before she was offered a vacancy, she had an acute psychotic breakdown with florid delusions and hallucinations.

It is worth nothing that although this interpretation was clearly *correct*, it *did not produce a deepening of rapport* – almost certainly the patient was not prepared to acknowledge her hidden anxiety at this time, presumably because it was too intense. A therapist needs to be warned by this not to press his interpretation further.

The Military Policeman

A third example is taken from one of the therapies conducted for Balint's Workshop for brief psychotherapy. The patient was a married officer in the Military Police, aged 38, who had always regarded any show of strong feeling – including love or anger – as a weakness, and had prided himself on his ability to cope with any situation. He now came complaining of an acute and severe anxiety state, in which he was often near to tears and was afraid he was on the point of breaking up. He was seen for a total of four therapeutic sessions, during which time he succeeded in confiding in a fellow officer who, he discovered, had suffered at one time from symptoms similar to his own. It seemed that this had been an important therapeutic factor, and from that time he felt better and his symptoms began to recede. The therapist therefore suggested that they should stop treatment at this point, but that the patient could come back at any time if he felt the need. The patient accepted this, and the therapist then deliberately remained passive in order to see what communications about the proposal might emerge.

The therapist wrote that 'a very relaxed, quite intimate atmosphere developed between us, in which he would be silent for, say, a quarter of a minute at a time and then come out with some remark about what was in his mind'. One of these was to say that 'There was a sergeant in his Unit who was always "flapping". Whenever anything went wrong he was always getting in touch with one of his superiors and asking what he should do. Yet he had many years' service and he, the patient, often handled this by telling him he could perfectly well do it himself.'

Again it is worthwhile for the reader to consider the nature of the unconscious communication, which should be obvious, and what the therapist should do about it.

What the therapist said in fact was, 'Surely you're trying to tell me that you don't want me to think you're like the sergeant who has to come running to me for help whenever anything goes wrong?'

The confirmation of this interpretation came during the later course of the session, when the patient made the following remarks:

(1) that he always had the feeling on arriving at a session that the therapist thought, 'Christ, it's that chap again';
(2) that the therapist must feel about him that at his age he oughtn't to allow himself to get into a state like this;
(3) when the therapist emphasized that in his opinion the problem wasn't solved, the patient said, 'Well, I hope I'll prove you wrong';
(4) at the end of the session, even though the therapist had said that he would

get in touch with the patient if the patient didn't get in touch with him, the patient said, 'Well, in a way I hope I don't see you again.' (For further details see Malan, 1976a, pp. 165 – 71.)

The characteristics of unconscious communication

Of course unconscious communication is a much broader phenomenon than is covered by these examples, as will be discussed in detail in Chapter 10. Nevertheless it is worth summarizing the characteristics of a particular kind of communication by which the therapist should immediately be alerted:

(1) The patient – often with an abrupt change of subject – speaks with evident interest and spontaneity about something whose relevance is not immediately obvious.
(2) On more careful thought, a clear parallel can be seen with some other subject whose relevance and emotional significance is much greater.

It should be added that the communication is not necessarily about the here-and-now, though it often is.

Once more it needs to be said that such communications should be noted – and indeed are ignored at one's peril, whether they occur in therapy or in everyday life – but should not necessarily be translated into words. Often, however, they should be, and the confirmation will come from a deepening of rapport and the emergence of the hidden feelings closer to consciousness. The perception and translation of this kind of communication is an essential part of the therapist's day-to-day work.

4

Elementary, though not necessarily easy, psychotherapy

Recapitulation

In the three previous chapters I have illustrated many of the basic principles of psychodynamics and dynamic psychotherapy: the adoption by human beings of various devices to avoid pain and conflict, the potentially damaging consequences, and therapeutic effects that result from bringing the hidden feelings into consciousness and expressing them.

The example of the Economics Student as told so far represents perhaps the simplest possible psychotherapeutic situation – the realization by the patient herself of a single piece of insight about her own hidden feelings, without the intervention of a therapist, within the actual situation that was causing them, followed by their free expression to the actual people involved and the resolution of the situation. Correspondingly, the example of Roberta in Hospital represents the simplest possible situation involving the *giving of insight about hidden feelings by a therapist* – otherwise possessing the identical characteristics of the first example. Yet the moment we introduce this new factor we come upon extraordinary profundity and complexity, which arise from the very special qualities possessed by the therapist that made his intervention possible. In fact, this example can be used as a paradigm to illustrate not only these qualities but important aspects of the understanding of human beings before and after the impact of Freud.

Qualities needed by a therapist

First of all, until James Robertson made his first film, *A two-year-old goes to hospital*, in 1952, it was not generally recognized that the temporary separation of young children from their mothers had any particular damaging effect. Everyone could observe that after an initial stage of distress children became quiet and well behaved, and it was natural to suppose that they had got over the separation and settled down. The subtle indications, shown so clearly by the film, that this was by no means the situation, were very easy to ignore. Thus the physicist had to possess a very considerable degree of *theoretical knowledge* – that children do not get over separation so easily; that quietness, and particularly exaggerated quietness, does not necessarily mean that all is well, and might well hide feelings of the utmost intensity; that the consequences of allowing the situation to develop unchecked would certainly be distressing and might well be serious; and that the way to deal with it was to bring out the hidden feelings there and then. That is four pieces of theoretical knowledge to start with.

But there is much more to it than this. He had also to possess an *attitude* to human reactions and emotions like the attitude of a physician to human physiology – that these internal processes are a subject fit for study, that an understanding of them is possible, and that rational interventions based on this understanding can have predicted effects. What he should not have, of course, is the plain physician's attitude to *human emotions*: for feelings need to be dealt with by feelings, and not by reversing their physiological effects – the correct treatment for Roberta in this situation was hardly the immediate prescription of anti-depressants (for which, I should say, I have the greatest respect in their proper place). But this in turn means something even more: the reason why the signs of distress in young children in hospital had been so easy to ignore was that *nobody wanted to see them* – it was so much easier to believe that all was well, and not everybody wants either to remember what it feels like to be so utterly bereft and abandoned, or to have to face the expression of such feelings in someone else. The physicist was an exceptional person, ideally suited to the situation, being someone with the profoundest insight which had been enhanced by many years of personal analysis, and who was only too painfully aware of the consequences for himself of being left in hospital at the age of six. He was thus able to *use his knowledge of his own feelings* in a process of identification with the little girl; to know not only *theoretically* but *intuitively* what was needed; and, having faced his own feelings in the same situation, not to be afraid to face those of someone else.

Yet even this is not all. It is so easy, in this kind of situation, to obtrude one's own personal feelings into what one says to the patient, which very quickly goes over into seeking sympathy rather than giving it. Patients are not interested in one's personal tragedies; certainly not when they are in the midst of their own. Thus the therapist's feelings can be shown, but must only be shown *objectively*, under complete control, entirely in the service of the patient.

When all these complex qualities came together, the result was an intervention of the utmost simplicity, with therapeutic consequences that have already been described.

Everyone who undertakes psychotherapy needs to have these qualities – not necessarily to the degree possessed by this exceptional person – but to some degree at any rate. Not everyone has even the potential to possess them, though they can be taught; and the best way of learning them, of course, is by undergoing psychotherapy oneself.

The Geologist

The example of Roberta in hospital represents a single intervention within a situation of acute current conflict. The following is an example that is similar except that the current conflict had been going on for some time and the intervention was made, away from the actual situation, in a psychiatrist's consulting room. The patient was a young man of 24, a post-graduate student in geology, who came asking for advice about a specific problem concerning his mother.

He is the younger by 5 years of two children, his sister now being married and living in Australia. His father died 3 years ago. Since then his mother has been in a state of chronic depression which has not responded to ECT, and she is still in hospital, unable to care for herself outside. Because of her incapacity, their home in Bristol has had to be sold, and she is now isolated in hospital in Bristol while he is doing his PhD at Birmingham University.

In the discussion with the psychiatrist who saw him for consultation, the patient said that what his mother needed was to be given more attention, more support, and more interest in life. He expressed a good deal of anger against the hospital for not supplying these things. The psychiatrist saw at once that this was at least partly an example of *displacement of blame*, as illustrated by the story of the mother and the spoilt son in Chapter 2, and led the patient to the point of agreeing that, with his father dead and his sister in Australia, he was the only person left to take responsibility in the situation. He then said that he had realized this, and that he had thought that in many ways the best thing would be for him to get his mother transferred to a hospital near Birmingham, to set up house near her, and gradually to ease her out of hospital into his home. What he had come for, he said, was to be *advised* whether or not this was the right thing to do.

The question of advice

Now advice is something that it is absolutely correct to give in its proper place, particularly when one has expert knowledge not possessed by the other person. This is so, for instance, when a psychiatrist is asked to recommend a suitable form of treatment; and even more so when a solicitor is asked to recommend a course of action involving complexities of the law. But in emotional situations advice is beset by pitfalls, and there are several reasons why giving it may be a mistake, at least before the feelings involved have been clarified. One of the reasons is that no one can be omniscient and foresee all the consequences of a given line of action; another is that it is far better for a patient to take responsibility for his own decisions. But the two most important reasons are simply that the advice is likely to be ineffective, and that clarification of the feelings may make advice unnecessary.

A superficial view of the situation just described might suggest that the obvious thing for the psychiatrist to say is simply, yes, the line of action that the patient suggests is utterly sensible and he should go ahead. Yet if one stops to think there is something quite paradoxical about what the patient is saying. If he has thought of this himself – and indeed it does seem the obvious thing to do – why does he need to ask advice about it, and from a psychiatrist at that? This suggests that there is more to his request than meets the eye. If so, what is it likely to be?

A little further thought may now suggest that the first answer to this question is that there is some reason why the patient cannot do what he knows to be sensible; and moreover, because it is so sensible, the reason must be fairly powerful. If the psychiatrist simply tells him to go ahead, the likely consequence is that the patient will superficially agree that this is what he should do, go away, come up against his inability to do it, and then be left in exactly the same situation as before.

This now raises another paradox. If the above formulation is correct, then why has the patient not simply said, yes I know this is the sensible thing to do, but I cannot do it? Instead he has come asking for advice.

The answer is almost certainly that he has not quite faced the reason why he cannot do it, and his request for advice from an expert in emotional problems – though he does not know it – is really a request to have his feelings clarified for him.

At this point we may bring in some of the qualities needed in a therapist and described in the previous section. The psychiatrist needs to identify himself with the patient and try to see what he himself would feel in the same situation. It may be worth while for the reader to do the same before going further.

The answer is utterly obvious; but, unless one has a certain capacity for ruthless honesty, it is not necessarily easy to reach. The first reaction that comes to mind might be that of course one's love and loyalty to one's mother would lead one to take the decision easily; but this conventional answer might be tempered by the realization that the prospect of being burdened for some years with an emotional invalid might not be a very inviting prospect for a young man at the beginning of his career. But why did the patient not simply say so? The answer is almost certainly that he feels too *guilty* to admit it, perhaps even to himself.

The psychiatrist therefore told him that the real problem he was bringing was not so much the question of what he should do, but his own *conflicting feelings* about having to take the responsibility, and having to pay a price, one way or the other, in dealing with his mother's situation.

The patient's response illustrates once more several of the ways in which an interpretation may be confirmed as correct – the patient speaks openly of the hidden feelings implied in the interpretation, elaborating and going beyond what has been said to him, and speaks with greater feeling and less conflict than before, giving a clear indication of deepening rapport. Here the guilt (which had not been specifically mentioned by the psychiatrist) emerged openly, together with relief, as the patient now confessed that last year he had gone off for 6 months on a geological expedition to Iceland, leaving his mother with no one outside the hospital to care for her; and moreover that many times during the past two years he had made excuses that he was too busy to see her during the university term and had left her unvisited for as much as two months at a time.

We may now try to see what lies behind this neglect of his mother, using the principles described in Chapter 2. Obviously it serves a *defensive* function, in the sense that if he keeps away from his mother he can more easily pretend that the whole situation doesn't exist. Yet is it also possible that his neglect serves an *expressive* function? It is here that the kind of ruthless honesty that is acquired by personal psychotherapy is needed even more. This situation, in which one has to balance one's own needs against those of ageing parents, is something that most of us have had to face at one time or another. Suppose the psychiatrist himself was currently going through this very conflict, and was unable to face or resolve his own feelings about it? He would be hardly likely to be able to help the patient. In particular he might well not be able to see that in the patient's confession are strong hints not merely that he is unwilling to make sacrifices, but that what he really feels guilty about is that he has hidden *resentment* about the demands that his mother's illness makes on him, and is expressing this by neglecting her. This is the part of his feelings that almost certainly is giving him more trouble than any other.

Emboldened by the favourable response to the previous comment, therefore, the psychiatrist gave him the full interpretation, speaking of the *resentment* and *guilt* that got tangled up whenever he tried to take a decision. The patient responded with great relief, and now said that it was obvious that what he had to do was what he had originally suggested. This is a striking illustration of the power of a correct interpretation, since it is almost certain that to have *advised* him to take this course of action would merely have intensified his conflict, whereas a clarification of the feelings involved has enabled him to face the idea of taking the decision relatively smoothly.

It goes without saying that to have taken a moral standpoint would have been even worse. This has no place whatsoever in psychotherapy – no one can face his true feelings within an atmosphere of being judged, still less confide them to the person judging him. This patient in particular had enough guilt without its being reinforced from outside, as was illustrated by his next communication.

With further deepening of rapport, the patient now said that while he had been thinking about the problem previously, another possible solution had entered his head, namely that he should throw up his work in Birmingham and go down to live near his mother in Bristol. This is an example of a very important psychodynamic principle: that where one meets what one may call the *neurotic all-or-nothing phenomenon* – here excessive neglect on the one hand, and excessive self-sacrifice on the other – one must look for two powerful and incompatible forces, neither of which is entirely accessible to conscious awareness, which cannot be integrated by the patient, but instead either leave him stuck in an ever-repeated pattern of alternating between the two (which is what happens in obsessional doubt), or else drive him towards a *neurotic compromise*, which is damaging to all concerned. In the present case the incompatible forces are *resentment* and *guilt*. Since the patient cannot quite admit the resentment, he cannot fully admit the guilt, as this would mean admitting what he feels guilty about. Thus both feelings are partly unconscious, though both are very close beneath the surface. What now happens is that his actual behaviour, which represents the neurotic compromise expressing hidden resentment by neglect, arouses his guilt, which leads to over-compensation and expresses itself in fantasies of excessive self-sacrifice. The idea that he ought to put these into practice almost certainly intensifies his resentment, and so the alternation begins again. The alternation is like the movement in the balance wheel of a watch – whichever way the wheel moves it mobilizes a force which reverses the movement, and although there *is* an equilibrium position the movement is kept alive by the mainspring.

One can now see why in this kind of situation advice is so useless. It is like an attempt to stop the balance wheel in *any* position. *Whatever* course of action is advocated, there will be a force opposing it, just as whatever position the balance wheel is stopped in, there will be a force that re-starts its movement.

Although the analogy now becomes a bit fanciful, the equivalent of the mainspring is the fact that the opposing forces are unconscious. It is an empirical observation that the way of unwinding the mainspring and breaking the pattern is to bring these forces into consciousness, thus enabling the patient to integrate them and reach a *realistic* rather than a *neurotic* compromise. This was illustrated here by the fact that the patient was finally able to admit that *he did not want to pay any price at all*, and patient and therapist agreed that he had better pay a price that was reasonable (the realistic compromise) rather than throw up his career – which clearly would leave his relation with his mother spoiled by so much resentment that in the end he would not be helping her at all. Thus at *this* point – once the true feelings had been clarified, some sort of implied advice was at last appropriate.

The patient ended by shaking hands and holding the therapist's hand for a long time, saying how grateful he was for the interview.

This story illustrates very clearly the theme of elementary though not easy psychotherapy. It was *elementary* in the sense that the conflict was utterly simple and involved nothing more than everyday feelings which all of us have experienced time and again in our daily lives. It was *not easy* for many reasons. The psychiatrist had to know that the patient's request for advice concealed an unconscious conflict; he had to restrain such natural human reactions as the impulse to give advice immediately or to react moralistically; he had to have faced his own feelings in parallel situations so that he could identify those of his patient; and he had to put the conflicting feelings to the patient in such a way that the latter would accept them, exploring stage by stage: first simply mentioning 'conflicting feelings', then speaking openly of resentment and guilt, and finally helping the patient with some realistic implied advice.

The influence of the past

As always, detailed examination of these stories leads to apparently unending complexity. It might be supposed that the patient's conflict has by now been fully identified – certainly the components that have been discovered are enough to have caused him considerable pain, his own recognition of them has afforded him great relief, and by the principle of economy of hypothesis there would be no need to look further. But, as already mentioned in Chapter 3 (see p. 17), in this field the principle of economy of hypothesis should be regarded with the utmost suspicion.

In fact if we forget about the principle of economy of hypothesis and simply regard the story from an empathic point of view, we can raise the question of why the patient was burdened with *so much* resentment and guilt about the self-sacrifice that his mother's illness demanded of him. Was there perhaps some *predisposing factor* making this conflict especially painful and difficult to face? If we now examine the history of relationships within his family in the past, we find the following: first, that he felt close to neither of his parents; second, that his mother had to look after his father, who was always ailing; and third, that no strong feelings – certainly not anger – were ever expressed in his home. We can speculate, therefore, that the patient himself felt somewhat neglected and resentful about it, that the resentment could never be expressed, and that this conflict was greatly intensified when he was called upon to care for the mother who had inadequately cared for him.

This leads to yet another point. Did these predisposing factors lead to detectable disturbances in the patient's life in addition to the disturbances caused by the immediate conflict? The answer is, probably yes. It was clear from an exploration of the patient's current relationships that he himself – like his family – had considerable difficulty in getting close to people, and in social relations in general. His choice of geology as a career, which involves a relation with nature rather than with people, probably was not entirely coincidental. Every single detail of the story has now fallen into place.

The question of therapeutic effects

The situation described here represents one almost universally encountered in psychotherapy, namely that (1) the patient is brought to seek help by a current conflict, but that in addition (2) this is within the background of longstanding emotional difficulties, and (3) both clearly have origins in the distant past. The fundamental question is now whether it is sufficient *therapeutically* to bring out the current conflict, or whether it is necessary also to make the links with the past.

This is an empirical question to which there is no general answer. In the present case it is clear that the patient received considerable immediate relief from his single interview, but whether this was of any lasting value to him can only be shown by subsequent events.

In fact we have a 3-year follow-up, from which the following became clear:

(1) The patient's mother consistently refused to be transferred, but the patient reacted constructively to this, reaching a reasonable compromise between his needs and hers.
(2) The patient overcame to a considerable degree his difficulties with people, and made what sounds like a happy marriage.

The evidence suggested that the first was a therapeutic effect, while the second was an example of emotional growth independent of therapy ('spontaneous remission').

For further details the reader is referred to our report on one-session patients (Malan *et al.*, 1975, pp. 118–23).

Thus in this particular case the link with the past was apparently unnecessary. This leads directly into the subject considered in the next chapter.

5

Elementary psychotherapy (contd): Symptoms, precipitating factors and psychiatric consultation

In the case of the Geologist described in Chapter 4 the patient knew perfectly well what the situation was that was causing him to seek help. Perhaps more often the patient presents with a *symptom*, which as far as he knows has just 'appeared' and has no connection with anything else in his life. In this case it is the therapist's task to discover the connection.

Now the origin of neurotic symptoms is a mysterious and controversial subject on which there are hardly any universally accepted views. It is a problem to which Freud devoted much of his energy, and to which he made overwhelmingly important contributions. Obviously, virtually the whole of psychodynamic theory, on which the present book is based, was formulated by him. Yet many workers in this field still maintain theories of the origin of symptoms, particularly phobic symptoms, that take no account of the psychodynamic point of view whatsoever. How is this possible?

The answer to this question is very complex, but a major part of it derives from the extreme uncertainty of therapeutic effects. If it were regularly possible to show that the emergence of hidden feelings rapidly and usually led to the disappearance of symptoms, the evidence in favour of psychodynamic formulations as at least part of the truth would be incontrovertible.

The Geologist, who both conforms to the usual pattern in one way, and represents an exception in another, can be used as an illustration. Although he presented with a request for advice, he was in fact suffering from symptoms, namely neurotic anxiety and indecision in the difficult situation with which he was faced. As already described in the previous chapter, an examination of the total situation revealed: (1) a current conflict; (2) other more general and more chronic disturbances; and (3) evidence for the origins of both of these in the past. This is the pattern that a careful psychodynamic assessment almost invariably reveals.

Now what usually happens in psychotherapy is that the current conflict can be identified by the therapist and clarified for the patient, but that this does not lead to any great therapeutic effect; and the therapist then has to set out on the long road of dynamic psychotherapy, in which the link is made between the current conflict and the general disturbances, and between both of these and the past. This is complex and time-consuming, and exceedingly unpredictable in terms of therapeutic outcome. Even if important therapeutic effects are observed, it is very difficult to say what factors they were due to. The final result is that the relevance of psychodynamic thinking to neurotic disturbances is by no means obvious. Dramatic examples like the Geologist, in which a single well-aimed intervention, concerned solely with the current conflict, is followed by improvements that prove to be sufficient, are the exception rather than the rule. Naturally, we all wish it were different.

Nevertheless this possibility should always be sought. Here there is a very interesting and favourable circumstance, unique to psychotherapy, which may be introduced as follows: in both medicine and psychiatry, the first step when a patient presents himself is to *take a history*, and where appropriate to establish *precipitating factors*. In medicine this is an essential preliminary to choice of treatment; in psychiatry it may of course be the same, *but sometimes it may constitute the treatment itself.* The psychiatrist who takes a careful history may therefore find that he has effectively begun a therapy or even have completed it; and thus the subject of *elementary psychotherapy* may be used to introduce and illustrate that of *psychiatric consultation*, a vast subject that is considered in detail in Chapters 18 to 23.

In medicine the question, 'How long have you had it?' is second nature; and this is very often followed by an exploration of the circumstances surrounding the first onset. Often the patient may be quite unaware of any causal connection between a particular symptom and recent events, and it may take considerable theoretical knowledge, clinical experience, and detective intuition on the part of the doctor to establish the diagnosis and the precipitating factors. A simple example might be a woman complaining of a rash on her body, where the *appearance* suggests a contact dermatitis, the *distribution* suggests a connection with her clothing, and the resulting *directed questions* reveal that she had done her washing with a new detergent two days before. Exactly the same kinds of principle apply in psychiatry and psychotherapy, though the reasons why the patient is unaware of the causal connections, the ways of establishing them through history-taking, and the connections themselves, may all be very different.

In psychiatric and psychotherapeutic consultation, therefore, the interviewer must almost always ask the question, 'How long have you had it?' and must follow this by such questions as 'What was happening in your life when it first came on?'. The establishment of these coincidences in time, and hence of probable causal connections, may occupy a very large part of the interview (see the Nurse in Mourning, pp. 137ff., for a further example).

There follow a series of examples where the *discovery of precipitating factors*, followed if necessary by further working through of the feelings involved, resulted in clear therapeutic effects. Several comments are worth making: first, that case histories of this kind represent important empirical observations which need explanation, and that psychodynamic theory offers an explanation which needs to be taken seriously; second, that in all these cases the conflicting feelings involved are readily accessible to everyday introspection; third, that although this is so, the inner mechanisms leading to the exact nature of each symptom are obscure, and no one should pretend otherwise (but therapeutically this does not matter); and finally, that the degree of empathy and skill needed to bring out the precipitating factors may be of a very high order indeed.

It is important, however, that this last condition does not always apply, and that the simple taking of a history may be sufficient. The following is an example.

Therapeutic effects from history-taking, the drama student

This was a young married woman of 22, complaining of a fear of travelling by underground which manifested itself as sweating, trembling, and awareness of her heart. This symptom was of acute onset about 3 months ago. When asked what she associated it with, she said that at this time she was beginning to face a feeling that had been there as long as she could remember, that she was insignificant and might 'disappear in a cloud of dust'. The interviewing psychiatrist could naturally make little of this communication; but the patient also added that hitherto she felt she had controlled her husband's life and that now he was beginning to strike out for his own independence. She did not emphasize this and he did not ask her exactly what she meant by it.

From her background we may pick out the following: she was the youngest of three, with two older brothers. Her mother had once complained about the way in which her father, a solicitor, controlled certain aspects of family life. The patient's childhood seems to have been reasonably happy, but after puberty she began to feel she was being 'swamped' and started a period of rebellion, which eventually involved staying out all night with boy-friends. Her parents seem to have been unable to set limits to this, and she remembered wishing that they would talk to her about it without laying down rules.

At the age of 17 she had a fairly severe depressive breakdown probably brought on by rejection by a boy-friend. She described weeping and a sense of isolation, with the feeling that she had no one with whom she could 'cross-check on her own identity'.

At case conference much of this story was obscure, and a psychologist was asked to see her. She now revealed that the onset of her symptoms had occurred in the following circumstances: She and her husband had an agreement, that as long as they were open with one another they could do what they liked, and if they wished they could have extramarital relations. In complete accord with this, one evening her husband had told her that he was going to put their agreement into effect. The result had been that she was much more upset than she had imagined possible, and her symptoms had started shortly afterwards. However, after the first interview, and presumably simply in response to having her attention drawn to the circumstances surrounding the onset of her symptoms, she had now talked it all over with her husband and her symptoms had disappeared.

Now we can see why this event might well have resulted in conflicting feelings that might express themselves in the development of symptoms. She is likely to have been overtaken by feelings of anger and jealousy, but to have felt that she could not voice them because her husband was doing no more than they had agreed he could. Once more, by the principle of economy of hypothesis there is no need to look further.

Before we reach any final conclusion, however, it might be as well not to be too hasty. The recent crisis contains the theme of *control* versus *freedom* and for her this clearly goes back a long way into the past. Moreover, in the interview with the psychologist, she added some further details. She feels that her feminine development was never noticed by her parents, though the masculine development of her brothers was. She clearly has considerable problems about accepting her own femininity, envies men and tries to emulate them, and wishes that her body was 'androgynous'. Thus, as will be discussed in more detail below, her problems are clearly not as simple as may at first appear.

This story, illustrating (like that of the Franciscans in Chapter 2) some of the possible consequences of 'trying to be better than you really are', may be used to illustrate several of the features described in the previous and present chapters, and also a difficulty not yet encountered.

First of all, the main theme of 'elementary' psychotherapy is illustrated by the fact that the simple procedure of taking a history was enough to draw attention to hitherto unconscious links, even though these were not seen by the psychiatrist at interview; and that this in turn led to open discussion with her husband (a parallel with the Economics Student in Chapter 1), with important therapeutic effects.

Second, it is now possible to make reasonable inferences about the feelings brought out by her husband's enlightened infidelity, and hence presumably about those involved in the genesis of her symptoms. *Anger* and *jealousy* have already been mentioned, together with the conflicting feeling that she was not justified in speaking up for herself. Yet there appears to be much more to it than this. With her husband she is involved in a conflict over *control* and *freedom*, which repeats (with roles reversed) a major conflict between herself and her parents that has been going on since her teens. In addition she has conflicting feelings about her own femininity, which may well have been intensified by the thought of her husband's relation with another woman. And finally there is something to do with a *lack of a sense of identity* and *not being noticed* ('disappearing in a cloud of dust'), which she herself associated with the onset of her symptoms and may possibly be related to her parents' over-permissiveness – which in turn appears to be the other side of the coin to a tendency to excessive control.

But in the excitement of complex psychodynamic insight on the one hand and effective simple psychotherapy on the other, something has been forgotten: what is the connection between all these mixed feelings and *fear of travelling by underground*? The answer is that no one knows.

This is an example of both the strength and weakness of psychodynamics, namely that it takes symptoms seriously as an indication of conflicting feelings and that it is prepared to identify and concern itself with these feelings in all their complexity, but that it may be quite unable to explain some of the inner mechanisms involved. It has to be said, however, that learning theory could not do much better, if as well.

Thus, as almost invariably happens – and just as in the case of the Geologist – an examination of the total situation in which symptoms have been precipitated results in a spreading of roots *laterally* into the patient's whole current life and *downwards* into the distant past. This is the main reason why psychodynamics is so difficult theoretically and dynamic psychotherapy is so difficult practically.

The Adopted Son

The second example is of phobic anxiety in a man, where because of the patient's resistance the intervention had to be much more forceful. Nevertheless the principle was exactly the same as in the previous example, namely the *discovery of a hidden precipitating problem*.

The patient was a man of 26, married for 2 years, who was referred to the Tavistock Clinic from the psychiatric department of a general hospital. His main complaint was of attacks of panic when away from home. These had first come on when his father had a stroke 5–6 years ago, but had threatened to become crippling since his mother died 4 months ago, often preventing him from going in to work.

He presented a bland picture of everything being rosy, but the fact that he only discovered by accident at the age of 14 that he was adopted, and now had no memories before this time, suggested that all was not as well as he wanted to make out.

Since the interviewing psychiatrist could make no contact with his deeper feelings whatsoever an attempt was made to refer him for behaviour therapy, but no vacancy could be found. Because of his urgent need for help, he was therefore taken on for six sessions of brief psychotherapy, which was all we had to offer.

In the first session (with a male psychologist) he again presented this bland front: everything had been fine with his relations with his parents and was now fine with his wife and at work – the only trouble was his symptoms. The therapist, in a determined attempt to break through the defence, became very forceful with him, saying first that he did not believe that symptoms of such severity could appear in such perfect circumstances. The patient reacted with a pleasant smile, saying he could not think of anything wrong apart from his symptoms. The therapist then confronted him with the fact that no vacancy for behaviour therapy could be found, we had no vacancy for long-term treatment, and if he didn't get better he would certainly lose his job. At this the patient became visibly anxious but volunteered no further information.

What then followed was an example of an utterly simple intervention, yet one based on deep intuition and much previous experience. The therapist wrote 'His innocent baby-like face led me to ask a question concerning his sexual life'. Now in fact the patient had said to the referring psychiatrist that there was something unsatisfactory in this area, but since then he had admitted nothing further. Now he first tried to answer that 'everything is all right', and then with great difficulty admitted that, because of his wife's complaint of pain if he tried to enter her, his marriage remained unconsummated. Moreover, although he had been married for 3 years, he had known her for 5 years, so that his relation with her more or less coincided with the duration of his symptoms.

In a later part of the session he described the building up of frightening tension in his body, moving his hands upwards over his ribs. The therapist pointed out that this gesture might as easily describe the building up of anger inside him (an interpretation of the *hidden feelings*, here an *impulse*); to which the patient said that if he expressed any anger to his wife she would leave him (a statement of the *anxiety*).

By the end of this session it had therefore become clear first that, in addition to whatever problems the patient may have had with his parents in the past, there was a severe current problem likely to cause him considerable pain; and second, that his wife might well need help in her own right.

The sequel to this is an example both of therapeutic effects, on the one hand, and of the kinds of difficulty that are likely to emerge in such a situation, on the other: from the time of this first session the patient's symptoms were reduced to the point at which he was able to go to work every weekday for the next 2 months, and in the sixth session he said his symptoms were no longer a problem. He discussed the whole situation with his wife, who at first laughed at him. He then *expressed some of his anger* to her and she began to take what he said seriously, but she still would not allow intercourse and steadfastly refused to see anyone herself. This was the situation on the expiry of the six sessions. We have no further follow-up.

It is important to note that his feelings about his parents, which must have contributed to his symptoms, were never dealt with in this therapy at all.

The Farmer's Daughter

This was a woman of 29, separated from her husband and awaiting divorce, whose unusual complaint was a deep preoccupation with guilt about the fact that she had given away her two children. It was clear that these self-reproaches were part of a depressive illness, the onset of which had been relatively sudden 14 months ago, and which at one time had been severe enough to keep her off work for 5 months.

The relevant history was as follows. She had fallen in love with her husband at 16 and married him against her parents' wishes less than a year later. He was a labourer working on a farm near that of her parents, in Shropshire. Everything went all right until about 3 months after her marriage, when she became pregnant. From this point, and especially after the birth of her first child, Geoffrey, her husband turned against her and started coming home drunk and beating her up. He was particularly resentful about the loss of earnings resulting from the pregnancy and birth; and the result was that she gave away first Geoffrey to her mother and then a second boy, Andrew, to a childless couple who lived next door, who subsequently moved away to an unknown address. Both her mother and this couple proceeded to bring up the respective children as their own. Giving away these two children did not improve the relation with her husband in any way. His behaviour became more and more psychopathic and 5 years ago she finally left him.

The interviewing psychiatrist chose to explore the background first, but could find nothing in it that might account for a predisposition to a relatively severe illness. He therefore turned to trying to find out the more recent precipitating factors. Invited to talk about events since she left her husband, she said that she had been perfectly well for 3 or 4 years. She had had jobs that she enjoyed very much, and 3 years ago she had formed a relation with a married man called Len. Then, 14 months ago, quite out of the blue, she had begun to get depressed.

Of course one of the major mysteries in this story was why her depressive symptoms had come on *4 years after* the break-up with her husband and not before. The most obvious explanation seemed to be that it had something to do with the relation with Len. This inference was reinforced when she said that one of the symptoms that she had at the beginning of her depression was bursting into tears at some disappointment, such as finding that Len wasn't able to take her out after all. In further discussion, she said that he was a Catholic and could not get a divorce, and that she herself had a lot of doubts about him and would never marry him while these doubts remained. The interviewer then made a guess, saying that at the time when her symptoms began perhaps she had begun to feel more deeply attached to Len than before, and therefore had to face the hopelessness of her relation with him (an interpretation guessing at the *hidden feeling*). This made her think, and she eventually brought out the following: that in August of that year she and Len had planned to visit her home in Shropshire, and he had made the passing remark, 'Perhaps I'll like it and we might start a new life there.' In fact he hadn't liked it, and it was clear that he had raised her hopes and then dashed them. In further discussion it became clear that her symptoms had started soon after their return to London, in the September, and both interviewer and patient became convinced that the precipitating factor had been found. Moreover, she by now admitted that she felt more for Len than she had wanted to acknowledge earlier in the interview.

This is an example of a very important general observation: that when symptoms are precipitated by a given event, this is very frequently not the first time such an event has occurred, but is a repetition. In this case the disappointment with Len repeated what must have been a previous severe disappointment, namely with her marriage.

She was now taken on for individual psychotherapy with a highly experienced social worker, a woman, who gently led her to discuss the present and the past and to think about emotional problems. After three sessions she wrote that she felt it was 'no longer necessary to attend the clinic. I am now able to understand far more about myself, and am able to live with the past and look forward to the future.'

Our final follow-up was 8 months later. The exact sequence of events is not absolutely clear. She clearly felt very relieved by her contacts with the clinic and described this in retrospect as 'like a cloud lifting.' At some point during the follow-up period it now transpired that the barriers preventing Len from getting a divorce were not as absolute as had appeared, and he and she were now planning to get married. Moreover, she had now told her first boy, Geoffrey, that she was his mother, which seems to have improved both her relationship with him and with her own mother; and she had also decided – I think sensibly and realistically – that it was best for her second boy, Andrew, to be left as he was, with the couple who had adopted him.

Her feelings about her previous marriage were never gone into during therapy, and we cannot tell what may still lie buried in her from this part of her past, or whether it may lead to further trouble when things go wrong in the future. Nevertheless, for the time being the therapeutic result from a very limited intervention seems to have been favourable – but since she refused further follow-up we do not know even whether Len did finally marry her, let alone whether they lived happily ever after.

The Daughter with a Stroke

This patient, a single woman of 27, was seen for consultation by an experienced and psychoanalytically qualified social worker, a woman, attached to a General Practice in London. All the interviewer knew was that the patient was complaining both of depression and of anxiety about going out, and that the GP was quite at a loss to account for this.

She asked the patient the standard question, how long had she had it? The patient began to answer, saying that she used to get stomach pains on going to school, but the question got lost in her anxiety, and she went on to say that she had asked her doctor if she might be physically ill, and although he had assured her that she was not, instead of being reassured she had felt increased panic. (This, incidentally, is an example of the frequently observed phenomenon of the ineffectiveness of reassurance, which will be discussed further on p. 87). She said she just wants to stay at home and curl up. The interviewer asked her what home consisted of, to which she said that she shares a flat with a friend – *her mother died of a stroke* two years ago and her father lives away from London.

It became clear that the patient's anxiety was very severe, and the depression was close enough to the surface to make her tearful during most of the interview. She said that she wants help before she goes beyond the point when she can no longer communicate with anyone – she is afraid of going mad. The interviewer asked if she had mad thoughts? She said that she had attacks of 'redding out', in which everything goes red before her eyes, and she feels out of communication with everyone for as much as a quarter of an hour.

In further discussion it emerged that her mother had been an extremely possessive, clinging, reproachful woman, and the patient had had to fight for her independence.

At this point we may take stock. It is worth noting that the patient's anxiety and confusion have been such that the basic fact in her history of exactly when her symptoms started has never been established. My own inclination, as a psychiatrist, would perhaps have been to have taken her back to this question and to have pressed her to answer it. At the same time I would have been watching for evidence of precipitating factors arising out of sources of conflict in her life, and the death of a loved and hated mother two years ago is an obvious candidate. It is well recognized that the death of such a person may intensify guilt to the point of preventing the natural process of mourning, and that this in turn may be one of the major factors leading to reactive depression. The interviewer, as a social worker whose training is concerned more directly with human relations, rather than the history of symptoms, chose to go for this at once. Had the patient wept over her mother's death? The patient immediately confirmed the above tentative formulation by saying that she had had 'the usual guilt dreams', an example of which was that her mother was still alive and the patient was telling her that she *shouldn't be there because she was dead*. If ever there was an example of a dream saying out loud the kind of thing that could not be said in waking life, this was it. The patient went on to describe a precarious sense of teetering on the brink of something, adding that her GP just prevents her from 'falling into something'. This image kept recurring, and as she spoke of it she pointed to the ground in front of her chair.

Here the interviewer had the confidence born of long experience to enter empathically into the patient's world, and to risk voicing a thought that may seem at first too fanciful to be entertained: was she perhaps afraid of falling into her mother's grave – of being as unseparate from her in death as she was in life? This had no dramatic effect, but the patient seemed relieved and interested. Encouraged, the interviewer now added a second empathic association of her own, and asked whether the 'redding out' was like what she imagined the experience of *having a stroke* to be. To her amazement the patient now said that *the first attack had occurred on the second anniversary of her mother's death, and indeed at the very same hour.* Nevertheless she still wondered how making such links might help, though she also said that the discussion brought her a sense of physical relief.

The interviewer therefore went further into the patient's personal history and the relation with her parents. The patient spoke of her mother's domination of the whole household, including the patient's father; of her own open rebellion against this; and attempts to side with her father against her mother. At one point she said that on the Sunday before her mother's death she had disregarded a plea from her mother to come and visit her; and she said quite calmly that possibly worry about her may have caused her mother's stroke. Later in the interview, however, she said that after her first attack of redding out she had sat in the corner of the room and had realized with terror just how one might be driven to commit suicide. To this the interviewer said that surely she really did believe (out of guilt) that she should be with her mother in the grave. Now for the first time the patient wept uncontrollably.

Briefly the patient was now seen five more times and the process of working through her feelings about her mother's death, particularly her anger with her mother and her guilt about it, was continued. She felt much relieved and was able to go back to work. As so often, however, it became clear that she had very considerable personality problems long antedating the precipitating factor to her recent illness, but – perhaps sensibly – she felt enough was enough and declined further help.

This is an example where the connection between one of the patient's symptoms and the precipitating factor can hardly be doubted. At the same time the kind of imaginative free-association used by the interviewer is not recommended to anyone who is not considerably experienced – the result is often just being clever at the patient's expense, confusing the issue rather than clarifying it.

Table 1   Summary of clinical examples

Patient	Page	Symptoms	Nature of conflict
Economics Student	1	Depression	Inability for face jealousy
Geologist	26	Anxiety	Resentment about demands, conflicting with guilt about not fulfilling his obligations
Drama Student	34	Phobic anxiety	Jealousy and anger conflicting with idealism; dependence and independence; control and rebellion; feelings of sexual inferiority
Adopted Son	35	Phobic anxiety	Sexual frustration and humiliation, anger; fear of loss if these feelings were expressed
Farmer's Daughter	37	Depression	Inability to face her feelings about a second disappointment
Daughter with a Stroke	38	Depression, phobic anxiety, acute anxiety attacks	Guilt about hostile feelings towards her mother who had died

Retrospect of clinical examples

During the course of telling these clinical stories evidence has gradually accumulated about some of the kinds of conflict leading to neurotic symptoms, and therapeutic effects that may sometimes follow from bringing these conflicts into consciousness. The main examples are shown in *Table 1*.

As was mentioned at the beginning of the present chapter, all these conflicts involve everyday feelings readily accessible to introspection. The kind of brief therapy described here can perfectly well be performed by anyone willing to be honest with himself about what he would feel in similar situations, and to use this self-knowledge *entirely in the service of the patient*. It is this last point that is not easy if he himself has unresolved feelings about such situations – or unresolved feelings about patients – which, once more, is why personal psychotherapy is so important. Another reason, however, is that there are also large areas of feeling, and other mental mechanisms, that are not by any means accessible to ordinary introspection, an understanding of which will sooner or later become necessary to any psychotherapist as his work proceeds. We can now only go further by entering this other world.

6

A note on the observations of psychoanalysis

Ever since its beginning in the 1890s, psychoanalysis has suffered from two major sets of barriers obstructing the general acceptance of its views and observations. The first set consists of the very nature of the observations themselves, many of which are concerned with feelings that are far indeed from what civilized man would like to believe about himself. This is intrinsic, and little can be done to mitigate it. The second set, however, is concerned with Freud's personality and background and the tradition to which these two factors have given rise; of which we may list many features, such as the divorce from the methods of experimental science and from contemporary biology, the esoteric language, highly questionable and most un-biological concepts such as primary narcissism, the libido theory, and the death instinct; and above all the intense identification between analyst and analytical trainee, which has led to the ossification of ideas into rigidly held ideological beliefs, instead of tentative theories that need dispassionate consideration and await experimental confirmation or disproof. Barriers of this kind are unnecessary and urgently require dismantling.

What is needed above all is a return to the most elementary of first principles, namely that psychoanalysis, like all sciences, deals in *observations;* and that, however improbable these may seem, if properly made they are incontrovertible and are quite independent of any theoretical framework that may be built around them.

One of Freud's most important contributions was a particular tool for making observations, namely the method of *free association*, according to which the patient is instructed to say everything that comes into his mind, or in other words to be totally honest. This was the first essential step that led to the possibility of Man's looking at his true nature – something that had never been done before in his history. It is now clear that anyone who had used this method would have made similar observations, many of which – as mentioned above – are very different from what civilized thought, expressed in such idealistic concepts as Reason and Progress and Enlightenment, would have us expect. Some of the phenomena observed are therefore both very strange intellectually, and very disturbing emotionally. They can only be explained as the products of our evolutionary history, which have become buried but not weakened by the veneer of civilization, and which still very powerfully affect our lives. Many of them can be summed up in a statement of the primitive, literal, and intensely physical nature of some components of such ordinary human emotions as love, hate, jealousy, and feelings about manhood and womanhood. They will not be made to go away by pretending they do not exist, nor will they be prevented from recurring again and again by dismissing each individual case as an isolated aberration.

In some people these feelings become fully conscious spontaneously, in some they are brought into consciousness by the process of psychotherapy, but more often they never become more than partly conscious and their presence has to be inferred. This is another of the difficulties in the way of their general acceptance. But psychoanalysts have not helped their cause by speaking as if such feelings were all *universal*, which is by no means certain, and were the *only* feelings present, which is obviously untrue. On the other side it needs to be said that whereas scepticism is a correct and scientific attitude, blinding oneself to evidence is not, and the observational basis for these inferences is in fact very wide indeed.

In the following pages I present some clinical examples in which the evidence is particularly clear. In this sense they are exceptional, but in no other way – they are part of a vast body of clinical evidence all leading in the same direction. Throughout the rest of this book, I would therefore ask the reader to approach the evidence with an open mind, and while retaining a healthy scepticism, to take seriously any theory that accounts for the observations, and to find alternatives if he can. But one thing is certain, that the true explanations cannot be any less strange than the phenomena themselves.

7

Common syndromes I: Problems of femininity and sexuality in women

The Economics Student (contd)

It will be remembered from Chapter 1 that this girl suffered a depressive attack while on holiday with a young man and another girl, and that her symptoms disappeared when she was able first to realize that she was suffering from *jealousy* in this competitive situation, and then to express her feelings to the other two people involved. Another important fact was that her depressive symptoms included a feeling of self-hatred, which was tentatively interpreted as an expression of *guilt*.

This story provides some very strong evidence for the nature of the main conflict causing her symptoms, which comes from three sources: (1) the precipitating circumstances; (2) the clear emergence of a powerful hidden feeling; and (3) the immediate therapeutic effects. Yet careful thought will reveal at once that there is something missing: why should this girl have been especially sensitive to – or guilty about – jealousy, which after all is a very ordinary human emotion? It is this that will be considered now.

An answer to this question may be approached through further details of her story. The depressive attack described above had in fact occurred during a follow-up period. The event that had originally brought her to seek treatment had been a previous attack showing very similar features. Shortly before her second-year exams at College she had been in her room, had become aware of the sound of music and laughter from neighbouring rooms, and had had another uncontrollable fit of weeping in response to the thought that all the other girls had boy-friends and she hadn't. This had been the beginning of a depressive attack similar to the one that she had suffered in Spain. In addition, as her exams approached, she had had a number of premonitory depressive attacks, with the feeling that she was worthless, a fraud, and that people wouldn't have anything to do with her if they knew her real self. Once more the themes of jealousy, feeling left out, and guilt, were prominent features in the whole story.

In the period described now, however, there had been one additional detail, namely that she had begun suffering from nightmares. Of course this is not surprising – most people suffer from examination anxiety, and this is likely to be intensified in anyone who finds it difficult to face jealousy and competition.

So far we have been guided by nothing more than emotional common sense. But in the area of psychodynamics common sense is a treacherous guide, by whom we may be led through familiar paths to turn a corner and suddenly find our guide and ourselves totally lost. For the nightmares were not about examination anxiety at all. What were they about? I almost hesitate to reveal the answer, but they consisted of *thinly disguised sexual dreams about her father*, in the latest of which – just before her final depressive attack – the disguise had been so thin that she had been unable to hide their true theme from herself any longer.

This is the point at which there is a great temptation to give up altogether, and to fall back on saying that of course we all have strange dreams for which no one has ever provided a satisfactory explanation – probably the brain's computer is clearing itself of useless thoughts in preparation for the next day. But in any area other than psychodynamics this would be seen at once to be a most extraordinary attitude, because it amounts to not taking observations seriously and in effect saying that they are without explanation. In the previous chapter we met a dream that might well be regarded as saying something that could not be said in waking life. Could this be true here? If it were, of course, we would be forced into the position first of admitting that a girl of 20 may have sexual feelings for her father, which is disturbing, and then of saying that there must be some connection between this and examination anxiety, which seems far-fetched and improbable.

Nevertheless, if we do dare to pursue this line of thought, an explanation emerges that is not so entirely far-fetched after all. If we accept the possibility that there were sexual feelings for her father, then naturally this would be likely to bring her into hidden competition with her mother. Obviously the whole situation would be laden with anxiety and guilt, and this might well be activated by *any situation involving jealousy and competition*. In fact once the initial step has been made, every detail of the story falls into place: the intensification of anxiety by the competitive situation of exams, the severity of the guilt, the theme of the nightmares, and the events leading to her two attacks of depression, the first at College and the second in the triangular situation in Spain.

Finally, if we now enquire into her background, we can see reasons why all these problems might have arisen. Her father worked for the Foreign Office and much of her childhood was spent in various capitals abroad. Although she had one very much older brother, he went away to boarding school in England when she was small, so that she was brought up virtually as an only child. Because of frequent moves, she had few companions of her own age and she and her parents were very much thrown together. She was extremely close to her father, who treated her more as if he were an elder brother. The family also had very advanced views, and she was treated as an adult from an early age. Thus, if problems ever do arise from triangular situations between a daughter and her parents, all her circumstances would certainly conspire together to highlight them.

This girl in fact was part of a series of untreated patients who were followed up more than two years after their initial assessment (see Malan *et al.*, 1975). At follow-up the interviewer felt it right to interpret to her the link between the triangular relation in her home and the situation in Spain. The patient's response was to tell how her father and mother had different views about her appearance. Her mother wanted her to dress in such a way that she looked smart but somehow not attractive to men; whereas the way her father wanted her to dress made her look much more beautiful. In fact, she tried to dress in a way that resembled neither of these, but if it resembled either, it was the way her *mother* advocated. The apparent paradox, in a girl who so obviously longed for close relations with men, is of course immediately resolved by the theme of her nightmares. In fact it looks as if her feeling of guilt had inhibited her from competing by making the best of her attractiveness, which in turn had exacerbated her loneliness and jealousy of other women.

This is an example in which, if the hypothesis is correct, circumstances and relationships within the home intensified the guilt-laden sexual element in the relation with the father and equally guilt-laden rivalry with the mother, with consequent inhibitions and anxieties both in the direct relation with men and in triangular relations involving another woman. This is usually referred to as the 'Oedipal' problem or 'Oedipus complex' in women, by analogy with the corresponding problem in men, which will be discussed in the next chapter. (The term 'Electra complex', derived from another Greek myth, seems never to have caught on.)

In this example the evidence for actual and literal sexual feelings for the father was absolutely clear. The question arises, how widespread are such feelings, and how literal are they in general? Equally, how widespread, how literal, or how primitive, are the competitive feelings directed against the parent of the same sex? If competition is taken to its logical conclusion, after all, it involves getting rid of one's rival altogether.

The answer is that the idea of the Oedipus complex is an inference or extrapolation from a large body of evidence, most of which – in individual patients – is partial and indirect. Yet the cumulative circumstantial evidence is very strong that in many people some such constellation of feelings does exist. This evidence comes from such observations as the choice of a sexual partner possessing features clearly resembling those of the parent of the opposite sex; and the profound anxiety and guilt associated with situations of jealousy and rivalry, and particularly with the actual death, or thoughts of the death, of the parent of the same sex. This kind of evidence will be repeatedly illustrated in the following pages.

As for the question of how widespread such feelings are, analysts often speak as if they were universal and an essential part of human development. This is a thesis that cannot be proved, and I suspect it ignores a large sample of therapies of women – and perhaps to a lesser extent, of men – in which such problems play hardly any part. Negative evidence is so much easier to ignore, or to explain away by saying that the feelings are really there and would have been brought to light by further analysis. Let us simply say that these problems are common, and should be looked for in one form or another in all patients, particularly those showing difficulties concerned with sex, competition, success, failure and femininity (or, as will appear in the next chapter, masculinity).

Mixed feelings about men

In the example just described, problems seem to have arisen from over-close relations within the family. A second large category of problems in women is concerned with intense mixed feelings about men, which often appear to have been derived from the relation with a father who has been distant or rejecting. In such patients inhibited longing for a good father is usually found as well; with accompanying hidden Oedipal feelings, which appear to have been merely intensified by the unsatisfactory relation with the actual father.

The following patient illustrates these features particularly clearly. She was one of those rare people who, though not at all sophisticated psychologically, have the gift of rapidly becoming in touch with their deepest feelings and of putting them into direct, simple, and everyday language. As will be seen, she therefore illustrates many features in the clearest possible way, which include deep anger against men, Oedipal feelings, direct evidence bearing on the origin of symptoms, and primitive impulses that lie very far away from common sense.

The Director's Daughter

Background and complaints

She was the youngest of three sisters. She had always been close to her mother and could share all her feelings with her. The problem lay in her father, who, although kind in every way, seemed always to have been at a loss when it came to softer feelings, and who consequently had little idea of his daughters' emotional needs and had never allowed himself close to any of them.

The patient came to psychotherapy at the age of 30, complaining of various gastro-intestinal symptoms, a fear of eating in restaurants, and an inability to form close and stable relations with men. She was also mildly depressed, had contemplated suicide, and was at present living at home with her parents, unable to work. She was seen by a male therapist first at three times a week, and then once a week, over a number of years.

As in an analysis, she lay on the couch and was asked to say everything that came into her mind. Her material will be presented under various headings, simply by quoting events of therapy, where possible in her own words.

Anger with men and the origin of symptoms

The first of her symptoms to give way to the therapeutic process was her inability to work. Two-and-a-half years after therapy began she at last felt able to start work again and was interviewed and accepted for a job. She rang up her therapist to tell him about this. One might think that her feelings would have been of pleasure and satisfaction – not a bit of it. The main feelings were of distress and anger. She said she had felt sick throughout the interview for the job, and she *wanted her therapist to suffer as much as she had*. She cried all the way home in the train, went to her GP, and had a terrific scene with him, saying, 'I hate all you men'.

The above episode illustrates an extremely important feature of neurotic symptoms, namely that *they are there for a purpose*, they fulfil an important function, and the giving up of them, so far from being a relief, may be accompanied by a feeling of loss and anger. In this case the inference is that her inability to work represented some sort of protest, or living reproach, about the failure of her relation with her father; and that the giving up of this entrenched position represented an act of forgiveness, and the renunciation of an attempt to get what she had never had from him, which she carried out with the utmost regret and anger. Let therapists be warned to keep their satisfaction to themselves when such a renunciation occurs – or at least, if they fail to do so, not to be surprised by the patient's immediate relapse.

It is also worth noting that the row with the GP is an example of the phenomenon of 'acting out' (for further illustration see the Imaginary Therapy, p. 97; and the Mental Welfare Officer, p. 155). What this means is that feelings stirred up by the therapy – and particularly feelings about the therapist – get expressed in an intense way towards people or situations in the patient's life outside.

During the next few years of her therapy there emerged quite explicitly some very strong hostile feelings towards her father and other men, and on a number of occasions the open expression of these feelings resulted in the immediate disappearance of an attack of symptoms. About 3 years after the start of therapy she met a man called Brian who was clearly very attracted by her. One day she said that she now realized that as soon as a man said he loved her she lost all feeling for him, and this was now happening with Brian. She knew that she was attractive to men, and she felt she must deliberately play up to them and get them in her power – it must be some sort of revenge. She now realized that she had done this with all her boy-friends in the past.

The following is one of many examples of the immediate disappearance of symptoms when she expressed her true feelings: 'The other day, when Brian said to me, "Can't you be nice to me? We have so little time together", for a moment I tried to be and I immediately felt sick; and then I said, "No!" and the sickness immediately went away.'

A second example is when she and Brian were talking about the news in the papers of a series of prostitutes being found dead in the river. As they spoke about this she began to feel sick, and Brian, said, 'Yes, it is a bit sordid'. With intensity she replied, 'it isn't that at all. If I were a prostitute there'd be a lot of naked *men* found dead in the river.' Her nausea immediately disappeared.

The link with her father only appeared explicitly some time later, as in the following example: She had managed to enjoy a party, something that would have been impossible in the old days. She described her former feelings as consisting of feeling alone and jealous of the other people, and how she would get abdominal pain and the need to open her bowels. Nowadays, she said, it would be *feelings* rather than symptoms that she experienced and one of these would be the wish to *shout out abuse about her father*.

The ability to express hostile feelings of this kind led directly to her steadily increasing ability to express warmth and love, particularly in the sexual relation with Brian, whom she eventually married. Previously, she said, she had been 'like a robot' in her relations with men.

Oedipal feelings

This patient provides an excellent and fascinating example of cumulative evidence for Oedipal feelings.

About two years after starting therapy she said that she had recently been preoccupied with feelings of *jealousy* and *remorse*. After some interpretations about Oedipal feelings she said that amongst these feelings there had been the irrational idea that *if her mother died* she could *have her therapist for herself*. (This, of course, is an example of *transference*.)

During the course of therapy she repeatedly reported waking up in the night with some anxiety-laden feeling, which over the months she gradually came closer and closer to being able to identify. At first it was that she *mustn't think of something*; then that she mustn't think of something *about her mother*; then that she mustn't think about her mother *in a particular way*; then that she mustn't think of her mother *in a jealous way*; more recently she had had a similar feeling involving Brian, but it wasn't an adult feeling, she wanted him to *come and comfort her*, but she *mustn't think of needing him*.

A long time later she was able to continue this series: the fantasy seemed to be of *having one of her parents to herself*; then there seemed to be in it something about *having a baby*; and then there was the feeling that *she went off with a man and left her mother alone*, which was associated with guilt and remorse.

As the reader will see, the fantasy of separating her parents, taking her father sexually for herself, and leaving her mother alone, was never explicitly stated; yet the inference seems very strong that this was the basis of the above series of feelings, and that these feelings had arisen – perhaps quite unconsciously – in childhood.

A piece of insight leading towards the same kind of conclusion can be quoted in the patient's own words: 'It seems as if my mother is always interrupting me in some fantasy that I am trying to work out for myself. And of course I can't express any of my sexuality in her presence, and it seems as if life with her consists of nothing but washing up and making jam.' Here it must be said that the feeling of guilt and remorse about leaving her mother was very strong, and indeed it was quite clear that her love for her mother was deep and genuine, and led to the feeling that she could not leave her for a man, which in turn led to utter despair. She described one of the situations in which she tended to get abdominal pain, as 'going shopping with my mother without hope of ever doing anything more exciting'.

There is strong evidence that, in spite of repeated working through, these feelings were never completely eradicated – this is an indication of their depth and power. Several years after termination, when she had already been married for some time, she asked for a further session because of an attack of severe anxiety and physical symptoms. This had occurred after a party at which a male friend of her boss was 'going it pretty strongly' with her boss's wife and the patient overheard someone saying that the boss had had a previous wife who had died 25 years ago. In a letter describing this incident she wrote: 'Rationally of course, though I like my boss very much I would not want him to make love to me or to live with him, but I wonder if this was rather a vulnerable situation for me and evoked some feelings which I may have thought too frightful to express and then felt guilty about … I remember thinking the next morning. "I must not tell my mother about this, and thank goodness I am not having a baby". ' The situation at the party was one packed full of triangular relationships, both real and symbolic, and in her fantasy she seemed to bring her mother into it as well; and the symbolism of a man having a relation with another and younger woman – and a forbidden woman at that – after the death of a previous woman, has obvious Oedipal implications. It is indirect yet powerful evidence of this kind that leads to the construction of the basic hypothesis of the Oedipus complex in both sexes.

Primitive feelings

As was mentioned above, Freud's use of the method of free association has led to the discovery of many facets of human nature, some of which – like the intensely physical quality of human emotions – would be obvious if there were not a strong tendency to deny them; while others are very far from obvious and can only make sense if they are regarded as residues left over from Man's evolutionary history. It is not surprising, for instance, that *eating* should be of immense importance – in Western society we tend to take eating too much for granted – but it is surprising to find impulses to do with eating playing a fundamental part in human relationships. Yet this does seem to occur.

It may be remembered that one of this patient's principal symptoms was an inability to eat in restaurants, which applied particularly when she was with a man. When a patient presents with such a symptom, one needs to approach it empirically, with an open mind about what it will turn out to mean. As with Oedipal feelings discussed above, each individual piece of evidence is often indirect and inconclusive, yet – as they accumulate – the final inferences are almost unavoidable.

This young woman's intuitive understanding, both of her own mental processes and of her instinctual nature, is illustrated by a passage that occurred fairly early in therapy. She spoke of an incident in which her parents had been asked out to a *meal* by a woman, and her father hadn't wanted to go. She had thought this *terrible*, as the woman would be so disappointed – 'I suppose that's how I'd feel, so I think other people feel the same' (describing mechanisms of 'identification' and 'projection' in simple and direct language). She went on to say that probably out of revenge, because she had been so disappointed herself, she wanted to disappoint other people. The therapist tentatively made the link between this and her *inability to eat* when asked out by a man, implying that she wanted to disappoint him. Her response to this was to say that only recently she had been saying to her mother that if one received a present one could *pretend* to be grateful, but this would not be possible over the *fundamental things like eating and making love.*

We may now ask the following question: If a woman is disappointed by a man, what is her way of expressing her anger and need for revenge? Or, put in another way, what impulses tend to be found as the expression of the quotation, 'Hell hath no fury like a woman scorned'? One could give a series of answers, starting with the most civilized and ending with the most primitive. One could start by saying that, if she gets an opportunity, she will reject him back, or will flirt with another man in his presence, or will try to humiliate him as a man, or will want to hit him, or to scratch his face. But one can continue this series to the ultimate in primitiveness, as the following will show:

In one session this patient reported that she had had a dream in which she was with an older man and she had had the impulse to *grab his penis*. This was accompanied by the feeling that she was *possessed by something evil*. The therapist tentatively interpreted to her that, because she felt rejected by men, she had the impulse to retaliate by attacking a man's penis. Shortly after this she spontaneously associated to a remark made in her presence by her father about a woman 'wanting to bite a man's balls off'. Nothing had been said to her about such impulses by the therapist.

One day after Brian had been making love to her he said he had to go, and she immediately said to him, 'If you go now I'll bite you', and, to herself, 'and spit it out'. The therapist interpreted the exceedingly primitive attack on a man who disappointed her, and tentatively linked this with her eating difficulty. Her response was to say that she felt this must be right, and then that she *couldn't have eaten* with Brian at a previous dinner unless she had *got all the bad feelings out of her first*.

On a later occasion, after many circumstances had prevented Brian and her from being together, they at last had an opportunity to make love. She was full of angry feelings and tried to include them in the love-making by being as fierce as possible. She also felt, and said, that actual intercourse was at that moment the last thing she wanted, and she began to *feel sick*. Suddenly the following image passed through her mind: that she ate Brian, and then *vomited him out* red and dripping, like steak.

Here it must be said that red meat, and particularly steak, lay at the top of the hierarchy of her anxiety about eating. Moreover, one of the feelings that she became aware of during her therapy was that, whereas she couldn't eat in a restaurant, 'other women could do it', and that his made her feel in some way inferior as a woman; and one of the situations that aroused her anxiety was seeing another couple at the next table *eating steak*, i.e. presumably expressing freely primitive aspects of their nature which she felt she could not do herself.

The above evidence is less conclusive than that concerned with the connection between her anxiety and aggression against men in general, but nevertheless it is highly suggestive. The essential indications are of primitive aspects of eating and the connection between these and sexuality.

At the end of this therapy, and throughout many years' follow-up, this patient's symptoms had entirely disappeared. She has committed herself fully to marriage with Brian, whom she deeply loves, and their sexual relation is free and passionate.

Envy of men

The previous patient illustrates very clearly the anger against men aroused in a girl who feels rejected by her father. What this patient was fortunate in *not* suffering from is a problem that tends to be much more intractable to therapy, namely a hatred and envy of *everything masculine*, and a corresponding competition with men, which forms the principal feature in certain other women who have suffered similar rejection. Behind this there often lies a deep sense of inferiority both to men and to other women, and a hidden depreciation of everything feminine. Such women are in a most unenviable position, because they (obviously) cannot be men, and at the same time do not feel themselves to be proper women, and they tend to fall between the two, unable to function properly in either role.

It would be an interesting research project to try and establish which kinds of early relation lead simply to anger against men because of rejection, and which lead to explicit envy and competitiveness. It is tempting to suggest that the latter feelings arise particularly when the father has been dominating or overbearing – certainly this was so in the following example.

The Pilot's Wife

This recently married young woman came to treatment at the age of 25 because of a severe distaste for sexual intercourse, persisting after an operation on an exceptionally tough hymen which had prevented consummation of her marriage on her honeymoon. Her case was complicated by the fact that she suffered from irregular periods and some degree of hirsutism, which was diagnosed as being due to mild adrenogenital syndrome. Endocrinological evidence, however, suggests that this would be more likely to increase her libido than to decrease it, so that in a psychological assessment the endocrine factor can probably be discounted.

She almost refused to be seen in consultation by a male doctor, on the grounds that no man could understand how she felt. When she did come, she could talk of little else but comparisons between men and women – how she had always been a tomboy and the boys had not dared to attack her on the way back from school because she could give as good as she got; how furious it made her to see rows of men in the Underground who would not give up their seat to her (when women got equal pay, *then* this could be justified); how, apart from carrying heavy things, there was nothing that a man could do that a woman couldn't; how she had always wanted to be a man; how in sexual intercourse the man produced the mess but put it all over the woman, and how she had to have a bath the next morning; how the arrangement that she had finally come to with her husband was that he went to bed first and 'used his imagination' and then 'got it over with as soon as possible'; and so on and so on.

At consultation she showed a great admiration for, and identification with, her father; but during therapy a somewhat different picture emerged: that her father had said that if she behaved like a boy then she should be treated as a boy, and consequently whenever she did anything naughty he beat her (the last time being when she was thirteen); and eventually she spoke of the struggle between the two of them and how 'he always came off best, and I'm still afraid of him'.

Therapy was characterized at first by her continuing the battle of the sexes by contradicting everything the (male) therapist said, thus largely defeating his attempts to function as a therapist; but it culminated in her finally admitting that, if therapy was being unsuccessful, it was *she* who felt she was failing – i.e. she was failing in her role as patient. This looked as if it exactly paralleled the sexual situation: by preventing her husband from functioning as a man she failed to fulfil her role as a woman. This is of course another excellent example of *transference*, and the parallel was repeatedly interpreted to her.

There followed a good deal of material indicating a contempt for women rather than men, and the fear that men (including her father and the therapist) found other women more attractive than she was. However, in the end therapy was a failure, and she did not change at all. A final vignette that characterized her attitude to femininity comes from a letter that she wrote several years after termination: at the age of 32 she was found to be suffering from fibroids, and she wrote of this, 'There was some talk of a hysterectomy (to which I was agreeable, as you may imagine) but although my husband readily signed for this, it was not found to be necessary.'

8
Common Syndromes II: Problems of masculinity and sexuality in men

There is a group of problems in men in which anxiety, often severe, is aroused by a wide variety of situations, some of them obviously related to one another and some apparently unrelated. Such situations are as follows: competition and rivalry between men, particularly in triangular situations involving a woman; heterosexual situations, particularly if guilt-laden; hostility towards, conflict with, or disapproval by, male authority, particularly in situations involving sexuality; being put to the test (e.g. exams); failure, downfall, punishment, retribution; physical injury, real or symbolic; *success*; the death or downfall of other males, especially authority figures, or injury to them, or other forms of triumph over them; taking another man's place; being let down or rejected by men; and finally, stealing something that can be seen as symbolizing power, strength, or masculinity.

There follow a number of clinical examples.

The Concert-goer

A man of 24 asked for treatment complaining of (1) difficulty in dealing with other men, especially in the presence of women; and (2) feelings of hostility in the presence of male authority.

Five weeks ago there had been an acute exacerbation of his problems, which had occurred in the following circumstances:

He had gone to a concert with his woman friend and a male acquaintance of hers, a Norwegian, whom he described as good-looking and a very forceful personality. Although he found the Norwegian fascinating as an individual, he immediately took a dislike to him because he sensed that his woman friend was attracted by him and he felt the two of them were in competition for her attention. As the evening progressed he became more and more agitated and eventually had to go home. He described his anxiety as so severe that he was in a daze for 72 hours afterwards.

Exploration of the current situation revealed that the patient was living with this woman friend, who was in fact married, was old enough to be his mother, and had a son roughly the same age as he was. Moreover, her husband, who was crippled with multiple sclerosis, was living in the same house. Nevertheless she and the patient carried on their sexual relation, apparently with the husband's connivance.

Specific features

(1) Unsuccessful competition with another man in a triangular relation,
(2) Successful competition with an injured man, and
(3) A sexual relation with a (much older) woman.

The Dental Patient

A man in his mid-thirties was admitted to a neurosis unit for very severe anxiety and panic attacks which had been precipitated by the extraction of a tooth. Part of his anxiety took the form of a fear that he would die of a heart attack.

Exploration of his current and recent past revealed the following. Some years ago his best friend had married a girl by whom he (the patient) had become extremely attracted. He was much too loyal to his friend to have made any advances to her, and the three of them kept up a close and warm relation. About three years ago, however, his friend had died suddenly and quite unexpectedly of a coronary thrombosis; and, to cut a long story short, the patient had eventually married his friend's widow.

Further exploration revealed that, just before the extraction, the dentist had said, 'Some people have bad hearts; some people have bad teeth'.

Specific features

(1) Physical injury,
(2) Fear of retribution,
(3) The death of a male friend, and
(4) Taking the friend's place with his wife.

The Articled Accountant

This young man of 22, who had previously been largely unaware of sexual feelings, suddenly began to experience an uncontrollable urge to watch homosexual contacts being made. On one of these occasions he himself got picked up by another young man, and he experienced a great sense of relief when the latter touched his genitals. He was arrested for indecent behaviour in public.

At interview it emerged that a girl in the office where he worked had been showing some interest in him, and he remarked that 'homosexual feelings seemed easier somehow'. The interviewer suggested that he must have felt in some way frightened by his feelings for the girl; and in response the patient told the following: that (1) the chief clerk in the office was unpleasantly disciplinarian; (2) for some weeks the patient had been afraid of making small mistakes, which the chief clerk would discover, and as he later said, he had also experienced a constant 'sense of foreboding'; and (3) there was also a middle-aged woman in the office who, he was afraid, 'would talk' (presumably to the chief clerk) if he took the girl out.

Specific features

(1) A heterosexual situation,
(2) Fear of disapproval by a male authority.

The Minicab Driver

This young man of 26 was referred because of severe phobic anxiety in crowded places, which had come on suddenly about two years before. Although the exact time sequence was not clear, he associated the onset of his anxiety with the following two situations:

(1) He had formed a very good relation with a boss, who had made a number of promises about promotion. The boss, however, was himself promoted and transferred, the promises became forgotten, and the patient felt betrayed.
(2) At around the same time as the above was occurring, another and more acute situation arose, as follows. One evening, when he tried to start his car to go home, he discovered that the battery was flat, and he exchanged batteries with one of the firm's cars. He did not mean this as a theft, and always had the intention of replacing the defective battery later. However, the exchange was discovered, and he had to confess. Although the firm treated the matter quite leniently, he said he had never felt so guilty and ashamed in his life. A few weeks later he left the job.

Among background problems he mentioned:

(1) A repetitive pattern of leaving jobs because of his inability to restrain his anger with his bosses, and
(2) An inability to commit himself in his relation with women.

Specific features

(1) Hostility towards male authority.
(2) Anger with a male authority because of being let down over the question of advancement.
(3) A situation which could be construed as symbolizing the stealing of power or strength.
(4) Inhibition in heterosexual situations.

Discussion

Examples of this kind could be multiplied over and over again. So far the emphasis has mainly been on *precipitating factors*, but the examples could also be considered from the point of view of demonstrating a *constellation of apparently unrelated disturbances*, continually recurring. This constellation, or syndrome, seems to contain four main components. It would be another interesting and important research project to use statistical methods to demonstrate that the four components are more frequently associated with one another than could be attributed to chance, but this has never been done; and for the time being clinical impression will have to suffice.

The four components are as follows:

(1) Symptoms (usually anxiety in some form);
(2) Difficulties over competition and/or achievement;
(3) Difficulties in relation to male authority figures (usually involving fear and/or hostility);
(4) Inhibition or anxiety in relation to the opposite sex.

There are now two questions that immediately spring to mind:

(1) What is the underlying reason for the clustering together of these four components?
(2) What on earth is the source of the anxiety which is frequently so severe, and so apparently out of proportion to the often comparatively trivial and everyday nature of the precipitating events?

Thus, the Concert-goer was devastated for 3 days because his woman-friend showed what was probably no more than a passing interest in another man; the Dental Patient reacted as if he deserved retribution for having killed his best friend and stolen his wife from him, whereas in fact his behaviour had been above reproach; the Articled Accountant may or may not have been right in thinking that the chief clerk would disapprove of his relation with the girl, but in any case all he had to do was to make the choice of whether to ignore the chief clerk's disapproval or the girl's interest; and finally, while the Minicab Driver was certainly unwise to exchange the car batteries, this was not the terrible crime that it seemed to be in his imagination. Once more, what is the source of the anxiety?

Of course we all know the answer that Freud gave to this question, but what I want to do here is to approach the question purely empirically, using Freud's answer only as a guide. So far, as mentioned above, the only evidence presented has come from precipitating factors. Three other categories of evidence may now be introduced, namely *response to interpretation*, the *emergence of hitherto buried feelings*, and *therapeutic effects*.

The first answer to the question of the source of the anxiety comes from considering the second and third of the four components of the syndrome, namely; (2) problems of competition; and (3) hostility to male authority. It is an empirical fact that many patients respond with confirmatory material to the basic interpretation that *both the competition and the hostility are ultimately directed against the father*. Since the relation with the father is likely to involve far more intense and deep-seated feelings than, for instance, that with bosses or rival peers, this immediately begins to make some sense of the intensity of the anxiety and – where present – the accompanying feelings of guilt. Much of this can be demonstrated in the following case.

The Indian Scientist

This was a man of 29 who showed the syndrome under discussion in the clearest possible manner. His immediate complaint was concerned with an instance of component (4) combined with component (1), namely a tendency towards *premature ejaculation*, about which he was very *anxious*. Because this was not very severe the interviewer made an attempt at reassuring him, but he brushed this aside, said he wanted to know what the trouble was, and launched into a series of unconscious communications, which, somewhat simplified, went as follows:

(a) 'Perhaps I am too sensitive. I often say rude things to people, which worries me for a long time afterwards' – thus, apparently irrelevantly, bringing in the subject of *anxiety about aggressive feelings*.
(b) He went on to say that there was a time when he used to lose his temper with people, but this didn't happen any longer.
(c) One of the forms that this took was to get into fights with men in the street in India, but one day he met a man who punched him on the nose and knocked him down, and from then on he stopped fighting altogether. This was at the age of 17.

Thus the spontaneous transition has been from a sexual difficulty in relation to women, to the apparently quite unrelated subject of *suffering retribution for aggressive feelings towards men*, or, in other words, from component (4) of the syndrome under consideration, to component (3).

The interviewer, being of course aware of the four components of the syndrome, then introduced component (2), saying that perhaps from the moment of losing the fight with the other man he had had difficulty in *competing* with other men. The patient immediately added the subject of *achievement*, which is of course related to competition, saying that although (as had emerged previously) he had done very badly in his Finals, he had previously come out top in an intermediate exam. It was therefore absolutely clear that at some point there had been a change from doing well to being unable to fulfil his potential. He was in fact at present working in a very humdrum job from which he got no satisfaction whatsoever.

The crucial moment in the interview, from the point of view of the present discussion, came in now. The interviewer used his theoretical knowledge to take the bull by the horns and say that perhaps the man that the patient was in competition with all the time was *his father*. Was his father perhaps a very able person? The patient immediately confirmed this to an amazing degree, revealing that his father had got many medals for his work, was a good artist, had represented his state at cricket, and in addition was a *very pugnacious man, had got into a lot of fights, and had never been beaten*. In a later part of the session, the patient brought in another aspect of component (3) of the syndrome, saying that he often felt he wanted to rebel against male authorities, or even to *punch them on the nose*. He added that his father fairly often used to lose his temper and thrash him, and he was always determined not to cry.

Here, once more, we may pause and both review the evidence and ask questions. This patient has shown evidence of serious inhibition over achievement and competition, and appears to have confirmed that he is in competition with his father. Now we may ask: what is he in competition with his father *for?* Is it achievement, or supremacy – both of which seem to be implied in the above story – or is it for something deeper?

The first answer, which can be given not so much from this patient as from an accumulation of responses to interpretation (and other evidence) given by other patients, is that the basic object of competition is a *feeling of manliness*. What the patient is showing is a general inhibition of aspects of manliness as seen in his society (here Eastern society is no different from Western); and this at once makes sense not only of the inhibition of *achievement*, but also of *sexuality*, which is (obviously) one of the most important aspects of manliness.

As always the questions never end. Why should he be in competition with his father over manliness? The answer to this question is by no means obvious, except that one can say that sons, as they pass puberty and begin to grow up, certainly begin to want to think of themselves as men, may openly resent their father's superior position, and may begin to challenge their father's authority.

However, the answer is more dramatic than this. Here we may continue the story of this particular patient. In a subsequent session he began to speak (1) of going around with a constant feeling of guilt, and then (2) of having at the age of 17 (it is worth nothing the second mention of this age) *become interested in a girl cousin*, which was absolutely forbidden in India, and having been told off for this by his father.

A selective account of the next session is then as follows:

(1) He spoke of having sometimes thought that his *father might die*, but he was *afraid of taking over responsibility as head of the family*.
(2) He mentioned for the first time that he suffered from anxiety attacks, with the feeling that there was something he should or shouldn't have done, such as writing home to his father (thus bringing in another aspect of the first component of the syndrome, namely anxiety symptoms).

The therapist said that it looked as if *guilt* was at the centre of his trouble, and that it probably had something to do with his *father*. To this the patient suddenly said, 'Yes, you know, once I read his love letters to my mother'. He went on to speak of the great love he had always had for his mother, and how this recently seemed to have become somewhat blunted.

After this session the patient experienced the most extraordinary sense of relief ('I felt I wanted to leap in the street from relief'), and in subsequent sessions he reported that not only had his *anxiety attacks disappeared* but he had found himself *getting on much better with men*.

Further discussion

The point that I now want to make is that the above account is not a piece of psychoanalytic ideology, presented – as is usual – with little or no evidence; it is an account of a series of *observations* made on a particular patient. When almost any scientific area starts to be investigated, unexpected and startling observations begin to be made, which cannot be denied, and for which some explanation needs to be found. The area concerned with what patients say in psychotherapy, and how this affects them, is certainly no exception.

Now the accepted explanation for observations like these just described does not automatically follow from this one case. It follows from cumulative, overwhelming evidence from thousands, even tens of thousands, of cases, and overwhelming evidence from many other sources as well. In this particular case, however, a large number of the elements of the explanation are present or can be inferred, and can be listed as follows:

(1) Inhibited competitiveness towards other men;
(2) Hostility towards male authority;
(3) Evidence of competitiveness towards the father;
(4) The hint of incestuous feelings, overtly disapproved of by the father, in the relation with the girl cousin;
(5) Anxiety based on guilt towards the father; and finally
(6) The confession of an incident which on the face of it appears relatively trivial, leading to relief that seems quite out of proportion, but which is intelligible and not out of proportion if the incident is seen as an indirect expression of *incestuous feelings towards the mother*.

At once every element in the story falls into place: if the father is seen as a *rival for the mother*, then a conflict between intense competitive feelings and deep-seated hostility on the one hand, and profound guilt and fear of retribution on the other, is a natural consequence. This is what is meant by the Oedipus complex in males.

The Oedipus myth and the male Oedipus complex

This term is of course derived from Sophocles' tragedy, which embodies an earlier Greek myth. The elements of the story are as follows (for details of this and other Greek myths mentioned below, see Graves, 1955):

(1) There was a prophecy made by the Oracle at Delphi that any child of Laius and Jocasta, the King and Queen of Thebes, was destined to kill his father.
(2) When their son, Oedipus, was born, they therefore exposed him on a mountainside, but he was rescued and brought up at Corinth.
(3) When he was grown up, he met a chariot on the road, and provoked into a quarrel, killed both the charioteer and the passenger, without knowing that the latter was his father, Laius.
(4) Going on to Thebes, he solved the riddle of the Sphinx and was granted the hand of Jocasta, the recently widowed Queen – the identity of the King's murderer being of course unknown.
(5) When he later discovered that he had killed his father and married his mother, out of remorse and self-punishment he blinded himself.

Now on the face of it there is nothing particularly special about this story, chosen from among many Greek tragedies, a surprisingly high proportion of which are concerned with the murder of relatives of one kind or another, and/or sexual impulses towards blood relations. Although, as mentioned above, the term 'Electra complex' was used at one time, no one speaks of the 'Clytemnestra complex' to refer to a wife's murderous feelings towards her husband (which have been known!), or the 'Orestes complex' to refer to a son's murderous feelings towards his mother (which also certainly occur). Why, therefore, is the Oedipus complex by now more or less a household phrase?

The existence of the Oedipus complex was of course postulated by Freud as a result of his own self-analysis, and he quickly came to realize that this constellation of feelings was embodied both in the Oedipus myth, and in the myths and customs of many races of men (see *Totem and taboo*, first published in 1913). Later he came to realize the central importance of this complex in many neurotic disturbances in men and boys, and he regarded its development and resolution as an essential part of normal male development. In the end its very universality made him believe that it was a 'race memory' left over from a primitive stage of primate evolution, when (presumably) sons really did murder their fathers (or let them off with mere castration?), take over the leadership, and bear children by their mothers. But this seemed to imply the thoroughly discredited idea of the inheritance of acquired characters, and although Freud never abandoned his view, it led to a great deal of controversy; and it certainly seems now to have represented yet one more example of Freud's ignorance of, or indifference to, the findings of modern biology.

Nevertheless, Freud had good reason to put forward some kind of theory involving evolution. As in all science, it is *observations* that matter, and here the essential observation is the universality of the Oedipus complex. This is the answer to the question posed above why this particular Greek myth, rather than any other, has given rise to a household term.

Of course, as mentioned above, it is impossible to prove that it is really universal, and I know of at least one long analysis of a male patient in which it played *no* part. Nevertheless, there is something almost uncanny in the way in which the Oedipus complex seems to appear *regardless of the actual family situation*. In the example given above of the Indian Scientist there was the classical – and simplest – situation of a powerful and successful father, who exercised authority over his son, and who clearly aroused his son's hostility and competitiveness, with accompanying feelings, certainly of guilt, and probably of fear of retribution as well. Moreover this fear often quite clearly takes the form of a fear of *genital injury* called loosely and often incorrectly 'castration' – since the main fantasy appears to be the loss of the penis rather than the testes.

'Castration'

Corresponding to this fear of being castrated, the impulse in the son appears often to take the form of fantasies not so much of killing the father as castrating him. (This is embodied in another Greek myth, in which Cronus cuts off the genitals of his father Uranus with a flint sickle given to him by his mother – it was not the Greek style to leave much to the imagination). It is amazing – and for the father exceedingly distressing – to see, even in a son who has had a warm and close relation with his father, the envy of his father's strength, achievement, and manhood, and the wish to depreciate and destroy it. This impulse can be of the utmost bitterness and malignance; and it is made all the more unbearable, but in no way weakened, by the amount of guilt with which it is invested. Because of the guilt the impulse often takes the form of *failing* rather than having to give the father the satisfaction of feeling that he has imparted manhood to his son (for an example see the Man from Singapore, p. 264, whose father seems to have been wholly admirable and kind). In this way the son's malignant impulse to 'castrate' his father, and his need for retribution by 'castrating' himself, become fused together in a single line of action.

Sometimes, in addition to the malignancy and the guilt, there is deep sorrow. Here I am thinking of a highly intelligent professional man, who could not allow that his father had been successful – though he plainly had been – and who broke into bitter weeping whenever he thought of the prospect of his own success. The reason gradually emerged: namely that he could not get away from the feeling, how ever much he knew it was utterly irrational, that he could only achieve success by somehow diminishing his father. He showed a pattern of changing jobs, with the inner feeling that he was throwing back in his senior colleagues' faces all that they had taught him. He alternated between the wish to succeed and the wish to fail, breaking down under the intensity of this conflict into a state of severe indecision followed by depression. He thus represents an example of *Oedipal depression*, a subject which will be considered further in Chapter 13 (see pp. 148ff.).

Weak fathers

So far the emphasis has been on envy of the father's strength. What happens if the father is seen as weak? Then it seems we find *guilt about successful competition*, leading to the same inability to compete, and behind this again intense competitiveness. Moreover, the most extraordinary thing is that, when we examine the patient's fantasy life, we very often find an imaginary, powerful, authoritarian, punishing father, who apparently cannot represent any aspect of the real father, and towards whom the son has the same constellation of feelings as that shown by the Indian Scientist, whose father really was like that. Moreover we may well find the son taking up against *himself* the authoritarian and punishing role (corresponding to Oedipus' self-mutilation), acting as if he deserved to be castrated for his crime, and even showing literal fantasies of injuring his own genitals – fantasies that indeed may occur whatever the family situation. Thus the Paranoid Engineer (see Malan, 1963, p. 106) tried as a boy to burn his penis with a red hot iron because of his guilt about masturbation (but, as he said, 'fortunately it hurt so much that I had to stop'). This was a near-psychotic patient, and in such patients one may well find a much more literal and conscious expression of impulses that appear only as unconscious fantasies in 'ordinary' neurosis.

Dead or absent fathers

What happens if the father is dead? If the father dies when the son is old enough to realize he had a father, and particularly around the son's puberty when he is beginning to grow into a man, this may be one of the most traumatic events of all. The reason is of course that the natural Oedipal impulses and strivings may become enormously more guilt-laden. The son may well be faced with the actual situation of his father having been 'got rid of' and having to take his father's place. Thus the Son in Mourning (see pp. 71ff.) suffered a severe exacerbation of his anxiety when he *had to give his sister away in marriage*, in his recently dead father's place. Another patient (see p. 120) said to his therapist that he *could not touch* his weeping mother at his father's funeral – 'It was as if there was an electric current around her' preventing him from doing so. The Concert-goer's father had died when the patient was 11, and he had had to help look after his widowed mother; and this almost certainly was a major factor in the later extraordinary situation in which he found himself – living with a woman old enough to be his mother, and suffering the most intense anxiety when this woman showed interest in another man.

And then the final question: what happens if the patient *never knew his father?* The most extraordinary observation of all is that in such patients one frequently finds exactly the same kind of feeling, usually incorporating a fantasy of a ruthless, strict, authoritarian man who disapproves of the patient's sexuality in any form, towards whom the patient feels the most intense mixture of fear on the one hand and hostility on the other. Thus one young man (the Refugee Musician, see pp. 199ff., and 249ff.) was illegitimate and had no memory of ever meeting his father, nor (even after years of psychotherapy) of his mother's ever having had a relation with any other man. In the earlier stages of his psychotherapy, if he ever got near to having a relation with a woman, the fantasy became greatly intensified that he would be attacked by *men in the street* and he used (literally) to have to carry a knife around to defend himself. Another young man had no memory of his father, who left his mother when the patient was 15 months old and was never seen again. He had never been able to speak to his mother about his father and knew only that his father was now dead. Nor – like the previous patient – had he any memory of his mother's having a relation with another man. The patient had an extremely tense and unsatisfactory relation with his mother, for whom he expressed great contempt. He was homosexual, being interested in boys of his own age or younger, but he also had intense mixed feelings about other men, which included feeling that in his fantasy there was always another man with whom he was *in intense competition*. This patient later described a remarkable improvement in his relation with his mother after he had had a *sexual dream about her*.

The Oedipus complex and evolution

The observation that, even when the father is weak or absent, male patients tend to have a fantasy of a powerful and punishing father, forces one into thinking seriously about theories involving evolution. This is one of the many examples of the way in which psychoanalysis provides evidence about the evolution of human beings – a link between two areas that has been very little explored, and needs to be explored in collaboration with scientists familiar with modern theories.

The relation with the mother

In the first edition of this book I wrote, referring to the end of the last paragraph but one, as follows:

The final mention of sexual feelings towards the mother may provoke a question: if the central problem derives from feelings about the *mother*, why has practically all the emphasis in the foregoing description been on the relation with the *father*? The answer seems to be that, at its simplest – as in the case of the Indian Scientist, whose feelings about his mother apparently consisted of uncomplicated love – the relation with the mother in itself is in a sense no problem, and then the conflict is always seen in terms of the effect of this love on the relation with a father, whether the latter be real or imaginary. It is these feelings that need to be brought into consciousness. Undoubtedly the mother herself may intensify the feelings, e.g. by being seductive to her son, or by favouring him above the father, but in such cases the barrier to the relation with the mother appears always to be seen in terms of the father. Nevertheless I have the impression that it is often important therapeutically to make explicit the sexual element in the feelings about the mother. In addition, of course, the relation with the mother may be complicated by buried hostility, but that is a separate problem.

As I see it now, this passage under-emphasizes the direct relation with the mother. I think it is probably true that the idea of erotic or sexual feelings for the mother is itself invested with profound horror and guilt, quite independently of the feelings about the father – Oedipus, so to speak, was as horrified at the very idea of having married his mother as he was at having killed his father. Moreover, another problem which is often extremely important in psychotherapy is a hidden, eroticized, *pathological tie to the mother*, which may seriously interfere with the relation with other women. Both these types of problem will be illustrated by the next three patients whom I shall go on to discuss.

The relation with the mother and the triangular relation involving the son and his mother and father

The first question that springs to mind is: how literally are we to take the son's incestuous impulses, or erotic or sexual feelings, towards the mother?

In most cases the evidence is indirect, as it is with one exception in the examples given above. In the case of the Concert-goer, for instance, we can say with certainty that he had sexual feelings for a *mother-figure*, but this is not the same as having sexual feelings for his *mother*. Similarly the Indian Scientist became sexually interested in a cousin – which in India is regarded as incestuous – and was curious about his father's intimate relation with his mother, but the evidence goes no further than this. The exception, of course, is the man whose relation with his mother improved after he had had a sexual dream about her.

While I was searching for clinical material to illustrate these themes, I thought of a leading worker in the field of brief psychotherapy who has concentrated his energies on Oedipal problems in both sexes, namely Sifneos. I am indebted to him and to the Harvard University Press for permission to quote the following two examples, which appear in his book *Short-term therapy and emotional crisis* (1972).

Sifneos's 'Phobic Patient with Dyspnea'

This was a young man of 28 who asked for help in order to be able to face his wedding. He had suffered for 2 years from symptoms of anxiety, but these had become greatly intensified and accompanied by attacks of difficulty in breathing ('dyspnoea' in English spelling), soon after he set a date for his wedding in 2 months' time.

The aspects of his story relevant to the present theme are as follows. His father, with whom he had a basically good relation, died when the patient was 4. The mother re-married when the patient was 8. Not long afterwards his stepfather, who was about to leave for the war, said to him, 'Now *you* will be the man of the house.' That night he had an anxiety attack. Here we may note one of the precipitating factors listed at the beginning of this chapter, namely *taking another man's place*, and in this case quite literally taking a father-figure's place with his mother. As a result of his anxiety his mother allowed him for a time to sleep in his stepfather's bed next to her, which was also the bed in which at the age of 4 he had witnessed his real father *barely able to breathe* as he was dying from heart failure. Now at the age of 28 he masturbated in this bed with *fantasies of sexual intercourse with much older women*.

In the sixth and last therapeutic session before his wedding he suddenly recalled a memory, as follows (for brevity the words have been somewhat condensed and paraphrased, and the italics are mine): 'The day my stepfather returned from the war, I had an appendectomy, I was 12. I missed my mother while in the hospital and I was angry with her and with my stepfather for keeping her away from me. After my stepfather told me I was going to be the "man of the house" I was sure that I was never going to see him again. It was going to be like my real father. He would also die. I wished that he would never come back, but he did. I remember, in the hospital, having that *shortness of breath* and the *fear that I was going to die* whenever I thought of my mother and stepfather together.'

Comment

Here the evidence for sexual feelings for the mother, though still indirect, is stronger than in most of the other examples given so far. Surely it is not far-fetched to make the inference that the boy was sexually stimulated by the presence of his mother in the next bed, and that in his fantasies he substituted other older women because – obviously – to have thought directly of his mother would have been too anxiety-laden. Moreover, the evidence for (1) the literal wish to get rid of a father-figure so that he could have his mother for himself; (2) jealousy of his mother and stepfather's relation with each other; and (3) the anxiety with which these feelings were invested, is direct and conclusive. Finally (4) we may note the obvious link between the patient's symptom of dyspnoea, accompanied by fear of death, and the condition from which his father died. This symptom can clearly be described as 'taking his father's illness on himself', and thus can probably be interpreted as expressing either a fear of retribution, or a need for self-punishment, for wishing his father's death – perhaps indeed both together. Here there is an exact resemblance to the Daughter with a Stroke, described on pp. 38–40. The subjects of retribution and self-punishment will be discussed in more detail later (see pp. 146 and 174).

After the session in which he recalled this memory he went through with the wedding without serious anxiety, and the final therapeutic result at 2-year follow-up was excellent.

Sifneos's 'Pseudo-homosexual Student'

This was a young man of 21 complaining of homosexual leanings and a lack of interest in girls, from which he had suffered since puberty.

He described his mother as young, demonstrative, and very beautiful – 'a stunning redhead'. He said he was close to her, but he also felt rejected by her in favour of his older brother and younger sister. His father was seen as intolerant and critical.

His masturbation fantasies were of frontal intercourse with a boy, whose face he never saw, but who in some ways resembled a girl and was dressed in women's clothes.

Selected moments from his brief therapy are as follows.

On several occasions the patient expressed resentment when the therapist questioned him about his relation with his mother;

PT: You meddle in my affair. I mean affairs.
TH: With your mother!
PT: ... during all week I thought it would be very nice to run away with my mother as my mistress.

The patient went on to speak of 'all this tension and frightening feeling inside. It is as if my father knows my secret.'

TH: What is this secret of yours all about? Have you committed some kind of offense?
PT: Well, yes ... [in] all these things that I read in those sex magazines – the image of my mother always comes to mind.

In a later session the following dialogue occurred:

PT: If there were girls and I was interested in them it would be wronging the only one, my only one ...
TH: Who is that?
PT: My mother of course.

In this same session the patient said he felt tired; and later he spoke with great embarrassment of being attracted by a girl whom he had seen leaving the therapist's office. The therapist made the link between the patient's anxiety in two triangular relations: those involving (1) the patient, the girl, and the therapist, and (2) the patient and his mother and father; and he went on to speak of the patient's tiredness and his homosexuality, linking them together as defences intended both to disarm the male figure in these triangular situations, and to preserve the attachment to his mother. 'You use your weakness and your homosexuality as a kind of excuse not to go out with girls, so as not to be unfaithful to your mother, as well as to fool your father.' We may note here the use of the loaded word 'unfaithful', with its sexual implications, which is entirely justified on the evidence.

In the next session the patient brought a dream in which he was kissing a girl wearing a beautiful dress belonging to his mother. The therapist linked this with the masturbation fantasies of a boy resembling a girl and wearing a woman's dress. This had a tremendous impact:

PT: Oh my God – Oh no! ... sex with my mother in that way! It is horrible.

Therapy was terminated a few sessions later. The patient had already begun to take a girl out and to be intensely attracted by her, and his relation with his father had improved. At follow-up one year later he was married, and his homosexual feelings and anxieties had disappeared.

Comment

(1) In this second patient the evidence for direct erotic feelings for the mother, and jealousy of the father's relation with her, is overwhelming.

(2) It is of interest that the patient had a remarkable capacity for what may be called 'dissociation', in the sense that he was able to speak of wanting to go away with his mother as his 'mistress', yet was horrified at the thought that his feelings for her were sexual.

(3) There was also conclusive evidence for a pathological attachment to the mother which interfered with his relation with girls. This leads to the following generalization: When a male patient is found to suffer from anxiety in relation to members of the opposite sex, or to be repeatedly destroying such relations, the immediate interpretations that come to mind are concerned with Oedipal guilt in relation to the father in the first case, and buried hostility towards women in the second. Each may be true, but the clinician also needs to think of the possibility that the patient is avoiding heterosexual relations because *he secretly wishes to preserve the eroticized relation with his mother for ever*.

(4) This patient also illustrates a clinical phenomenon that is frequently encountered in both sexes, namely that certain details of sexual fantasies can be unequivocally traced to erotic feelings about the parent of the opposite sex. This is illustrated equally clearly by the Reluctant Hunter, to be described below.

(5) In this patient the mechanism underlying his homosexuality became absolutely clear as a defence against heterosexuality. Here one could exclaim: If only patients wishing to get rid of homosexual leanings could usually be helped so easily! But homosexuality is a mysterious phenomenon and many different kinds of homosexuality probably exist, including those partly or largely due to genetic factors. Even when its defensive function unequivocally appears identical to that in the above patient, the therapeutic task may be extremely difficult. This applied, for instance, to the Articled Accountant described on pp. 55–56, who apparently ran away into homosexuality because he was afraid of the chief clerk's disapproval of his interest in a girl in the office. His Oedipal anxieties were extensively worked on during the course of 27 sessions of brief psychotherapy, and

yet at 3-year follow-up his homosexual leanings had merely receded without being resolved, and he remained withdrawn from relations with the opposite sex.

(6) It is important to note the following: that just as anxiety about retribution from a powerful father seems independent of the father's actual characteristics, erotic and possessive feelings towards the mother are not confined to sons whose mothers are physically attractive – as the mother was described in the case of this second patient. Of course these feelings may be intensified by the mother's attractiveness, and may be intensified even further if she is openly seductive towards her son. Yet a 40-year-old son may still describe his aged mother in the most glowing and idealized terms; while after the pathological tie has been resolved by psychotherapy he may see her quite differently – realizing, for instance, that she is now an old woman and that she has always been selfish and manipulating.

Both of these patients were relatively healthy emotionally. The following patient of Davanloo's, on the other hand, suffered from severe obsessional anxiety, which was not quite incapacitating but still all-pervasive, and in addition he was extremely mixed-up in all his personal relations, especially those with women. He is described in Davanloo's book *Basic principles and techniques of short-term dynamic psychotherapy* (1978, pp. 345 – 88).

The Reluctant Hunter

The patient was in his early thirties. In the sixth therapeutic session he described an incident in his teens in which, although on the surface he very much wanted to go away on a hunting trip with his father, he pretended to be asleep and so was left behind. Davanloo brought out that this meant that he would be left at home alone with his mother.

Not long afterwards the patient described a childhood fantasy in which he put a woman's breasts and genitals – he didn't know what the latter looked like – into a sort of cement-mixer, where they would get churned up. He couldn't see the woman's face and didn't know who she might be.

In his therapy Davanloo brought out that although the patient was intensely attracted by large-breasted women, he had twice married women with small breasts. Part of his obsessional disturbance was manifested as severe indecision. He alternated between small- and large-breasted women, being quite unable to make up his mind which he wanted – the moment he was attached to one he wanted the other and *vice versa*. Davanloo linked the obvious conflict expressed in this with the fact that the mother had large breasts, and that as a child the patient had witnessed, with great fascination, his younger brother being breast-fed by her.

In this therapy it was also necessary to work through the patient's hostility towards his mother – after all, churning-up someone's breasts in a cement-mixer cannot be regarded entirely as an expression of love! One of the origins of this hostility was his resentment at his mother for being attached to his father rather than to him.

At follow-up, after a highly successful brief therapy, the patient said he now realized that in the cement-mixer fantasy *he was trying to avoid seeing that the woman's face was his mother's.* He said that now he could accept it easily and it was no longer threatening.

In this remarkable therapeutic result the patient also described a major lifting of his obsessional attitude to his whole life. Formerly he had to live his life according to a pattern set by somebody else. Now, if he wanted to do something, he just did it.

This illustrates with great clarity one meaning of obsessional symptoms, namely the need to avoid *impulsiveness* – which might lead the patient into doing something that his conflicts would make him regret (see pp. 113 and 120 for a further discussion of this issue).

Final comment on the son's erotic feelings for his mother

The above three patients illustrate a crucial principle of the therapy of male Oedipal problems: usually the therapist must not only bring into consciousness the hostility and jealousy felt towards the father, which is loaded with anxiety and guilt, but also the deeply pleasurable, highly defended, and intensely guilt-laden erotic attachment to the mother. *Mutatis mutandis*, as already described in Chapter 7, the same applies to the corresponding problem in women.

Mixed feelings towards the mother

So far I have concentrated on the simple Oedipal situation, in which the son feels eroticized love towards his mother, and hostility, guilt, and anxiety in relation to his father. It must be obvious that the opposite kinds of feeling – hostility towards the mother and love for the father – often form an essential part of this complex triangular relationship. In illustration we may begin with the following patient.

The Architect who Loved Kipling

This 50-year-old man had suffered for 9 years from attacks of depression, the first of which had been precipitated by the failure of his relation with his wife, and subsequent ones by the failure of relations with other women. Although these failures did not seem to show any obvious pattern, the interviewing psychiatrist suggested that the patient must have covered up his hostility towards women, but that in each of these relationships in some unknown way it caught up with him. This produced a quintessential unconscious communication in the form of an abrupt change of subject. The patient told of an incident a few years before in which his mother had – yet again – begun telling him what a terrible man his father was. 'I very rarely lose my temper, but I exploded. I said vile things to her. I told her how much I had hated her for turning me against my father.'

Thus this communication expressed the very opposite of the Oedipal situation, namely hostility towards the mother and grief and anger about the loss of the relationship with the father. It would be easy to conclude that this was a clear exception to the universality of the Oedipus complex, but one cannot count on anything being simple in the field of psychodynamics, and in fact his intense and living attachment to his mother was not far to seek. During his therapy he described with deep and sensuous feeling the pleasure of being put to bed at night by his mother when he was small, and the warmth and closeness of her body as she sat on the bed and read to him. It then emerged that to this day he still reads Kipling's *Just-so Stories* every night before going to sleep, which was his favourite of all the books that formed part of this nightly ceremony.

During his therapy he also told of an incident in which he had tried to confide his anxieties about his forthcoming marriage to a male friend, who had responded in a way that failed to take his feelings seriously. This was another of the times when he had lost control of his temper, and he had shouted at his friend in public. In therapy he responded with acceptance to the interpretation that this anger really derived from his father's failure to give him support and understanding.

Finally we may return to hostility against the mother. It seems that around the age of puberty his relation with her had changed. Possibly – as happens so often, and *mutatis mutandis* with fathers and daughters as well – his mother sensed that now that he was beginning to turn into a man the nightly ceremony was becoming too intimate, and she gave this up. Moreover she now became extremely demanding of her son's success. He was very good at football, and he told of an incident in which he had come home and announced with pride that he had been chosen for the school's second eleven. Her response had been: 'But Mrs Brown's son down the road is in the first eleven.' His therapist pressed him repeatedly to describe how in fantasy he might have reacted, challenging each of his evasions as it appeared. Eventually, with chilling intensity, he said: 'There was a bridge over a river not far from home. The parapet was low, and we used to walk there quite often ...'

Love and longing for the father

Until describing this last patient I had mentioned only what may be called 'negative' feelings for the father – fear, guilt, hostility, rivalry – and I must have given the impression that this is all a son ever feels about his father. Of course such a view is nonsense, and in fact the intensity of a boy's love for his father often matches in depth and intensity that for his mother (see e.g. the Man with School Phobia, pp. 225ff.). This further complicates what is probably the most complicated area in the understanding of human beings. A boy needs love and support and physical closeness from his father, and needs his father as a model on which he will base his own feelings of manhood; and the question is then whether he can derive his manhood smoothly from identification with his father, or whether the Oedipal hostility and rivalry mean that this process becomes in fantasy something that damages his father and depletes him. The development of the son's manhood then becomes in fantasy a sort of theft, and this is the reason for the importance of the theme of *stealing* which is so often met in patients with Oedipal problems. The conversion of the *smooth identification* into a *theft* is greatly intensified if the son feels his father has *withheld* support and strength from him – hence almost certainly the precipitation of the Minicab Driver's anxiety by the *theft* of the car battery within the setting of being let down by his boss over the question of promotion.

All this means that, even when the feelings initially presented by the patient about his father appear to consist largely of hostility, the therapist needs to watch for, and be prepared to bring up to the surface, intense underlying love and longing, including the feelings of loss of closeness if the relation has gone wrong, and grief if the father has died.

One final example will illustrate the kind of complexity that may be met in practice.

The Son in Mourning

The patient was a young man, the eldest of three children, complaining of a fear of going out and meeting people, particularly in the company of a girl. The initial onset had been 8 years ago, when he thought he had made a girl pregnant, and had had a severe attack of anxiety and nausea at the thought of her father's reaction ('he would have gone berserk'). Three years ago his father had died suddenly of a heart attack, and since then the patient had become increasingly hypochondriacal and anxious about dying, like his father, 'in the prime of life'. Four months ago he suffered an exacerbation of anxiety when he had to *give his younger sister away in marriage*, in his father's place.

The amazingly mixed feelings that emerged may be illustrated by the following:

The father was portrayed on the one hand as a strong man who acted as disciplinarian in the home, allowed no one to talk back to him, and was described as the 'village tyrant'; and on the other hand as a weak man who suffered from anxiety symptoms like those of the patient himself: the patient recalled an incident in which his father had not been able to go into a pub and he, the patient, had had to bring him sandwiches to eat in the car. During therapy the patient's dress and appearance varied in the most extraordinary way: for one session he arrived dressed entirely in black (as if in mourning) and beginning to grow a beard; for the next session he was very smartly dressed and clean-shaven; for the next he was dressed in a really flashy suit and shirt. It emerged that his father (1) was bald and strongly disapproved of long hair, moustaches, and beards; and (2) himself had to dress smartly for his job but strongly disapproved of flashy clothes. The mixture of mourning, identification, and symbolically flouting his dead father's authority, is absolutely clear.

His father had a similar attitude to cars to his attitude to clothes – he had driven expensive cars but strongly disapproved of cars painted in bright colours. The following dream makes reference to this and in addition has a clear Oedipal symbolism:

'His father is coming home after a long absence. The patient is upstairs and has parked a Hillman Imp painted in bright orange colours outside. Though this is a small car, he has installed a big racing engine inside it. His father is very angry – he is not quite sure why, but perhaps it is because he has parked it in his father's parking place in the driveway.'

In spite of the obvious 'negative' feelings of hostility, fear, and rebellion implied by most of the description so far, the patient's love and longing for his father were equally if not more intense: for instance he spoke of how his sister got more attention from his father than he did, and in the same session spoke of a *wish to be a woman*; and in other sessions there were frequently tears in his eyes when he spoke of his father, culminating in the most heartfelt direct statement, 'Oh how I wish he were alive' (for further material on this theme see Chapter 9, pp. 80ff.).

Conclusion

In the first eight chapters we have thus started with simple problems that are easily accessible to emotional common sense, and have ended with some of the deepest problems left in human beings by their evolutionary history, which have needed the psychoanalytic microscope for their discovery. This still leaves vast areas not yet mentioned, but many of these will be covered through clinical examples in the following chapters. In the meantime perhaps enough has been said to enable us to consider the whole area of the technique of dynamic psychotherapy.

9

The relation with the therapist: 'transference'

Recapitulation

In Chapters 4 and 5 I gave examples of some of the types of current conflict that may bring patients to psychotherapy. In at least three of these it became clear that the current conflict had overtones involving the patient's family of origin and going back into adolescence or childhood. In two cases (the Geologist and Daughter with a Stroke) the current conflict itself involved *parents*, so that the current and past conflicts were concerned with the same people; while in a third (the Drama Student) aspects of the current conflict, which concerned the marital partner, had clearly repeated, or *originated in*, or *been transferred from*, past conflicts which concerned both her parents and siblings, namely her brothers.

Similarly in Chapter 7 the Economics Student's current conflict over jealousy was shown to have probably originated in the past in her feelings about her parents, and this was used in a therapeutic intervention; and in Chapter 8 the main theme of the Indian Scientist's therapy was that his current conflict over competition originated in his rivalry with his father. It is clear that making the links from current to past, or from non-family to family of origin, especially parents, may constitute an important part of psychotherapy.

We have thus formulated two different categories of *person* towards whom conflicting feelings are directed, those in the original family and those outside it. The two have different significance, because conflicts about the family of origin are likely to have deeper roots, or go farther back, and to involve feelings more clearly belonging to an adolescent or a child than to an adult. As a piece of shorthand I shall use the symbol P (for 'parents' or 'siblings' or 'past') to refer to the family of origin, and O to refer to people 'outside' or 'other than' the family of origin. In both the Economics Student and the Indian Scientist the link (represented by an oblique stroke) was between Other and Parents, which is thus represented by O/P.

However, this does not exhaust the possibilities. In Chapter 3 I gave two examples of patients who communicated feelings about the therapist. The first example (the Neurological Patient, see p. 20), where the feeling seemed to be *gratitude* about what had been done for him, was probably simple and straightforward; but in the case of the Military Policeman (p. 23), who was afraid of being despised by the therapist for not being able to cope, the feeling expressed had profound implications permeating his whole life. Moreover, in

Chapter 7 this series was continued: for when the Director's Daughter told her therapist that she hoped he was suffering as much as she was, and then had a row with her GP saying 'I hate all you men', the evidence was overwhelming that these feelings not only permeated her whole life but had originated in her relation with her father, who had disappointed her since she was a little girl. Her anger with men had thus been *transferred from* her father, and was an example of what Freud called *transference*.

Now in this phenomenon of transfer of feeling from one person to another, the two people involved can obviously be of any category, but the word *transference*, since Freud, has come to refer to a particular type of situation: namely that in which the feelings are transferred onto the *therapist*. Just as 'O' could stand for either 'other' or 'outside', and 'P' could stand for 'parent' or 'past', 'T' can be used to stand for either 'therapist' or 'transference'.

History of transference

What is the significance of this phenomenon of transference to dynamic psychotherapy? The answer is that it is absolutely crucial. This can best be explained by a brief account of aspects of the history of psychoanalysis.

The original observations that led to the development of psychoanalysis were of course not made by Freud, but by the less well-known (but still well-known) Viennese physician and physiologist, Joseph Breuer, whose name has been perpetuated in the 'Hering–Breuer reflex'. He made his discovery through the treatment by hypnosis of a hysterical patient, who has become known as Anna O. Breuer came to recognize that Anna O's symptoms were associated with memories – which she had forgotten – many of which were concerned with her very intense relation with her father, whom she had nursed through a terminal illness. In the later stages of her treatment she developed intense erotic feelings for Breuer, culminating in her developing a phantom pregnancy – of which Breuer was clearly the phantom father – and eventually in her throwing her arms round him. There are hints that the amount of attention that he devoted to his fascinating patient even began to threaten his marriage; and this respected member of Viennese Society finally threw up such work altogether, understandably shocked and frightened by the situation in which he had become involved (see Jones, 1953).

It is a tribute of course to Freud's immense courage that in face of these phenomena he was still willing to persist. It became clear that erotic feelings were only one example of the kinds of intense feeling that a patient could develop for the therapist, which could in fact include the whole range of feelings that one human being can have for another; and moreover that these feelings could be accepted, 'worked through', and resolved, provided they were confined to verbal expression and were traced to their origins in the past, usually of course in the relation with parents. There followed a subtle but crucial change in the attitude to transference, which had first been regarded as an obstacle to therapy and a necessary evil, but was later regarded as the most important means of understanding and analysing the patient, since past conflicts were revived and arose in the here-and-now in front of the therapist's very eyes.

The modern position is therefore that although there are successful therapies that do not involve any interpretation of the transference whatsoever – see, for instance, the brief examples given in Chapters 4 and 5 – these are the exception rather than the rule. Every therapist must be prepared to recognize transference the moment it arises, to accept it uncritically, to interpret it to the patient when appropriate, to perceive the relation in which it originated, and to interpret this to the patient as well. Moreover, it is by now clear that such feelings arise almost inevitably during a therapy lasting more than a few sessions, and may arise at once – sometimes even before the patient arrives at the consulting room. There follow a number of examples.

The Falling Social Worker – two different kinds of transference

This single woman of 27 came to therapy complaining of a moderately severe phobia of falling down when she was exposed to public situations like hospital meetings. She had been treated with psychotherapy by a previous (male) psychiatrist, who had at one point attempted pentothal abreaction with her – which, if anything, had made her worse.

In his initial interview with her the second therapist (also male) gave her the interpretation that she was trying to tell him about both her good and bad parts and was anxious about how he would react to them. This was an interpretation of the relation with himself, and the power of such interpretations was at once demonstrated, for with great difficulty she now confessed to some of her sexual impulses, which she had not dared to reveal to her previous therapist even during a therapy lasting over two years.

In the third session, after speaking some more about sexual impulses, she said that she had become very relaxed and felt like going to sleep in the therapist's presence. The therapist recognized the possibility of sexualized transference but said nothing.

This possibility was amply confirmed when in session 10 the patient reported with great guilt that over the week-end she had woken up in the night feeling lonely, and had then had a vivid sexual fantasy about the therapist. It now emerged that something very similar – perhaps not fully conscious – had happened with the previous therapist; and that in the pentothal session with him they had ended up by having an intense conversation in which she was describing the kind of man she wanted to marry, who was just like him, and he was saying this was quite the wrong kind of person for her to marry – the here-and-now significance of which was apparently lost on both of them.

During the course of her present therapy, both before and after this session, it emerged that she was suffering from a serious split in her relations with men, which hitherto had entirely prevented her from finding a man whom she could marry. This consisted of her being able to allow sexual activity only with disreputable men – which was highly exciting to her but strongly guilt-laden – while she had to keep relations with marriageable men pure and platonic. On the other hand, under the influence of therapy, she was now experiencing the breakthrough of powerful and guilt-laden sexual fantasies for her therapists, with whom sexual relations were obviously forbidden and (one hopes) unattainable.

One may now ask, what is the source of these powerful sexual feelings for the therapist? The naive answer is that perhaps both therapists were attractive men, and there is no need to look further. But in fact this is not an adequate explanation – such feelings arise with this kind of patient and a male therapist no matter what he is like, and they are usually found to contain powerful components originating in unfulfilled longings from the past.

How should the therapist handle them? First of all he should know that they are likely to arise – especially with phobic and hysterical patients – and he must be on the look-out for them from the beginning. Second, he must himself be secure enough on the one hand to accept them unconditionally without being shocked, and on the other hand to be immune to the flattery and sexual stimulation that they offer – which is not easy, especially as the patient is often very attractive – and to respond to them by bringing them out into the open at once, before (as with Breuer) they become explosive and constitute a danger to therapy; and then to trace them to their origin, just like any other feeling that the patient brings.

In this particular case the origin was not far to seek. Once more the problem lay in an over-close relation with the father, who himself was almost certainly too involved with his daughter, intensely possessive, and extremely jealous of her boy-friends. It looked as if the hidden flirtation and sexual stimulation in this relation had enormously intensified the patient's guilt about sexual feelings, to such an extent that she *could not envisage integrating love and sex* – which offers an immediate explanation for her sexual problems. This can now be formulated in terms of impulse, defence, and anxiety, as follows: the *impulse* consists of forbidden sexual feelings; the *defence* is a form 'splitting', i.e., directing sexual feelings onto disreputable men and affectionate feelings onto 'pure' men; and the *anxiety* is becoming aware that the feelings have an incestuous component. Finally, this formulation offers an explanation for the breakthrough of intense, guilt-laden sexual feelings for her two male therapists, who, obviously, can be regarded as father-figures. This is the return of the repressed feelings for her father, now transferred onto the therapist – hence the word 'transference'.

In any case, this was how the therapist handled these feelings, and he used them as a lever to explore the relation between the patient and her father, and the way in which she had used this relation to tease her mother and score off her. In this way the feelings could be tolerated, worked through, and to some extent resolved.

But we meet over-determination in the phenomenon of transference just as in other areas of psychodynamics. This was shown in a clear and dramatic way by some later events.

The patient had to be admitted to hospital with a brief febrile illness, thus experiencing a short gap in her therapy. On her return she had the feeling that the therapist was indifferent to her, about which she experienced a good deal of suppressed resentment – although in fact he had almost certainly not changed in his behaviour towards her in any way. This is a new feeling in the relationship with the therapist. How should he handle this? This answer, of course, is to treat it in the same way – to accept it unconditionally, not to respond with any of the normal human reactions such as defensiveness, reassurance, or counter-resentment, and to trace it to its origin. It then quickly emerged that she had long been infuriated by what she felt to be her *mother's* indifference. Thus suddenly we meet a new kind of transference, involving the parent of opposite sex to that of the therapist. Once more, this too is a kind of feeling for which the therapist should always be on the look-out. In this case he was now enabled to do a considerable amount of work on buried feelings about the mother, and also to help to resolve some of the patient's resentment about the fact that therapy had to stop. This is a crucial step, since unresolved resentment about termination is a potent source of subsequent relapse.

It is worth noting that the main work of this therapy was done through making the transference/parent or T/P link. There is a very great deal of evidence that this is one of the main specific factors in dynamic psychotherapy.

The ultimate outcome of this therapy was a considerable improvement in many areas, including her symptoms, and several years after termination we heard that she had married (for further details see Malan, 1963 and 1976b).

The word 'transference' has come to be used rather loosely for *any* feelings that the patient may have for the therapist. In the early contacts one of the feelings that the patient is likely to experience is anxiety about whether the therapist can be trusted. This of course is quite natural, though it may also have 'transference' aspects in the sense that the patient's trust had been misplaced in the past. In any case it is often important to bring such feelings out – the mere fact that the therapist is willing to accept that he is not necessarily to be trusted in itself may engender trust. The following is a beautiful and unequivocal example of this, taken from the second session with a patient called The Contralto (see Malan, 1976b). The therapist was a woman.

The Contralto: a question of trust

'The patient produced a book by Crichton Miller and asked me what school I belonged to. I interpreted this as her anxiety about my competence, which led her to say that she thought she would tell me what she would never tell anybody else. It turned out later that she had asked her sister if I was trustworthy, having told her sister what I had said in the first interview.'

The therapist was then entrusted with an account of sexual events that had occurred when the patient was a child, about which she felt extremely guilty and ashamed, and which she had never revealed to anyone else in her whole life.

Thus interpretation of the *anxiety* in the relation with the therapist led to the revelation of important *hidden feelings*.

The Mother of Four: transference in the initial interview

Whenever a patient seems not to be communicating, the possibility should always be considered that the difficulty lies in the transference. The problem is then how to reach a hypothesis about what these transference feelings are. This can partly be done through previous experience, and knowledge of the patient's history; but mainly it is done through watching the patient's communications and perceiving a parallel between something that the patient has said and the relation with the therapist. The following is a dramatic example taken from the initial interview with a married woman of 29 complaining of depression.

The situation that developed in the interview was one in which she seemed to expect the interviewer to do all the work, with the feeling that he had to prise information out of her. Although the GP had made the diagnosis of post-partum depression, her latest child (her fourth) had been born 18 months ago, and she denied that there was any connection with her depression. The main feeling in her depression was the self-reproach that she wasn't a good enough wife and mother. The interviewer asked if she had been depressed before. Her answer was that she had 'never felt well'. When asked what she meant she said that she had never got on well with her mother and had left home at 19. She went on to say that not long after this she had had a 'brainstorm' in which she had smashed a number of things in her flat. This had followed an argument with her boy-friend, who wanted a sexual relation with her without committing himself to loving or marrying her.

The interviewer wrote that although she had given important information, throughout all this she had created an atmosphere of steadily increasing sullenness and defiance, and he felt quite unable to go on with the interview unless something could be done about it. This was finally driven home when she became silent, and on being asked what was happening said that she thought the interviewer was playing some kind of game with her, expecting her to say something.

The interviewer put a number of things together in his mind. These were, first, previous experience: a woman who has herself not received good mothering may well suffer from an underlying resentment about having to give good mothering to her children, and a fourth child may well overtax her capacity to give. This is a very common problem and often accounts for depressive attacks occurring around the birth of a child. Second, it can be put together with her symptoms: she is likely to suffer from considerable guilt, and this would account for the content of her depressive self-reproaches. Third, there is the most striking of her communications: a similar problem over giving and receiving seems to have operated with her boy-friend.

Finally there is the parallel with the situation at interview: the fact of making the interviewer do all the work, and the atmosphere of sullenness and resentment, suggests the possibility that she was playing out a similar problem with him.

He therefore said to her, first, that it was very difficult to give to one's children the kind of love one had not had oneself; and second, that like the man who wanted sex without giving love, she must feel that the interviewer wanted a lot out of her without himself giving anything back. Once more we have an example of the extraordinary power of interpretation. Muttering 'Oh I can't bear it' the patient crumbled into tears, and when she had recovered the interview proceeded without difficulty. One of the main features that emerged was of a dominating mother who used material things as a substitute for love and expected gratitude for this from everyone around her. This was an example in which the patient's *life problem* of giving and receiving manifested itself in the transference from the moment she entered the door.

It is also worth noting that the basic interpretation about giving and receiving implied all the *links* between 'Other' (her boy-friend), Transference, and Parent (her mother), represented in our notation by O/T/P.

The following is an example of the use of a transference interpretation to resolve a difficult situation in the early stages of therapy.

The Carpenter's Daughter: transference in the early stages of therapy

This young woman of 25, complaining of a variety of depressive and psychosomatic symptoms, was originally seen three times by a male interviewer. It seemed that her maturation had been held up at a number of stages of her life by a series of traumatic incidents, which had combined to convey the message to her of disastrous consequences, or parental disapproval, if she developed into a woman. She was assigned to time-limited therapy (30 sessions) with a woman therapist, with this problem as a 'focus'.

In the first two sessions she talked quite easily but somehow conveyed the feeling that therapy had not quite got off the ground. In the third session she opened with the rather double-edged ('ambivalent') statement that she had found the previous session *constructive*, although she *hadn't thought about it during the rest of the week*. One of the principal themes of her further communications was then how at home she had always had to be sensitive to her mother's needs. There followed a long account of the tensions at home caused by her rather difficult father, followed by the theme that she couldn't express her own feelings as freely as her brother and sister could; that her father had been critical of the way her sister dressed, calling her a 'tramp' and a 'gypsy'; and that if she, the patient, really dressed in the way she wanted she would be very original; and finally there was a return to the theme of having to be sensitive to her mother's feelings.

One of the most important qualities that a therapist needs is the ability to put a number of observations together that indicate when a theme has relevance to the transference. In this case the therapist put together (1) these communications about the mother, with (2) the feeling that therapy had not quite got off the ground, and (3) the whole issue of parental disapproval of self-expression (particularly as a woman). She said that *perhaps in therapy too she had to take care to be sensitive to what the therapist was feeling*. This was essentially an interpretation of the *defence* and the *anxiety*, since the implication was that the patient was *speaking guardedly* (defence) for *fear of the therapist's disapproval* (anxiety) if she were more open. It is also worth noting that since it leads towards *parental disapproval* it is essentially an interpretation on the focus chosen in the therapeutic plan.

The patient's immediate response was 'I didn't want to offend you'; followed by saying that at the beginning of the session she had started with the positive thing about the previous session being constructive, but of course she could have started with the less positive thing about the reasons why she had not thought about the session during the week. She went on to say that she had found it easier to talk to the (male) psychiatrist who had originally interviewed her, but she was very aware that her therapist was a woman and of the need not to cause any offence. In fact, she said, *she had resented this and had spent the first few days after the last session thinking that she could waste the whole therapy in this way*.

Once more, this passage illustrates some of the ways in which an interpretation can be judged as correct. It means nothing if a patient simply agrees with an interpretation, which can just be an example of compliance. Here, however, the patient not merely *agrees* but *elaborates*, going beyond what the therapist has said – the therapist had said nothing about *offending* her; she then confesses to a hidden anxiety-laden feeling, namely resentment; and finally she brings out something that she was obviously holding back as too difficult to say, that she had been afraid this would result in her wasting the whole therapy. It was obvious that until this *transference* feeling could be brought out, free communication would be seriously held up.

Further confirmation of the importance of this crucial piece of transference work came in the next session. The patient opened by saying that after the last session she felt that things were really different – she would even say that a therapeutic effect had begun. She then said that other things had come into her mind during the last session but she had not felt that they were relevant at the time. The first was the following story concerning the time of her brother's birth, when she was eight. Her mother had gone into hospital and she and her father were left at home with her younger sister. Her father said to her 'why don't you come in with me tonight, just for company?'. She remembered being worried by this suggestion and wanting to refuse and sleep in her own bed. She didn't dare refuse and she had spent the night with her father, lying at the very edge of the big double bed, with the constant uneasy feeling that it was wrong and her mother ought to be there. She said that it had always worried her that this was never discussed when her mother came home.

Why should she have been made so uneasy by this perfectly innocent episode in her childhood? It is quite clear that neither her father nor her mother thought anything of it. We know enough now, however, to realize that the child is aware of the sexual implications of such an event even if the parents are not.

Thus this work on *defence* and *anxiety* in the transference led quickly into the possibility of working on the *hidden Oedipal feelings*, which constituted the original focus and the theme of the rest of therapy.

Homosexual transference

The above example was one of what is called in the jargon 'negative' transference – the woman therapist being seen as the disapproving rival. The first example, the Falling Social Worker, was of course one of 'positive' transference, the feelings directed towards the therapist being of heterosexual love. Neither is easy for a therapist to face, and thus such feelings may very easily be mishandled or missed altogether. How much more difficult is it, therefore, if the feelings seem to have homosexual implications. The final example illustrates this very clearly.

The Son in Mourning (contd): love of a male patient for a male therapist

This patient, who may be remembered from Chapter 8, had suffered from agoraphobic symptoms for 8 years, and had developed hypochondriacal symptoms in addition 3 years ago after his father's sudden death from a heart attack. During therapy his intense mixed feelings for his father emerged very clearly. As has already been mentioned, he described how his sister got more attention from his father than he did, and in the same session he spoke of his *wish to be a woman*.

The following sequence occurred in Session 3:

One of the themes of the earlier part of the session was his need to prove his superiority to other men, which he did through the clothes he wore and the cars he drove; and the therapist gave an excellent interpretation of conflicting feelings in the transference – that the patient needed him and yet felt in competition with him. The patient responded by saying how unthinkable it was to compete with the therapist, who 'might have a Rolls Royce in the car park or a £400 suit in the cupboard'. The therapist linked this with the patient's feeling that he could never hold his own against his father (T/P interpretation). Soon after this the patient said: 'Tell me if my headaches are psychological. I wouldn't go to my own doctor about this because he thinks I'm a nut case. Even if I went to him with a boil on my bottom he'd tell me it was psychological.' This contains a mass of interlocking communications with very powerful implications. First, the patient asks a question of the therapist about headaches, which is revealed as almost certainly being a plea for warmth and care. The possible answer, yes the headaches are psychological, is revealed as implying that they are *of no consequence* which would be a *rejection*. And the sudden emergence of the remark about a *boil on his bottom* implies something much more intensely physical than mere headaches, and has clear homosexual overtones. Moreover, this communication following on the theme of competition implies a defensive as well as an expressive function – submission as a defence against challenge. Yet to interpret it as *only* a defence would be quite wrong, since this would be a rejection of the clearly expressed intense need for love.

It is clear that however the therapist reacts he must react with *implied acceptance* of the patient's need for love. For my own part, in order to do this, I would leave out any mention of the defence altogether. Moreover, since the patient's communication is essentially about the *hidden feelings* in the *transference*, it is important to trace these quickly to their origin in the relation with the *father*, i.e. to make the T/P link. Some such comment as, 'Yes, I think you had a great longing for affection from your father and felt he rejected you; and now you are still looking for it in other men such as your doctor and myself, and are afraid we will reject you', spoken in a very gentle tone, would perhaps have met the need of the moment. The T/P link softens the impact of the transference, and the word 'affection' softens any anxieties there may be about homosexuality.

In fact the therapist reported his response as follows: 'I said that either he had to show me his strength, like his clothes and his cars; or else, when he felt I wouldn't tolerate this, he had to turn round and show me his pains and boils and bruises.'

This is not an unsympathetic comment, but it is not sympathetic enough. The implied interpretation of submission as a defence against rivalry is rejecting, and so are the words 'had to'. Even worse, soon afterwards the therapist said it was the end of the session.

Many patients would react with greatly increased resistance in the next session, and both therapist and patient might be puzzled by this and waste many sessions in vain attempts to understand it. Not this patient, who simply came out with his feelings:

'Well I'll tell you and do whatever you want with it. I've had a hell of a week and haven't been able to think of anything else, and the reason is that at the end of the last session you rejected me. The tone of your voice when you said that time was up made me feel you didn't want to know me; and since you didn't say, "I'll see you next week", I just felt you wanted to get rid of me'.

Here the patient is almost certainly *displacing* part of his feeling of rejection from the therapist's interpretation to the way in which the session was ended.

The degree of intensity of transference feelings in a man starved of a father's affection can be judged from the following events.

In Session 12 the therapist broke the news that he would be leaving the Clinic, having got another job, and therapy would have to finish considerably earlier than expected. In supervision, after this session, the therapist was persuaded to withdraw this and to agree to continue therapy at his new hospital. In Session 13, before the therapist spoke of this revised plan, the patient said, 'There is no way I can stop just now. I feel like bursting, and last night I couldn't sleep a wink, dreaming all night that I was talking to someone in this room, and it was eerie because that person was you but you looked different, just horrible.'

In passing it is worth noting an important mechanism here. The fact that the therapist 'looks horrible' is of course an expression of the fact that he has behaved horribly to the patient, but almost certainly there is some kind of 'projection' mechanism at work also, in the sense that the patient has horrible feelings about the therapist, which he dare not face, and which in some way get transferred to the therapists's image. The Director's Daughter, who had a gift for the simple expression of such inner mechanisms, put it beautifully: 'First I *hate* him; and then I feel he's *horrible*; and then I'm *afraid* of him', thus expressing the way in which she seemed to become afraid of her own anger.

Anyhow, the therapist now told the patient that he could go on with therapy to the original termination date. The patient looked overjoyed, and not long afterwards admitted his anger: 'I was really very angry with you for going away, but I couldn't bring myself to tell you about it'. He went on to take this back by saying that it wasn't really 'he' that was angry, but his 'unconscious' – how could he be angry with the therapist for something he could not help? The therapist interpreted the *defence* and the *anxiety* as well as the *impulse*, that he *dared not experience* (defence), his *anger* (impulse) for *fear* (anxiety) that there would be no limits to it and he would explode. The patient said 'Oh, that is very true – the number of times I have felt like that', and he went on to tell of fixing the engine of a car with his father, and his father 'going on and on about it', and 'I remember shaking with anger and my father scolding me for my shaking hands'. (The patient thus made the T/P link for himself.)

The therapist by now had learnt his lesson about accepting the patient's love, and he was able to say, first, that 'his father never understood that he could fix the car, but he needed his father to know more than that, he needed his father to praise him for it'. The therapist then spoke of the patient's feelings about his father's death, and then went on, 'and there is a lot of this feeling here with me, that I don't appreciate how much you need me because if I did I wouldn't have been talking about ending the therapy'. At this point the patient became tearful and said, 'I don't mind you seeing tears in my eyes; what I mind is that I can't cry properly and I know I need to', and then, after a pause, '*It's good that you are there*'. This echoed one of the most moving moments in previous sessions, already mentioned in Chapter 8 (see p. 72), when the patient had said of his father, 'Oh how I wish he were alive'. The therapist had now really learnt his lesson, and his next comment opened with the words, 'This love for me is very precious to you ...'

We have thus ended with an example both of the intensity of the feelings that a patient may develop for his therapist, and of incontrovertible evidence that these feelings may be *transferred* from someone in the patient's past. As has been shown also, the therapist needs a very considerable degree of security and self-knowledge to face such transference and to handle it appropriately; but when he does so it constitutes one of his most important therapeutic tools, making possible the working through of feelings long buried and often reaching into the distant past.

10

The dialogue of psychotherapy and the two triangles

The basic principles of dynamic psychotherapy

The reader who has made himself familiar with the previous chapters has within his grasp all the principles of dynamic psychotherapy, which now need to be summarized.

Within an atmosphere of unconditional acceptance, the therapist establishes a relationship with the patient, the aim of which – usually unspoken – is to enable the patient to understand his true feelings and to bring them to the surface and experience them. For this purpose the therapist uses theoretical knowledge, guided wherever possible by his own self-knowledge, to identify himself with the patient; and puts his understanding to the patient in the form of *interpretations*, which constitute his main therapeutic tool.

Now of course the subject of how, when, and what to interpret cannot be learned from books. Clinical judgement is a kind of computer that gradually becomes programmed by experience, and, having taken into account and integrated a large number of different factors, delivers a ready-made response at the output terminal, which is the therapist's consciousness. The whole point of a computer is that, once it is programmed, it saves the mathematician the laborious process of calculating out each problem in detail. On the other hand, devising the programme may take months of work. In the same way, all I can do is to describe how the clinical computer is programmed, which will take many pages; but in the actual clinical situation the therapist obviously cannot go through this kind of elaborate calculation every time he wants to open his mouth – the process is essentially intuitive and subconscious.

The aim of every moment of every session is to put the patient in touch with as much of his true feelings as he can bear. The therapist therefore needs to make judgements of the following:

(1) The degree to which the patient is already in touch with his true feelings, a synonym for which – since he is talking to the therapist – is the *depth of rapport*;
(2) The nature of the hidden feelings of which he is not yet aware;
(3) How close these feelings are to the surface, i.e. how accessible they are;
(4) The degree of anxiety or pain with which they are invested; and
(5) The patient's capacity to bear it.

Of course, most of the time the therapist cannot know all these things at once. What he must do, therefore, is to initiate a process of step by step exploration, the whole time watching for feedback. The essential nature of this feedback consists of changes in the level of rapport, so that the capacity to judge this is one of the therapist's most essential qualities. Rapport is the universal indicator by which the therapist may be constantly guided. If rapport increases after an intervention, the intervention was appropriate and appropriately made; if rapport decreases, his intervention was inappropriate (not necessarily *wrong*) and he must wait until he can try something else.

This concept of rapport is so important that it is worth describing a single session in detail to illustrate its use.

The Interior Decorator (contd), illustrating fluctuations in rapport

Some details of this session have already been given in Chapter 3, in illustration of the concept of unconscious communication. The patient was a young man of 26 complaining of an inability to consummate his marriage. He had already been seen for consultation by a male psychiatrist, who was now seeing him for the second time with the aim of taking him on for brief psychotherapy. In between, he had had projection tests given by a psychologist.

The therapist opened by asking him how he felt now. The patient at once launched into a long story about recent events between him and his wife. The essence of this was that on one occasion he now claimed to have had successful intercourse, but that when he tried again a few days later, he had lost his erection, and later on the two of them had had a row.

Nothing had been said about whether or not he wanted treatment, so the therapist asked him this. His answer was 'yes', but said in such a tentative tone that the therapist asked him a second time, to which he answered the same, but in a tone little less tentative. The therapist decided to ignore this and offered him therapy with a time limit of *16 sessions*, which he accepted, and then invited him to talk.

So far rapport had been very shallow, and it became no deeper as the session continued. He chose to start by returning to the row with his wife, in which it transpired that she had said some very hurtful things about his manhood; but instead of examining his feelings about all this he rapidly veered away to saying that perhaps his impotence was due to fear of making his wife pregnant, or even simply to being tired.

This was obviously a *defence of superficiality* against *anxiety-laden feelings*, and the question is what the therapist should do. The answer is that he must gently point out or imply the *defence*, and suggest that the reason for it is *anxiety*. He cannot be more specific because he does not know what the anxiety is.

This he did by making the general comment that the patient had spoken much more freely about his inner feelings in the previous interviews (thus implying that he wasn't speaking freely now), and perhaps he had became *frightened of examining them further*.

The patient clearly took this as telling him to do better, and he set about doing so, with some success. The theme that emerged was how he had to *protect* his wife, and how he had *hurt* her in the past by telling her a lot of stupid lies in order to *make himself look big.*

It is thus interesting that the therapist's general *anxiety interpretation* has produced a clear response, in that it has led the patient to reveal one specific anxiety and a defence against another: i.e. the fear of hurting his wife on the one hand, and the need to look big, which almost certainly is a defence against a feeling of inferiority, on the other. Moreover, the fact that the patient is willing to reveal a feeling of inferiority to his male therapist sounds like an indication of trust – or could it be just an attempt at submission? Even if it is the latter, however, it indicates *heightened interaction* with the therapist. The whole adds up to a clear deepening of rapport.

The therapist then gave the clearly indicated interpretation of the *defence* and the *anxiety*, saying that if he needed to make himself look so big (defence), he must be very unsure of himself underneath (anxiety). The patient said that that was right, and went on to say that he had never achieved much in his life, again showing deepening rapport and increased trust; he then came out with the aforementioned amazingly clear unconscious communication, representing a further deepening of rapport: that the only time he really felt he had achieved something was when he was in the forces and had done a '16-week course in navigation'. He had really felt that this was a challenge, had been determined to do as well as the others – who had been older than he was – and he had succeeded.

It is worth a digression to speculate about the extraordinary way in which the unconscious makes use of coincidence. His 16-week course, it would seem, was by an amazing coincidence absolutely tailor-made to provide this important communication about his attitude to therapy – but, one may ask, had it really been a 16-week course, or did his unconscious change it to fit in with the number of sessions he had been offered? And, if it was a 16-week course and the therapist had offered him, say 20 sessions, what communication would he have made then? These questions are fascinating but unanswerable. The only thing one can be sure of is that his unconscious would have had no difficulty in finding a way round the problem.

In any case, the coincidence was too much for the therapist to miss, and he gave the obvious interpretation about the here-and-now. It is important to note that whereas the previous two interpretations mentioned have been general and *undirected*, i.e. not concerned with any actual person, this interpretation brings in at least a hint of the relation with the therapist, i.e. the transference (T).

The interpretation was that 'perhaps he regarded the course of treatment with me as a sort of challenge in which he hoped to do as well as possible.'

There was immediately yet another deepening of rapport, because the patient now spontaneously admitted an anxiety-laden hidden feeling, which had been clearly deducible from the way in which he had accepted the offer of treatment earlier in the session, namely that his feelings about treatment were very mixed. He went on to elaborate on this, saying that he was a *suspicious* sort of person and it wasn't easy for him to *trust* anybody. An example of misplaced trust had been when he was teaching in a school and he and some other teachers had formed a deputation to speak to the headmaster about some complaints. He had been appointed spokesman, but as soon as they all got to the door of the office everybody else had melted away, leaving him to undertake the task alone.

This again is clearly an unconscious communication, though it is not as easy to translate as the one just described. There seem to be two important elements in it: one is being let down (an anxiety) and the other is confronting an authority figure with a complaint (which is much nearer to an impulse). In any case, since the whole context is concerned with the patient's feelings about therapy, it cannot help being a communication about the transference.

The therapist tried the anxiety first, asking if he was afraid that the therapist would let him down. The patient said he didn't think so; so the therapist tried the impulse, bringing in the previously used word 'challenge' as well: 'Perhaps he felt that any man in a superior position was a sort of *rival*, and thus the relation between us might develop into a sort of *challenge*.'

A review of the session so far will reveal that there has been very considerable progress in content as well as in rapport: from general anxiety to *specific* anxiety, from *undirected* interpretation to *transference* interpretation, and now from transference *anxiety* to transference *impulse*, with the possibility of reaching Oedipal feelings not very far away.

The patient immediately said, 'You've really hit something there'; and his next remark, elaborating in a meaningful way, made clear that this was not simply compliance: he said that he did feel like that about other men, and that what he then did was to *try and find out their faults* – obviously to bring them down to his level, or below. Thus, once more, the leap-frogging process of dialogue between patient and therapist has continued: the therapist only mentioned rivalry and challenge, the patient has spoken of a considerably stronger *impulse* – to pick holes in the other man's superiority. Moreover, there may well be a projection mechanism at work here, leading to an anxiety, in the sense that the patient is afraid that the other man will try to do the same to him.

The therapist chose to make an interpretation about the anxiety rather than the impulse, continuing the leap-frogging by bringing in the stronger word, *humiliation*, and re-emphasizing that the whole dialogue was concerned with the *transference*: 'The trouble was that in this sort of treatment *I* was in a sense trying to find out *his* faults, and he would feel the treatment was a sort of struggle, and even that I might be trying to humiliate him.'

This resulted in the first high point of the session, with a moment of maximum rapport, in which the patient entrusted the therapist with a crucial piece of hitherto undisclosed information about which he felt anxious and ashamed: His first remark was, 'Yes, that's the heart of the whole thing', followed by, 'There's something I'd like to ask you. If my wife has a mackintosh on I could kiss her and never stop. I know this kind of thing does happen to people, and it's called a fetish. Is it very abnormal?'

The question of reassurance

This is a kind of situation with which a therapist is frequently confronted. The patient is asking for *reassurance* (compare the Geologist's request for *advice*, p. 27). Is it correct to give it? The answer is usually no, and for the following reason: It is the task of therapy to *bring out* the patient's anxieties and trace them to their origin, not to drive them underground by reassuring them. In this particular case the patient, whose complaint is impotence, is presumably suffering from sexual anxieties, and has just expressed an anxiety about his sexuality. The therapist must behave in such a way as, first, not to reject the patient, who has just entrusted him with a closely guarded secret, but then not to reassure the anxiety either.

The Interior Decorator (contd)

This therapist now showed a failure in therapeutic tact, refusing to give reassurance but doing so rather roughly, saying: 'I'm not going to answer your question; you're trying to tell me you're afraid there's something wrong with your sexuality, and it's much more important to find out what this means.'

This resulted in a plummeting of rapport. The patient was completely taken aback, became silent, and then said, 'Can you give me a lead about what I should talk about?'

How do you handle this new situation? In certain situations it may be absolutely correct to admit your mistake and apologize; but at the same time, if you can see what lies behind the patient's particular way of reacting, it may be much better to give an interpretation. This is what the therapist tried to do, saying, 'I think the reason why you can't go on and want a lead is because you are *angry* with me. You asked me to reassure you about something, and I wouldn't do it.'

'Defence should be interpreted before impulse'

This moment of therapy can be used to introduce a fundamental principle (for further discussion see below, p. 102): subsequent events showed that this was a correct interpretation, but it was wrongly given. The patient is showing a *defence* mechanism, submission as a defence against anger (the *impulse*), because of some *anxiety* (the exact nature of which is as yet unknown) about the consequences of expressing the impulse. The whole process is unconscious, and if you simply interpret the impulse without also showing the patient how he is defending against it, he will often respond as if you were offering a *non sequitur*. In this particular case it will certainly not be obvious to the patient what the connection is between wanting a lead and *being angry*.

Even better, you should if possible detect what the *anxiety* is and interpret this as well. The anxiety is often fantasy-based, and if the patient can be shown this, it is likely to be a great relief to him and to contribute more than anything to his being able to face his true feelings. In this case, however, the therapist neither knew the nature of the anxiety – though of course it can never be easy for a patient to express anger to his therapist in the second session – nor did he see the necessity for interpreting it.

The Interior Decorator (contd)

As might have been predicted, therefore, the patient reacted by not being able to admit any anger; and this time the therapist intuitively saw that in order to make any progress he must interpret the defence, though he still left the anxiety to take care of itself. He brought in some information from the previous interview, pointing out that when the patient was angry he tended to go a long way in the other direction and submit himself completely. When he and his wife quarrelled he did the housework for her; in the present situation, when he was angry about not receiving reassurance, his reaction was to submit himself completely and say he would go anywhere the therapist liked. It is worth noting that this interpretation makes the T/O link, i.e. the link between a mechanism operating in the transference (T) and one operating in his *life outside* (O). It thus begins the process of acquainting the patient, through the here-and-now, with mechanisms that interfere with his efficient functioning in his life in general.

It would probably have been better to have added some general remark about the anxiety, e.g. that perhaps the patient had some reason for being afraid of getting angry; but perfection is often not needed in psychotherapy, especially when − as here − a good therapeutic alliance has been established.

At this point the patient showed a marked deepening of rapport in two different ways. First, he began speaking spontaneously and with animation; and second, he showed one of the signs of active, unconscious, collaboration in the therapeutic process, namely that having received a partial interpretation he goes on to complete it. Here, having received an interpretation of the *defence* and the *impulse*, he went on to reveal the nature of the *anxiety* with the utmost clarity.

He said that he realized that this kind of submission was true of him − the trouble was that he was very afraid of his temper. He then went even further, beginning spontaneously to take the step that − as described above − is an essential part of almost every therapy, namely to make the link with his *parents* in the *past* (P). The essence of this was to say, first, that the only person who had ever seen his temper was his mother; and then to describe his *father's* outbursts of temper − which in fact sounded like the helpless violence of a weak man. As he described this he spoke in a tone of considerable contempt.

It was now near the end of the session, and the therapist decided to draw the patient's attention once more to the transference; which he did by reminding the patient of the moment when he seemed to be regarding the therapist as setting him a challenge, and adding that the relation between the two of them was probably going to be important in the future. This resulted in another moment of intense rapport. The patient immediately said, 'Yes, when I told you about the mackintosh, that was an opening', and he went on to say, 'I hope you don't mind me saying this, but I like your face. I like the way you look people in the eyes and give it to them straight. I want you to give it to me straight. If I'm mad then I'm mad and I want you to tell me so.' The faintly homosexual tinge to these remarks was not lost on the therapist, but of course he said nothing about this.

Instead he said 'Good', and then proceeded to draw some issues together. Amongst these was the fact that after talking about his difficulty over his temper, the patient had spoken of his *parents*; and quite possibly the relation that he had built-up with his parents was being repeated with other people now, for instance there might well be things about which he was angry with his *wife* which corresponded to similar things with his *mother* (the O/P link).

The patient clearly followed this line of reasoning and *interrupted several times* with his own comments, which was very different from his former passive behaviour when he had come to a halt and asked the therapist for a lead. Soon afterwards it was the end of the session.

The two triangles

Now although the above passage was intended to illustrate the use of *rapport*, it illustrates much more than this. Throughout the whole of the preceding chapters there has been repeated reference to what may be represented by *two triangles*: the first may be called the *triangle of conflict*, and consists of Defence, Anxiety, and Hidden feeling. This is related to the second triangle by the fact that the hidden feeling is directed towards one or more categories of the *triangle of person*, namely Other, Transference, and Parent or Sibling, represented by O, T, and P, respectively. It was Karl Menninger who drew attention to this second triangle, in his book *The theory of psychoanalytic technique* (1958). He named it the 'triangle of insight'; but both are triangles of insight and 'triangle of person' is thus a much better term. These two triangles are shown diagrammatically in *Figure 1*, each standing on an apex because one of the three elements can be regarded as 'lying underneath' the other two.

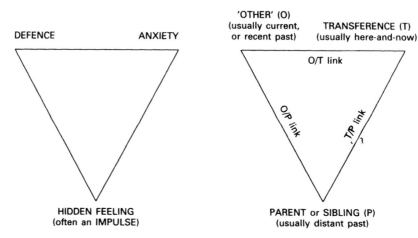

Figure 1   The Two Triangles

The fact that there are three categories of person in the second triangle also means that there are three possible *links*, which have repeatedly been mentioned in passing in the preceding pages, and are represented in the figure by the three sides. These are the O/P link, where feelings directed towards Other are derived from those directed towards Parent or Sibling, the O/T link, where some kind of similar feelings are directed towards Other and Therapist; and the T/P link, where Transference feelings are derived from feelings about Parents or Siblings.

As mentioned above, each triangle stands on an apex, which represents the fact that the aim of most dynamic psychotherapy is to reach, beneath the *defence* and the *anxiety*, to the hidden feeling, and then to trace this feeling back from the present to its origins *in the past*, usually in the relation with parents. As is shown in *Figure 1*, the triangle of person can also usually be represented by a *triangle of time*: the top left-hand corner referring to current or recent past; Transference to here-and-now; and Parent or Sibling to distant past. However, the term 'triangle of time' is not always accurate. For instance, transference feelings may be concerned with a previous session rather than with the here-and-now, while obviously the patient may also have *current* relations with parents or siblings.

This leads to a comment about notation. I have used 'O', for 'Other', to represent the top left-hand corner of the triangle of person; but Davanloo and most American authors use 'C' for Current, and my co-author and I have done the same in *Psychodynamics, training, and outcome* (Malan and Osimo, 1992). In the majority of therapeutic sessions this is accurate; and it remains accurate as long as 'Current' is understood to include the past other than the really distant past. The trouble is that it might include, for instance, a woman's relation with a previous husband – which could refer to events as long as 20 years ago – where the term 'current' is obviously inappropriate. For this reason in the present book I am sticking to the notation 'O'. However, it must be remembered that 'O' and 'C' are absolutely equivalent.

The importance of the two triangles is that between them they can be used to represent almost every intervention that a therapist makes. Much of a therapist's skill consists of knowing which parts of which triangle to include in his interpretations at any given moment.

Here I would have liked to take an actual example and to analyse it in detail in these terms. Unfortunately no real example shows either clearly or completely enough all the features that I wish to illustrate, and I shall therefore make up an account of a fictitious therapy. Nevertheless, everything that occurs in it is of a kind that has occurred in countless actual therapies throughout the world.

Of all the features illustrated, probably the most important is the *inevitability* of the patient's problem manifesting itself in the transference sooner or later as therapy proceeds.

Account of an Imaginary Therapy

The patient is a young man in his late twenties who is seeking treatment now because of a critical situation in his relation with his current girl-friend. In the past he has shown a repetitive pattern in his relation with girls: after an initial period in which everything seems to go well, he finds himself unable to feel deeply beyond a certain point, and sooner or later this results in the break-up of the relationship, which is followed by an attack of depression. He is now faced with the fear that history is going to repeat itself, and he realizes that something must be done about this pattern if he is ever to achieve happiness. Having been seen previously for a consultation by a male psychiatrist, he is taken on for once-a-week, face-to-face, treatment by a female therapist, under supervision. This therapist has a flair for psychotherapy but is at the beginning of her career.

First phase: completion of the triangle of conflict in relation to the girl-friend (O)

Told that all he is asked to do is to talk, the patient opens by forming a trusting relationship and describing his current predicament. The therapist sees that this inability to feel must represent a *defence*. She has ideas about what this is a defence against, but in accordance with the principle of exploring gradually and allowing the patient to do as much of the work as possible, she only gives a general interpretation: 'I think this inability to feel (defence) happens because you are afraid (anxiety) of something that might occur between you and your girl-friend if you were to become more deeply involved.' She has thus made an exploratory interpretation mentioning *defence* and *anxiety* (two corners of the triangle of conflict) in relation to someone in the patient's current life (one corner of the triangle of person, namely O). This interpretation can also be described as *asking a question of the patient's unconscious*: i.e. 'What is it you are afraid of?' and is part of the therapeutic dialogue between the two of them.

A good patient will allow his unconscious to answer the question, as this one does. Without being fully aware of the significance of what he is saying, the patient now mentions that he had become *more deeply* involved with his first girl-friend than with the present one, but that she had not really wanted him, and when she had left him he had become very depressed and had spent long periods crying, without fully knowing what he was crying about. After the break-up of a subsequent relation, however, he had found himself consciously indifferent, though he had suffered from a long period of work inhibition and early waking.

The patient's unconscious has now in a sense exceeded expectations, since it has not only supplied the *anxiety* but the *hidden feeling* as well. It has told the therapist very clearly that the patient's inability to feel is a *defence* against the *anxiety* of losing the girl and being exposed to overwhelming grief (the *hidden feeling*). The patient himself has thus *completed the triangle of conflict*, initiating a process of 'leap-frogging' in the therapeutic dialogue, in which each of the two participants goes one move beyond what the other has just said.

The therapist makes the triangle of conflict explicit, the patient shows that this is meaningful to him, and shortly afterwards the session comes to an end.

Second phase: the link with the past (O/P link)

In the next session, the patient opens by recounting how, in the early relation with his present girl-friend, he had woken up one Monday morning to find that he had lost much of his feeling for her. He has thus himself offered an opportunity for the discovery of the *precipitating factor*; which, as described in Chapter 5, often provides an important clue to the understanding of the psychodynamics. Alive to this, the therapist asks him what had happened that week-end. He says that the strange thing is that they had had a week-end in which they had felt particularly close to one another, and he gives some details.

The therapist is now given an opportunity to reiterate her interpretation of the *anxiety*, this time in relation to a specific event, saying that surely the very moment when he feels closest to her is the moment of greatest danger in case he should lose her. The patient is struck by this, and after a moment's thought says it has just occurred to him that much the same happened with the second of his two previous girl-friends, namely that he had lost his feeling just after they had been particularly close together. This is a clear confirmation of her interpretation. Then after a pause, he says, 'But why should I be like that?'.

This is an important moment in the therapeutic dialogue. Although he does not know it, the patient is directly asking the therapist to *make the link with the past*, here the O/P link. The therapist is well aware of the patient's history and offers him the interpretation, tentatively put, that perhaps he doesn't want to be exposed again to the kind of feelings he experienced when his mother died, when he was sixteen. The patient sees this, rapport becomes much deeper, and he begins to recount some memories of this traumatic event – how his mother out of the blue had begun going a strange colour and feeling increasingly ill, had been admitted to hospital, and had died of acute leukaemia complicated by pneumonia after three weeks. Both the patient and his father had been stunned by her death, and though the patient had cried, he did not seem to have cried enough, and not long after the funeral his mourning had been cut short by his having to go back to boarding school.

Third Phase: resistance, and the entry of transference

This now initiates a period of therapy in which the patient tells about his childhood and his relation with both his parents, to whom he had been very close. All this is told quite calmly, though with his feelings not far away. As the sessions go on, however, he seems to become less and less in touch with feeling and more intellectual, and he even begins to speculate about his psychopathology from theoretical ideas about the 'Oedipus complex' that he has picked up from books. The therapist tells him rather sharply that those ideas are a waste of time and he is not properly in touch with his feelings, at which he redoubles his efforts, but to no avail.

In supervision the therapist mentions this incident with some guilt. The supervisor now helps her out by telling her the following: that hitherto she has been in the 'honeymoon' period of therapy, but that this has now come to an end; that this is an almost universal occurrence; that now she is facing a particular aspect of defence known as *resistance*, in which the patient is fighting against becoming aware of painful feelings in the therapy; and that very probably these painful feelings are at least partly concerned with the transference. In fact there is little difficulty in seeing what the transference is: we know that the patient's pattern with girls is to withdraw after getting close to them; he has certainly felt close to his therapist during the early sessions, when he has been understood; and he is now repeating exactly the same pattern of withdrawal after closeness, with her. With hindsight we can see that this was always inevitable. Therefore the patients' main or 'nuclear' problem is now manifesting itself in the transference, which is something that she should not feel frustrated about, but should welcome – since she and the patient now have an opportunity to work it through as it happens before their very eyes. In fact this can be said to be the point at which therapy can really begin.

The supervisor goes on to say that she is now experiencing the kind of frustration that is experienced by the patient's girl-friends, who must be bewildered and angered by the way in which he withdraws after the relationship has appeared to be going so well.

Thus the supervisor points out to her that the feelings produced in her – for which the not very elegant and not always accurate term 'counter-transference' has been coined – can be used to understand the patient and to facilitate the process of therapy. What is needed is an interpretation of the resistance (defence) in the *transference*, together with an interpretation of why this defence is necessary to him, i.e. that he is afraid (anxiety) of becoming more deeply involved, in case he loses her and is exposed to grief (the hidden feeling).

Here the supervisor also points out to her the following: so far no transference interpretations have been given, and in accordance with the principle of proceeding gradually from what is nearest to consciousness to what is more deeply buried, it is probably best to start, not by interpreting the whole of the triangle of conflict in this way, but simply by making the T/O link, pointing out that the pattern that he is showing with her is exactly the same as the pattern he shows with girls.

Fourth phase: the interpretation of the resistance and the T/O link

The patient begins the next session by saying that he realizes all these intellectual ideas are no use, but he doesn't seem to have anything else to say. He adds that the situation between him and his girl-friend seems to be getting worse, and there is some danger that they are becoming estranged.

There is something of great importance happening here. The nuclear problem, which has begun to manifest itself strongly in the transference, is intensified by this and is now spilling over into the patient's relations outside, which are becoming endangered. This is a situation that cannot be allowed to go on.

However, there is something else that is also very hopeful. The patient himself has continued the leap-frogging by quite unconsciously juxtaposing his problems in the transference with his relation with his girl-friend. This means that he is almost making this T/O link himself, and therefore his unconscious has quite independently reached the same position as was reached by supervisor and therapist. The breakthrough of the therapist's feelings has in fact jolted all three of them – a situation not to be recommended, but in this case it appears to have been useful.

The therapist therefore states the T/O link explicitly, also making the link with the patient's nuclear problem: that after an initial period of trust and closeness with her he has withdrawn emotionally and retreated into intellectual talk, and that this is exactly similar to the pattern that he shows with girl-friends, for which he originally came seeking help. There is an immediate deepening of rapport, and the patient now says that during the past week he has found himself becoming angry with his girl-friend on several occasions, the cause for which appeared to be that she failed to understand him.

Since this is the first mention of anger throughout the whole of therapy, it is yet another example of leap-frogging, and it at once suggests that this may be another of the hidden feelings against which the patient has had to defend himself for many years – an example of over-determination. This the therapist sees, but the immediate point is that almost certainly the anger is displaced from the transference, and arises out of the therapist's sharpness in the previous session. This displacement is of course a defence, but the patient has admitted the hidden feeling openly, so that the defence can be bypassed, and all that is needed is to make the link with herself. She therefore suggests that perhaps he had felt she was telling him off in the last session for being intellectual, and had been angry with her. (Someone more experienced and more secure would quite possibly have openly admitted that she had been irritated with him, and have linked it with what his girl-friends must feel, but what she did was in fact quite sufficient.)

The patient looks relieved, but says nothing, and falls into a pensive silence. The therapist senses that this is a *productive* rather than a *resistant* silence, and after a few minutes helps him out by asking what had been passing through his mind. He says he was thinking of some of the times with his first girl-friend, before it went wrong with her. This, again, is almost certainly a communication about his warm feelings for the therapist. She sees this, but also realizes that it may well be embarrassing for him to acknowledge; and, with excellent therapeutic tact, just says, 'Yes, it's a relief to be understood, isn't it?'. He knows perfectly well what she means, but the issue remains unspoken between them.

In the next session the patient reports that, during the past week, for some unaccountable reason he has found himself feeling much closer to his girl-friend, and things have been going very well. Of course this is in fact because he is no longer displacing anger from the therapist, but she deliberately leaves this unsaid. The atmosphere is warm, and the session is largely spent in recounting recent events.

Fifth phase: crisis, the T/P link, breakthrough

Two days later the therapist goes down with jaundice. She phones the Clinic and asks her secretary to let the patient know that she is ill and will get in touch with him when she is fit to return to work.

Therapy is resumed three weeks later. The patient greets her with a constrained smile and begins to speak about trivialities. This goes on for some time, and the therapist then sees what is happening and gives him an interpretation completing the triangle of conflict about her absence: that he is avoiding feeling (defence), because he cannot face the pain (anxiety) of his loss of the therapist (hidden feeling) during her illness. Deepening rapport is shown by his becoming more animated, and he now says that over the past three weeks he had become preoccupied with the loss of his two previous girl-friends. This is of course a partial response to the interpretation, since he now admits the hidden feeling but does not admit that it relates to the therapist (he is still using the defence of displacement). However, there is no need to emphasize the defence, and she simply reiterates that this must have been set off in him by the loss of herself. The patient now says, 'Yes, it's funny, but the thought did cross my mind, "what if she never comes back?".'

At this point the coincidence with the past is so close to the surface as to be unmistakable. Very gently the therapist makes the T/P link, saying that if this had happened it would have been exactly the same as had happened to his mother. Suddenly the patient breaks down and sobs for ten minutes, then recovers, and begins to recount with deep feeling how his mother had died one night, much sooner than expected, and his father's in-drawn breath as he heard the news over the telephone, and how no words were necessary but the two of them went to opposite ends of the house for a time and then had breakfast together and just carried on with their lives in a stunned and frozen state. He has not thought of some of these details from that day to this.

The therapist here tries to make some interpretations of the defence of withdrawal at fear of loss which has been a feature of his life ever since, but the patient cannot take this in, and she falls silent, not quite knowing what to say or do.

Her supervisor, after congratulating her on the way she handled the first half of the session, tells her that trying to make interpretations later on was really an intrusion, that in any case it was unnecessary, and that what was needed at this point was something that will not be found in books on technique, namely for her to sit with him and simply *share his grief.* In her own personal psychotherapy her therapist weighs in with an interpretation, namely that she had not quite faced her own grief about certain losses in her life, and therefore was making use of *words* for the purpose of covering up her own feelings.

This session is followed by several in which the patient reports that he has been overcome by waves of crying and has been recalling further details surrounding his mother's illness and death. This, of course, is part of the process of *working through.* His girl-friend has been sympathetic and has shared his feelings with him, and she has received her own reward because he has now found himself kissing her in a way that he had never known before. This is as well, as her capacity to bear his feelings about another woman is not unlimited. Finally, he reports that they have decided to become engaged.

Sixth phase: the threat of termination, relapse

Things seem to be going very well, and a few sessions later, after consultation with her supervisor, the therapist suggests to the patient that they might think in terms of meeting less frequently – though not immediately – in preparation for stopping altogether, while emphasizing that she will be available in the future if he has a crisis or wants to talk anything over with her. The patient is pleased to think that he is getting well and readily agrees.

However, in the next session he reports that he has lost his feeling for his girl-friend, and he even mentions that he has had some thoughts about whether his engagement may be premature. After this he embarks on further intellectualization. This is a phenomenon of fundamental importance, now well known but most disconcerting to Freud and the early analysts, namely *relapse at threat of termination.* The reason for it is that part of the therapeutic effect has been due to the continued presence of symbolic love provided by the relation with the therapist, and that this fact is exposed the moment the love is withdrawn. The way of handling it is to interpret feelings about the loss and to work them through, and if possible to link them with the past.

The therapist had been warned by her supervisor to expect difficulties, and she interprets that once more he is being exposed to a loss, and that the old way of defending himself against his grief has begun to reassert itself. This does not help, so she interprets that perhaps he is *angry* with her (the second hidden feeling) for abandoning him. This doesn't help either. Since he has not responded to these interpretations about the relation with her, there is no point in trying to make the link with the past.

Seventh phase: acting out

Therapy continues in difficulty for several sessions. Then one day the patient reports the following: that there had been a misunderstanding with his girl-friend. He had assumed that they were going to spend the week-end together, but in fact she had arranged some time before to attend a conference in connection with her work, which he had forgotten. On hearing this he had been disappointed and resentful, and when she returned on the Sunday night had found himself unable to kiss her. She had become offended, it had blown up into a quarrel, and she had walked out on him. There had been no communication between them since.

The therapist (who, owing to troubles in her private life, is having an off day) here makes the O/P link, saying that he must have been angry with his girl-friend for failing him, and perhaps there had been some reason for being angry with his mother. The patient denies any recollection of being angry with his mother, rapport remains shallow, and no progress is made.

This moment in therapy can be used to illustrate two important themes. First of all, as subsequent events were to show, this is an example of a *correct* but *inappropriate* interpretation. The therapist, who had done well so far, had a blind spot – as usual, about the transference – and interpreted the wrong side of the triangle of person, making the link with the past (the O/P link) instead of the link with herself (the O/T link). The correct interpretation was of course that much of the anger against the girl-friend arose from his feelings of being abandoned by his therapist, who had recently suggested termination. Although this anger has been interpreted before, it is only now that it has become accessible.

Second, this is once more an example of *acting out* (first encountered in the Director's Daughter, p. 48). Here the patient expresses towards someone in his life outside feelings that are really directed towards the therapist.

Eighth phase: over-determination – an earlier trauma

All this is explained by the supervisor. In the next session the patient reports that he had phoned his girl-friend and had tried to apologize; but in fact it had been one of those 'I'm sorry but …' apologies which just continue the quarrel, and they had ended up on no better terms than they began. The therapist then gathers herself together and gives the correct O/T interpretation, mentioning *defence* and *hidden feeling*: that he feels abandoned by her for suggesting stopping treatment, is angry, and has been taking it out on his girl-friend instead of her.

Again there is no conscious acknowledgement of this interpretation, but he shows immediate deepening of rapport by becoming thoughtful and then saying 'I had a dream last night'. Encouraged to tell it, he says that he was in a building that seemed to be a cross between the Clinic and a hospital, and as he watched through the window a car drove away and crashed. He could not quite see the driver, but he thinks it was a woman and it seems she was injured, possibly killed.

This requires a digression.

The use of dreams in dynamic psychotherapy

Freud remarked that dreams represent the 'royal road into the unconscious'; and whenever a patient reports a dream it should be regarded as a potentially important communication. (Of course, like any other communication, it may also be used to divert attention from something else, which always needs to be borne in mind.)

Now some dreams are transparent and can be interpreted immediately as expressing some feeling that the dreamer does not wish to acknowledge consciously – examples were given in connection with the Economics Student (p. 45) and the Daughter with a Stroke (p. 39). But with the majority of dreams this is not so, and even when the therapist thinks he can see part of the meaning of the dream there may be many hidden details that he could not possibly know. It is therefore an almost universal procedure to *ask for associations* to the dream, which means directing the patient to say what comes into his mind in connection with the dream as a whole or individual details in it. If there seem to be significant details that he leaves out, then the therapist should direct him to associate to these as well.

Eighth phase (contd)

The therapist therefore asks him to give his associations to the dream, to which he says that he once saw the therapist driving away from the Clinic after a session. An idea occurs to her, and she asks, does he remember which session? He says that it was some weeks ago, but certain details enable him to work out that it must have been the session in which she had first mentioned the possibility of termination. He goes on to say that the car in the dream was the same colour as hers but it did not really resemble hers in design – in fact it was quite old-fashioned.

This is a moment of breakthrough of the patient's primitive feelings that are very far from consciousness indeed, and it needs to be neither shirked nor over-played. The therapist leaves on one side the detail of the old-fashioned car, which she does not understand, and goes for the most immediate interpretation. She says that since a car resembling hers crashes and the driver is at least injured, possibly killed, and since it is *his* dream, she thinks he may have *wished serious harm to come to her because she suggested stopping the treatment.*

In my view this wording strikes the correct balance – anything less strong would be watering down the true impulse and giving the impression of not being quite able to face it; whereas to say that he 'wanted to kill her' would probably be too far from consciousness to be meaningful to him. It is also worth noting that this is a direct interpretation of the hidden feeling, here a very disturbing impulse, without mention of defence or anxiety, which is correct because the impulse is so explicitly stated by the dream.

Again he makes no direct response, but tells of a story he had read in the papers of a woman who had been dragged out of her car and killed by hooligans after stopping at traffic lights in one of the poorer quarters of New York. The therapist notes the progression from accident to murder, which is a confirmation of her interpretation, but, correctly, says nothing.

In the next session the patient reports that he has again phoned his girl-friend and found himself able to apologize to her properly this time. They have made it up and all is well again. This is in fact almost certainly a response to the work of the previous session, but the therapist, again with excellent therapeutic tact, refrains from saying so.

The patient then returns to the dream and begins to puzzle over two features, the hospital and the old-fashioned car. The therapist offers her own association, pointing out that his mother died in hospital, but though this ought to be relevant the details of that hospital don't fit the hospital in the dream. Then another idea occurs to her, and she asks if the patient had ever been admitted to hospital when he was small. The answer is, yes, he had – he had his tonsils out at the age of four. This is a beautiful example of empathic guesswork on the part of the therapist, and also of therapeutic dialogue, for suddenly the patient realizes that the car in the dream reminds him of the car that his parents had at that time. The patient feels on the edge of some discovery but cannot quite reach it.

In between sessions the patient meets his father and asks what happened around the time of his admission for tonsillectomy. His father says that he doesn't remember about his son in hospital but does remember that they had a terrible time with him for several weeks after he came home. Quite apart from the soreness of his throat, he had been difficult and fractious, alternately sulking and throwing tantrums. His mother had had the greatest difficulty in coping with him and finally had been reduced to locking him in his room and leaving him to scream for a whole morning, after which he seemed to improve.

During the next few sessions, patient and therapist gradually reconstruct something of his experience in hospital. It comes back to him that his mother had meekly accepted the hospital regulations concerned with visiting hours, whereas the mother of a boy next to him had made such a fuss that she had been allowed to stay with her son for much of his admission. The therapist says that he must have been angry with his mother about this, and the patient agrees, without really being in touch with it. The patient says he can recollect going into the ward with his mother, but nothing more till after his operation; and the therapist says 'I think you saw your mother through the window driving away'. The patient is struck by this, but again can recollect nothing about it.

Final phase: working through termination, together with the T/P link

In fact, struggle as they may, they can get no nearer than this to recapturing memories and feelings of that time. During the next many weeks, the therapist returns to working on the transference, repeatedly making interpretations of herself as an *abandoning mother*, with whom the patient is *angry*. This is a different form of T/P interpretation – not in the form 'and this is what you must have felt about your mother', because actual recollections appear to be beyond the possibility of recovery. It is also a direct interpretation of the hidden feeling, which is now close enough to the surface to make interpretation of the defence and the anxiety quite unnecessary.

During the course of this work something new emerges about the past, namely that between the ages of ten and sixteen there had been a number of occasions on which he had quarrelled with his mother because of her failure to understand him. Moreover, her behaviour in the hospital now emerges as part of a more general phenomenon: putting conventional behaviour before her son's emotional needs. The therapist, recalling the dream, tries making some interpretations about death-wishes directed against his mother, at which the patient looks blank and there is a marked lightening of rapport. She is told off by her supervisor about this, since such feelings are clearly far too inaccessible to the patient to be interpreted, and only serve to disturb and upset him. She falls back on the correct level of interpretation, which is to emphasize how much more difficult these quarrels must have made it for him to face his true feelings about her death. He now recalls with guilt that one quarrel had occurred not long before she was taken ill, which makes this interpretation doubly meaningful. This again illustrates a general principle, that where there has been failure to mourn, one should always look for mixed feelings towards the person who has died (compare the Daughter with a Stroke, p. 38). Finally, this is yet another example of over-determination – not only was the mother's death traumatic because the grief threatened to be overwhelming, but because it greatly intensified guilt about mixed feelings towards her. Over-determination never ends and should be watched for constantly.

After this has emerged the patient seems to be in a stable position, the relation with his girl-friend is going well, and he accepts termination without difficulty. Therapy has taken just over a year.

Let us add a five-year follow-up. The patient is married to his girl-friend and they now have two children. The old pattern of withdrawal has gone and there have been periods of great closeness. At the same time he still has the feeling that there is some quality in the relation that is missing – he knows of its existence and yet has never been able to capture it. This outcome takes care of the obvious reality that therapeutic effects are usually incomplete.

Comment

I have found this piece of fiction extraordinarily easy to write, which has surprised me. I am sure that one of the main reasons is that if one understands the phenomena of unconscious communication and rapport, and the use of the two triangles, everything grows naturally and intelligibly. The truth is that I had only intended to illustrate the two triangles, and particularly the progression from completing the first triangle, step by step, to completing the second, but the therapy then grew of its own accord in such a way as to illustrate a very high proportion of the phenomena likely to be met in practice, and the principles of handling them. The detail of having the therapist inexperienced and under supervision also enabled me to illustrate some of the mistakes that a therapist may make, and how they may be corrected.

I think that this therapy may well repay detailed study, and to assist in this I shall now give a summary of the general principles that it illustrates.

Summary of principles illustrated by 'An Imaginary Therapy'

Phase 1: completion of the triangle of conflict in relation to the girl-friend (O)

Exploring gradually.
Interpretation of the defence.

Asking a question of the patient's unconscious, here about the anxiety.
The patient's unconscious answers the question, supplying not only the anxiety but the hidden feeling as well.
This is an example of 'leap-frogging' in the therapeutic dialogue.

Phase 2: the link with the past (O/P link)

The therapist asks a direct question designed to discover the precipitating factor.
The patient unconsciously asks for an interpretation.
Interpretation of the O/P link.

Phases 3 and 4: resistance and the entry of the transference

The patient shows resistance and the therapist reacts with irritation.
The end of the honeymoon.
Repetition of the nuclear problem in the transference.
Intensification of the nuclear problem by the transference leads to deterioration in relations outside.
The patient himself juxtaposes the transference with the relation with his girlfriend, thus unconsciously asking for an interpretation of the T/O link.
Interpretation of the T/O link.
Response in terms of a new hidden feeling, anger – an example of over-determination.
Interpretation of the T/O link in terms of anger.
Sensing the quality of a silence.
Therapeutic tact: things that can be left unspoken.
Improvement in relations outside in response to work on the transference.

Phase 5: crisis, the T/P link, breakthrough

The therapist's illness, by a coincidence typical of real life, repeats the trauma in a quite unforeseen way.
Interpretation of the triangle of conflict in the transference.
The response is to point directly towards the link with the past (the T/P link).
Interpretation of the T/P link leads to massive de-repression of feelings about the past.
The importance of sharing the patient's grief.
The therapist fails to do this because of her own unresolved feelings.
Working through the grief.
Result: improvement in relations outside.

Phases 6 and 7: the threat of termination, relapse

The therapist suggests cutting down on the frequency of sessions in preparation for termination.
Relapse in relations outside, restoration of resistance.

Interpretation of the triangle of conflict in relation to termination, including both grief and anger, is ineffective – it is necessary to wait until the feelings are more accessible.

Acting out in relation to the girl-friend – the feelings are now accessible.

The therapist misses the transference and wrongly makes the O/P link – an example of a correct but inappropriate interpretation.

Phase 8: over-determination: an earlier trauma

The correct O/T interpretation.

Response: a highly meaningful dream.

Asking for associations to the dream sheds considerable light on its meaning.

Breakthrough of the primitive unconscious impulse, which must be handled carefully.

Interpretation of the impulse in the transference.

Response in terms of an intensification of impulse – again, things that should be left unspoken.

Relations outside again improve in response to work on the transference.

More work on the dream leads to the suspicion of an earlier trauma.

The earlier trauma is reconstructed, but the memory and feelings are not completely recovered.

Final phase: working through termination, together with the T/P link

Return to working through the transference over the issue of termination.

A new kind of interpretation making the T/P link.

This leads to recovery of mixed feelings about the mother which have added to the burden of guilt in connection with her death – yet another example of over-determination.

Termination now proceeds smoothly.

Follow-up

Major improvement in the nuclear problem, but there is still something missing.

The two triangles: general principles

In the above account of an imaginary therapy the two triangles were used in a definite and logical order, as follows:

Since the patient comes complaining of a problem in his current outside life (O), it is natural to start by exploring the nature of the conflict in this area. Thus the first phase, which is completed very quickly, is to interpret the triangle of conflict in relation to this single corner of the *triangle of person*.

The order in which the triangle of conflict is interpreted is also logical, and is important as illustrating a general principle. The progression is from the *defence*, which is what is manifest, through the *anxiety*, to the *hidden feeling*, which is what is being defended against.

There are many reasons why this progression is usually necessary. The most important is that the *hidden feeling* is of course the most disturbing of the corners of the triangle of conflict, and needs to be approached gradually. It is important to weaken the defence to allow the hidden feeling nearer to the surface; this will probably result in an increase of anxiety, which in turn can be interpreted; then, as mentioned above, since the anxiety is often fantasy-based (e.g. that the expression of any kind of anger will result in the total destruction of a close relationship), and the interpretation can imply this, the anxiety is reduced; and finally these interventions result in the hidden feeling becoming close enough to the surface to be interpreted directly.

If this procedure is not observed, and, for instance, the hidden feeling is interpreted at once, the result may be incomprehension (for an example, see above, p. 88), because the connection between the defence and the hidden feeling is too difficult to perceive, or, worse, threatened increase of anxiety followed by an intensification of the defence, with the result that the patient withdraws, or even worse, that the hidden feeling is so difficult to face that the patient becomes very much more disturbed, and in the extreme case may be precipitated into breakdown.

Thus the general procedure is to interpret the defence, the anxiety, and the hidden feeling in that order, in relation to the particular corner of the triangle of person with which the patient opens – usually someone in his current life outside (O). Once the nature of the conflict has been clarified, *and not before*, it is the time to make the link with one of the other corners of the triangle of person. In a therapy in which the transference develops slowly this corner will be the *past* (P), so that the next step is to make the O/P link, to begin to clarify the triangle of conflict in this area, and to show the patient repeatedly that this past conflict is being re-enacted in the present.

As the work proceeds, the *transference* will then gradually intensify. At first this will be largely unconscious, and even if it becomes partly conscious the patient will try to avoid speaking of it. The result will be that it is sensed by the therapist as resistance. This is now a *defence* manifesting itself in the transference, so that the triangle of conflict needs to be interpreted once more, this time in relation to the third corner of the triangle of person (T). In many cases the conflict will be essentially the same as the patient's main problem with people outside (O), which has already been linked with the past (the O/P link); and thus the second side of the triangle of person, the T/O link, is obviously called for and is made quite naturally.

Since the O/P link has already been made, the T/O link will *imply* the T/P link (if T resembles O and O resembles P, then T resembles P), which also can possibly be made quite naturally at this point. It may, however, be better to wait until the transference develops a quality that is more obviously derived from the past. In the imaginary therapy just described this occurred through a coincidence, namely the therapist's illness, and resulted in a major breakthrough.

Although this kind of dramatic breakthrough of uncontrollable feeling does not happen very often in actual therapies, it does happen, and in any case what I have wished to illustrate here is that the moments of real therapeutic progress often occur when the T/P link is interpreted. In fact the main aim of most therapies – certainly those that last for more than a few sessions – is to reach the lower apex of the triangle of conflict, i.e. the *hidden feelings*, in relation to the lower apex of the triangle of person, i.e. *parents or siblings*, but for the most part the only route by which this can be reached effectively is via the *transference* and the T/P link.

Once more I must emphasize that no general rule of this kind should be over-valued or taken too literally. Nevertheless the possibility of making the T/P link should always be sought and should be welcomed when it occurs. In *Toward the validation of dynamic psychotherapy* (1976b) I present statistical evidence suggesting very strongly that those therapies in which this link can be worked through tend to be the most successful.

The reader might now expect some such statement as, 'Once this work on the T/P link has been completed, therapy can be terminated'. As was illustrated by this imaginary therapy, this is usually not true at all. Indeed, at this point *the possibility of termination can be mentioned*, but the patient's reaction then needs to be watched very carefully. Whatever the patient's main problem, *disappointment* and *loss* are likely to be important in his past; and the loss of the therapist – who has provided a unique kind of experience of symbolic love, in the form of real understanding and unconditional acceptance – is likely to revive such feelings with considerable intensity. These now need to be worked through and linked with the past. Only then can termination be considered safe in terms of the patient's future. In many cases, where feelings about loss constitute the main problem, work on the T/P link over the issue of termination may really be the crux of therapy.

Once more it needs to be emphasized that all this is only a rough guide, which may help the therapist to find his way through the maze of the patient's material, but which will certainly be a treacherous guide if followed slavishly. I have several examples of therapies in which termination is not an issue – the patient has received what he wanted and is happy to go out into life and use it, while in the final stages the therapist is frantically making interpretations about termination to which there is no response whatever. Indeed he should try them out, but should abandon them quickly when they appear to be irrelevant (see the Gibson Girl, p. 218, for an example).

Equally, in different therapies, the two triangles may be interpreted in any order. In the example of the Mother of Four, for instance, the opening interpretation in the *consultation* was not merely of the *hidden feeling* in relation to the *therapist*, but made the T/O link explicitly and the T/P link by implication. Equally, in other therapies in which transference arises early, the triangle of conflict needs to be completed in this area at once, and then may be linked first with O and then with P, or first with P and then with O. Sometimes the main issue concerns the *parents* in the patient's *current* life, and there is no one representing O, so that the triangle of conflict will be completed in relation to P and then linked with T, and so on and so on. The whole point of this exposition, however, is that if the therapist understands thoroughly the basic principles underlying these two triangles, and is constantly monitoring rapport, he will know where to go.

The universal technique

As the reader may have recognized, the technique that I have described is much more active than the traditional psychoanalytic technique, in which the therapist is supposed to act as a 'passive sounding board', and may say nothing for long periods at a time. I call it the *Universal Technique,* because I find that, no matter what part of the world a reasonably well-trained therapist comes from, this is most frequently the technique that he instinctively uses. Moreover, the language that he uses is that of everyday human interaction, entirely free from jargon. But above all, what he is doing is actively pursuing the two triangles, using rapport as a guide, instinctively knowing which corner or corners he is seeking, all the time using much of his own personality, which includes eye contact, questions, humour, and his own comments and associations – as always, entirely in the service of the patient. In this chapter I have formalized the principles, but in fact I will have described no more than what every such therapist already does.

11

Three linked themes: aggression, elimination of bodily products and obsessional phenomena

Recapitulation

In previous chapters I have presented a number of case histories in which symptoms could be seen as arising, at least in part, from inhibited resentment, anger, rebellion, hostility, or in other words aggressive feelings. A summary is shown in *Table 2*.

Table 2 Summary of problems of inhibited aggression in previous chapters

Chapter	Page	Patient	Situation arousing anger	Consequences
4	26	Geologist	Demands resulting from his mother's illness	Alternation between (1) neglect, and (2) fantasies of excessive self-sacrifice
5	34	Drama Student	Husband's infidelity	Acute onset of phobic condition
5	35	Adopted Son	Wife's frigidity	Acute onset of phobic condition
5	38	Daughter with a Stroke	Mother's domination	Acute attack resembling her fantasy of having a stroke
7	47	Director's Daughter	Distant father	Phobic anxiety and severe inhibition in relation to men
7	52	Pilot's Wife	Authoritarian father	Severe sexual inhibition, envy of men
8	58	Indian Scientist	Authoritarian father	Inhibited competitiveness
9	75	Falling Social Worker	Indifferent mother	Transference phenomena after break in treatment
9	77	Mother of Four	Mother who used material things as a substitute for love	Severe problems over giving and receiving
9	71	Son in Mourning	Indifferent father	Inability to mourn his father's death

Neurotic conditions of this kind are extremely common, and also, it seems, they respond more readily to treatment than almost any others. Dynamic psychotherapy is of course not the only method of treating them – assertive training, and even hypnosis and exhortation (see Browne, 1964), can also be effective. Nevertheless, dynamic theory, through the triangle of defence, anxiety, and hidden feeling (here aggression), together with the link with the past, often appears to offer a more complete explanation than any other theory of some of the phenomena observed. I shall therefore use the current chapter for the twin purposes of continuing to illustrate the use of the two triangles, while introducing some aspects of psychopathology that in previous chapters have remained as yet unexplored.

It is of course absolutely impossible to cover all aspects of such a vast subject, but each example will contain something new – whether in the situation that produced the aggression, the defences against it, or the means of expressing it.

Here it is important to make two further points. The first is that there are of course many problems of the opposite kind – not inhibited aggressiveness but excessive aggressiveness. Such problems tend to have more primitive roots and will be considered later (see the Cricketer, Refugee Musician, and Foster Son, Chapter 16).

The concept of constructive aggression

The second point is that (*pace* those with extreme pacifist views) aggression and self-assertion are a necessary and useful part of human interaction – and there are kinds of aggression that can be described as *constructive*, because they result in benefit not merely to the individual but to his whole environment as well.

This arises for many related reasons, which may be listed as follows:

(1) In accordance with the principle already mentioned many times, that ways of *avoiding* feeling often include a way of *expressing* the feeling as well, many ways of avoiding aggression are in themselves extremely aggressive – of which one of the best everyday examples is 'getting into a sulk' instead of becoming openly angry. Here the other person is indirectly invited to approach and restore the situation, and is consistently rejected when he or she tries to do so. There is a more chronic form of this, in which the individual is just unable to express love, an example of which was given in the imaginary therapy described in Chapter 10.

(2) In consequence, ways of avoiding and yet expressing aggression are often extremely destructive both to the individual and to his environment, since they have many consequences that just go on for ever, until the true expression of the original feelings can be reached. These consequences include permanent loss of spontaneity, creativeness, and efficiency, the development of symptoms such as phobias through which other people's lives are controlled and restricted, sexual symptoms such as impotence and frigidity, which result in the permanent stunting of the emotional life of the marital partner, and, in general, vicious circles set up with other people leading to the permanent poisoning of relationships.

(3) The almost universal fear on which these inhibitions are based is that the open expression of aggressive feelings will inevitably lead to disastrous consequences, such as ultimate rejection or the destruction of relationships. The truth is, of course, that it is the *failure* to express them that usually leads in the end to the same disastrous consequences. What such people do not realize, and need to be taught by experience, is that there are 'clean', non-destructive ways of being aggressive, which have the effect not only of freeing the individual, getting him what he wants, and earning respect, but of improving relationships all round, and hence of greatly benefiting his environment as well.

(4) It seems to be true that these considerations often apply in the sexual sphere, where over-considerate and tentative love-making – on the part of the man especially – has only too often resulted in the partner 'unaccountably' turning away to someone else.

(5) Therefore, no matter whether the problem is of *inhibited* or *excessive* aggressiveness, and no matter what the form of treatment, the aim is always that the patient should reach the same end point: a state of enlightened self-interest through the ability to express *effective anger or aggression* and *constructive self-assertion*. In our follow-up work on the results of psychotherapy, this is a criterion laid down for almost every patient.

There will be several examples in the following detailed case histories, but before that it is worth quoting a brief example that illustrates the concept in a particularly striking way.

The discovery of constructive self-assertion: The Almoner

This was a young woman of 22 who came to treatment complaining of mild depressive symptoms. Behind this lay a deeply ingrained pattern of being on her best behaviour and keeping everything 'nice'. There were in fact severe tensions in her home, which she admitted, but she expressed no anger against either of her parents, and in her projection test, whenever there was any possibility of aggression or resentment, she changed the story in such a way as to eliminate it.

One of the main foci of therapy was her hidden aggressive feelings against her parents, linked with the transference to the male therapist wherever possible. This bore fruit, and in therapy she rapidly became able to criticize her parents quite forcefully. The climax came when she visited them one week-end, had her first row with them since her early 'teens, and walked out. Therapy (11 sessions) was terminated soon afterwards.

Four months later the therapist received a letter from her father, from which the following is a condensed quotation:

'This is a note to thank you most sincerely for the help you have given my daughter. . . . My wife and I have seen her most week-ends. She is much more relaxed and cheerful and able to cope with her life very much better than when she first came to you.'

At 6-month follow-up she reported that not only was she now getting on much better with her parents, but *they were getting on much better with each other*. Thus her act of self-assertion seems to have cleared the air all round. This is an example of constructive aggression *par excellence*.

At 5-year follow-up it was perhaps true that she still had some residual traces of difficulty in demanding her rights, but otherwise she was living an essentially happy and normal life as a wife and mother. For full details see Malan (1976a), pp. 92 – 100.

A second example, illustrating a number of different points, is as follows.

The Maintenance Man and the meaning of a urinary phobia

The patient was a married man of 39, with little education but a considerable capacity for insight, who came to treatment because of panic attacks of acute onset five weeks previously. The immediate precipitating factor seemed to be that he had had a motorbike and sidecar, of which he was very proud, and his wife had made him give it up because she was afraid of travelling in it.

Exactly why he had married this particular woman would seem on purely common-sense grounds to be utterly mysterious. Before she consented to marry him she had made him promise that he wouldn't make many sexual demands on her, and she now allows him intercourse once a month or less. She is dominating and makes all the decisions.

The only possible explanation seems to be that he feels guilty about sexual feelings and needs his wife to keep them under control. There seems to be some relation between her and his mother, in the sense that his mother was also dominating and disgusted by sex. (This therefore seems to be an example of the *compulsion to repeat*, discussed more fully below – see p. 133). His father was promiscuous and had left his mother when he was 13.

In the third session there emerged a second event which seemed to have contributed to the precipitation of his symptoms. His wife meets a number of wealthy men, who own cars, at her work. The patient has always had an ambition to possess a car, but feels he cannot afford one. Two days before the onset of his symptoms his wife had brought two of these men home, apparently in order to show him he need not be jealous.

It is now worthwhile to try and formulate a hypothesis about the onset of his symptoms. The following facts in the history may be put together:

(1) His mother was disgusted by sex,
(2) He has married a woman who he knew in advance would ration his sexuality,
(3) He is very proud of his motorbike and would like to own a car,
(4) His wife has contact with men who own cars, and
(5) His wife made him give up his motorbike.

These facts would be expected to lead to a complex set of interlocking conflicts: guilt about sex, use of his wife to help control his sexuality, resentment about his wife's domination and his lack of sexual satisfaction, feelings of inferiority as a man, strivings towards manhood expressed in his attitude to cars and his motorbike, intense resentment and an increased sense of inferiority when his wife takes away his motorbike – an act of symbolic emasculation – but associates with men who have cars.

In Session 4 the (male) therapist made an interpretation of part of these feelings, mentioning his need to suppress his anger with his mother for not allowing him to be a sexual man (defence and hidden feeling), making the parallel with his wife (the P/O link), and, mincing no words, using theoretical knowledge of Oedipal feelings to interpret the motorbike as standing for his penis. The patient responded by revealing that ever since he was a child he had suffered from difficulty in travelling because of the *fear that he would have to urinate.*

Elimination of bodily products

We may now introduce a digression on the subject of the elimination of bodily products from the anal and urethral orifices. It is an empirical fact, that is quite incontrovertible, that in some people these processes take on a significance apparently out of all proportion to their simple function of expelling unwanted matter from the body. It is very difficult to know exactly why this should be so, but as far as I can make out there are at least two important roots. The first is some kind of primitive equation between the *inside of the body* and *feelings*, so that elimination of physical matter becomes equated with the expression of feeling. The second is that whereas a human infant is completely free to urinate and defecate at any time and place, there comes a point at which he has to give up this freedom. In our society this process is often – and 50 years ago was almost always – strongly reinforced with approval and disapproval, reward and punishment, by the parents. Thus the struggle of toilet training may come to represent the whole issue of *freedom versus restraint*; and incontinence which results in *making a mess* may become a way of expressing anger and rebellion. If in turn there is a later struggle over the right to express sexual feelings, then this may reawaken the earlier struggle, and the two may become associated.

The Maintenance Man (contd)

I shall now pick out from a complex therapy the material and interpretations relevant to these themes.

The therapist, who of course was fully aware of the above theoretical background, made the interpretation that quite possibly the patient's anxiety about urination symbolized a *fear of loss of control*, and that this probably included loss of control of sexual feelings (an interpretation of the anxiety and the impulse).

In Session 5, the patient spoke of being ill in terms of 'keeping things in' or 'letting them out', which the therapist linked with the patient's urinary anxieties.

In Session 6, he reported that his wife had refused him intercourse, and that he had been silent afterwards and unable to do anything about it. The therapist made an interpretation completing the triangle of conflict and making the O/P link: that he had to be a good boy (defence) for his wife, as for his mother (O/P link) because he was afraid of losing control (anxiety) of his rage (impulse) if he *let himself go.*

In Session 7 the patient brought out for the first time *impulses to defy authority*, e.g. how during the War he went to brothels and never told his wife, and a long-standing fantasy of having sex with a coloured woman.

In Session 11 the patient remarked that he was doing things in his own time instead of when his wife told him to. The therapist linked this first with the patient's rebellion against his wife's control of the sexual situation, and then with the patient's impulse to urinate when he wasn't supposed to, suggesting that this was a sort of defiance. Though this may seem at first sight to be a far-fetched interpretation, the patient said immediately that it had struck him that nowadays it is mostly when he is with his wife that he gets this symptom (as, one may speculate, as a child, it was mostly when he was with his mother).

In Session 12 it emerged that three times recently he had had *nocturnal emissions* when there were clean sheets on the bed. Thus, unconsciously, he might possibly be employing his sexual function to *make a mess* and make his wife clean up after him, which the therapist interpreted.

In Session 13 he reported that whereas he used to have a recurring dream of panic at *being unable to urinate*, after the previous session he had had a dream in which he was 'urinating to his heart's content', so much so that he couldn't stop, and had woken up afraid that he was wetting the bed. This dream would seem to offer confirmation of a number of previous interpretations: the hidden pleasure in urinating, the fear of loss of control, and the wish to make a mess.

In Session 16 the patient himself seemed to give confirmation of the parallel between elimination and 'letting go', when he said that he never knew what he was going to say before he came, but that it just 'poured out of him'.

In Session 23 he offered confirmation of *ejaculation* as a way of making a mess, when he said that twice recently he had woken up to find himself on top of his wife and ejaculating, and had had to apologize in the morning. The therapist asked him why he had to apologize, to which he said that he felt he was messing her up. He then went on to say that he felt that deep down she wanted sex as much as he did, and that he was depriving her by not giving it to her.

The climax of therapy came in Sessions 25 and 27. In Session 25 the patient reported with considerable anger that his wife would start lovemaking with such remarks as, 'Come on, get it over with, I suppose you want to perform now', and similar romantic endearments. The therapist suggested that behind this lay a hidden wish that he should dominate her.

In Session 27, the patient reported that to his own great surprise he had really blown his top with his wife last night. She had told him off for taking some money from the housekeeping that he was going to return anyway, and he had banged the table and shouted at her to stop treating him as a child. During the course of this he said that the thought had crossed his mind that he could come along and discuss it with the therapist the next day. The therapist therefore, perhaps insensitively, tried to make a link with the patient's pattern of compliance, saying that he had the row in order to do what was expected of him. At this the patient picked up his newspaper and shook it at the therapist, banged the chair with the point of his finger, and said that the therapist was trying to take this away from him now – he hadn't done it for the therapist but had really got wild with his wife and had done it for himself. Thus his moment of constructive self-assertion with his wife was followed by a similar moment with the therapist.

Termination came smoothly after 30 sessions.

At 4-year follow-up, the situation was complicated. His severe panic attacks had disappeared, but he still had some urinary symptoms. At one time these consisted of hesitancy, but now this has been replaced by some degree of precipitancy (he has had a cystoscopy and been told that there is nothing physically wrong). He and his wife seem to have reached a working compromise: where the issue is under *his* control, he takes his own decisions, if necessary against her wishes. Where it is under *her* control he states his position firmly and is satisfied even if he doesn't get his own way. The sexual situation has varied: soon after the end of therapy a major change occurred in his wife, and their sexual relationship became exciting, vigorous, and frequent. There has now been some relapse from this position. The patient said that he was determined not to get hurt by being rejected sexually, but he senses when she is willing and then it is enjoyable.

He bought a *car* against his wife's wishes, and now he drives her all over the place, much to her enjoyment. He was very proud of this.

For full details see *Toward the validation of dynamic psychotherapy* (Malan, 1976b).

Obsessional anxiety and fear of aggression: The Pesticide Chemist

In the Maintenance Man the anxiety, psychiatrically speaking, was essentially phobic; in the next case the anxiety was obsessional.

A married man of 31 was brought to therapy by a sudden uncontrollable outburst of rage – something apparently quite foreign to his nature. His job was as an industrial chemist, developing pesticides.

At consultation (Session 1) this event was reconstructed, as follows:

(1) He has always been perfectionist and over-conscientious at work. The assistants who work under him need a lot of supervision, and he finds it difficult to keep an eye on them. He worries that the materials he develops may not have been tested properly, and that this may result in a large claim against his firm. He is not able to relax at home because thoughts about work keep occupying him. He can never keep things tidy, though he tries very hard.

(2) He has been upset about the way his boss has not shown appreciation of his work and has been critical of small things instead.

(3) He has always suffered from premature ejaculation. In recent months this has been worse and he has been unable to satisfy his wife.

(4) It is clear that he had been mildly depressed during the past few months, and one morning he went to his doctor complaining of loss of energy. He returned home and his wife suggested that he might stay at home for the day. (He said that it had been a 'good-humoured joke' between him and his wife that his work is more important to him that his home – and in fact he had been late home the night before, which had annoyed her.) Despite his wife's remark he started off for work. His wife said that in

that case perhaps she might get on with treating the house for woodworm. (He had been doing this slowly over the last year. The first job he did wasn't satisfactory and had caused some staining.) This remark of his wife's enraged him. He got out of control and tipped a gallon of anti-woodworm solution down the sink – splashing a good deal of it over the floor. When his wife tried to intervene, he hit her. He then cried for three hours.

The patient was the elder of two children. His father was a travelling salesman who worked very hard, spent most of his time away and saw very little of the family. The patient remembers no warmth from him. The mother, on the other hand, was described as warm and kind.

During and after the consultation, some of the issues in the patient's life could be seen, but it certainly was not possible to understand the origins of his outburst completely, let alone why it was of such intensity. It is clear that his perfectionism would make him particularly sensitive to criticism; at consultation he agreed that he had taken his wife's offer to do the work as a criticism of the way he had done it himself; there is clearly considerable tension between him and her over the amount of time he gives to her; but exactly how these issues were linked, if at all, it was impossible to see.

In the first therapeutic session, with an experienced male psychologist, the patient started reviewing the present crisis. He now changed the emphasis and said that he thought it had to do with the fact that he was doing his best at *work* and his *boss* had been criticizing him quite unjustly. This statement may seem at first to deepen the mystery, since the outburst had been not against his boss but against his wife. In fact, however, it does offer important clarification, because it suggests that the central theme is *trying hard and yet being criticized*, which appears to be what had happened with his wife as well.

This link between the boss and the wife may make us reconsider the whole sequence of events, introducing in addition an important digression on the subject of *obsessional symptoms*.

This patient shows three related obsessional symptoms: (1) perfectionism, which he finds it difficult to maintain, e.g. in relation to the assistants working under him; (2) a need to keep things tidy, which he also cannot maintain; and (3) obsessional anxiety, in the form of preoccupation with the fear that he may not have done his work properly and this may result in a large claim against his firm.

There runs through these three symptoms the theme of *precariously keeping something at bay*. Once more we may ask, do we dismiss phenomena of this kind as something mysterious for which there is no point in looking for an explanation; or do we take them seriously, and try to explain them in terms of intelligible human anxieties? If the latter, then there is not much difficulty in bringing forward a piece of evidence that is staring us in the face, namely that when his control did finally break down, the result was an intense outburst of rage. Could it be that all three of these obsessional symptoms are symbolic ways of *controlling angry feelings*?

This hypothesis in fact makes some additional sense of the third of his symptoms. The symptom of having to perform some action in case harm comes to someone is a very common manifestation of obsessive-compulsive neurosis.

There is a standard psychodynamic explanation for this, namely that the compulsive action is a symbolic way of controlling, or undoing, a *wish* that harm should come to someone – once this formulation is made, the compulsive action begins to make complete sense. In many cases the action itself is quite irrational; but in the present case it is perfectly rational, namely that he must test his products properly to prevent harm from coming to his firm – the only part that is irrational being the intensity of his preoccupation with anxiety about this. The patient has told us by implication that he is angry with his boss, so that this preoccupation now makes sense if we translate it as a desperate wish to prevent himself from unwittingly expressing his angry feelings against the firm, and thus causing a disaster to them – and, of course, to himself as well. The whole can now be formulated in terms of the triangle of conflict: the *defence* is symbolic control, while the *anxiety* is his fear of the harm he may do if he expresses the *hidden feeling*, which is anger.

What is he angry about? This is not clear, although an element in it that applies both to the boss and his wife is *being criticized*.

How did all this originate? Again this is not clear. There is no evidence whatsoever that he is angry with his *mother*, but on the other hand he could have reason to be angry with his *father*, who seems to have neglected the family. The fact that this neglect was all in the interests of supporting them would only make the conflict more difficult.

Finally, we may note the fact that the particular way in which he expressed his anger during his outburst resulted in his *making a mess*. This may of course be quite incidental, but on the other hand it might represent a childhood way of expressing anger, for which there is strong evidence in other patients (see the Maintenance Man just described), and which – at any rate according to psychoanalytic tradition – appears to be a particularly common feature in obsessionals.

After this digression we may consider what is the appropriate course of action now that the patient has made the link between his outburst and criticism by the boss. According to the standard principles described in Chapter 10 (see pp. 102ff.), since the patient has started speaking about the boss, the natural procedure would be to start by trying to clarify the triangle of conflict in relation to the boss. However, this is an illustration of how each moment of therapy needs to be considered on its merits and treated with complete flexibility: since the conflict with the boss appears to be essentially the same as the conflict with his wife, and since the crisis occurred in relation to the wife and not the boss, it might well be better to make the link with the wife at once (an O_1/O_2 link); and, having done this, to clarify the triangle of conflict in relation to both these people together.

The style of the present therapist, however, did not consist of this gradual approach, but an attempt to go to the heart of the matter as soon as possible. This is something that I would strongly discourage in beginners, since it often results in interpretations made on guesswork and book knowledge, without the use of rapport as a check, and rapid loss of contact with the patient's feelings. If I were ever asked – which of course is unlikely – I would not really recommend it to experienced therapists either. No one, however experienced, can be sufficiently sure of what he is saying not to need constant feedback from the patient. However, it is acceptable if, as here, the interpretations appear to be both appropriate and essentially correct.

What the therapist did in fact was to make the link at once, not with the wife, but with the *father* (the O/P link), to ignore the defence altogether, only to hint at the anxiety, and to go straight for the hidden feeling: that there was a parallel between the boss and the father, 'with whom it was impossible to be angry'. The patient agreed that it was impossible to be angry with his father – 'he was never there as a father, but it would have been totally unjust to be angry with him because he was doing so much for them all. Anyhow, the boss has now stopped being critical, and this has put everything right'. The therapist ignored this defensive move and now made the link with the wife. The patient agreed with this also, saying that his wife is critical of him because he puts more energy into his work than his family.

Towards the end of the session the therapist offered the patient once weekly therapy, but the patient now said that he felt he could reorganize his life without therapy in such a way as to improve the situation. On closer questioning, however, it now appeared that what he was going to do would have the result of taking him away from home more than ever, and the therapist forcefully pointed this out. There was also an obvious parallel between the way in which the patient was treating his family now, and how his father had treated his own family in the past, which the therapist pointed out, although exactly what this meant did not seem to be clear. The patient went away saying he would think about the situation and decide what to do.

The result was that the patient arrived for Session 3 having decided that 'there was no point in coming for treatment'. During the course of most of the session the therapist made a series of forceful interpretations pointing out the patient's life problem and completing the triangle of conflict over and over again. Interestingly, these interpretations (as recorded by the therapist, at any rate) were largely 'undirected', though the patient's wife was mentioned in passing: 'I interpreted his fear of treatment in terms of the frightening things that might be discovered, that the recent outburst had been a great shock to him, and he was really quite frightened of what it might mean. I said that I thought he had come to realize that everything was not really all right even before the outburst, and that his fear of treatment was that things might be revealed that he might not be able to cope with, and that he did not want to know about'. All this is essentially an interpretation of the *anxiety*. Now the defence: 'I said that he had difficulty in knowing about his feelings, and that he had based his adjustment in life on control of feelings, that he had been severely shaken by his sudden outburst of feeling, which made him aware for the first time of a part of himself that he had not known existed, that what he was doing now was saying that he would deal with this part by clamping down on it even tighter than before. I said that his technique of keeping his feelings under strict control was acting as an impediment in his marriage, and I put it to him that although he might feel that his "recovery" was satisfactory to himself, would it be satisfactory to his wife?' Now the hidden feeling: 'I said also that the feelings that he was so terrified of were strongly aggressive feelings, and that they were to do with the part of him that wanted to let go all his controls and make a mess.'

The result of this was a volte-face. The patient now said he wanted to come into treatment, and he was grateful that his decision had been changed. However, he carefully prepared his line of retreat by adding the qualifying phrase, 'until we decide to discontinue'.

There is a very interesting phenomenon in psychotherapy which I have nicknamed Malan's Law. This is that where, as here, the therapist gets considerably ahead of the patient's emotional capacity, the latter may respond at the time, but will return for the next session in a state of resistance that is penetrated only with difficulty, if at all. When the therapist is recording sessions from memory, this is reflected in the amount he writes – the length of the record reaches a peak at the 'good' session, and shows a marked fall in the next session. As long as the therapist is not too far ahead, there is no evidence that this matters, since the patient usually recovers in the next session but one. (In this particular case the length of the records, measured in lines of type, was: Session 3, 48 lines; Session 4, 32 lines, Session 5, 52 lines – a ratio of 1 : 0.67 : 1.08.)

In accordance with this law, the patient spent Session 4 in a state of passive resistance – 'You give me a lead and I will follow'. I hope this excellent therapist will not mind if I say that the interpretations that he made in terms of dependence were largely inappropriate.

This did not matter, since major communication was resumed in Session 5. The patient now said that, if he had understood the therapist correctly, he had made a conscious attempt at putting aside childish feelings and growing up, and that this was the cause of his trouble. He didn't agree – everybody has to grow up and learn to be responsible and rational.

The therapist again ignored the defence and went for the hidden feeling, saying that the patient was angry with him for criticizing his best efforts, which is what the boss had done (T/O link). The patient went on to speak of the situation at work, where he had been criticized by the boss for *ignoring long-term projects* and paying too much attention to the *immediate needs of customers*.

The therapist took this as a communication in the transference and in addition introduced a crucial concept that later made sense of the whole situation, namely that of the *demands* that the patient felt were being made on him. He said that the patient felt impossible demands were being made on him in therapy, 'to achieve long-term aims in terms of changes in his whole way of life, whereas he has the task of coping with the immediate situation of keeping his anger under control. I related this to his childhood feeling that it was demanded of him to suppress his feelings and grow up.'

This interpretation of the T/P link (where P stands for 'past', since parents were not actually mentioned) produced an important response in terms of a long description of the patient's childhood and adolescence, from which it became clear that he had had hardly any home life. His father was constantly away, and the patient involved himself in activities away from home seven nights a week, where in fact he found a substitute father who took him under his wing. This meant that he did not miss his father, who of course did really love him and was doing everything for the best. At this point the therapist made a major interpretation of *defence* and *hidden feeling* in relation to the father, *completing the triangle of person* by making the links with the boss and the *transference* – and, though the *wife* was not mentioned, making sense at last in ordinary human terms of the intensity of his outburst: 'I interpreted his denial (defence) of his anger and despair (hidden feeling) at being unloved by his father – his unconscious wish to rebel and express his anger – *that it is the last straw when his efforts to control this become themselves the subject of criticism* – this linked with the work situation and also with the transference'.

Although in my view this was a brilliant interpretation, as usual the patient only made a limited response, saying he could see the relevance of this now but he was not aware of such feelings in his childhood.

Again we may review the situation reached at this point. In fact every clue that is needed is now present. The crucial word, once more, is *demands*. What has been happening is that the patient has been desperately trying to meet the demands of everyone around him, while finding himself unable to make any demands on his own behalf. His compulsion to satisfy everyone else is being used as a defence against becoming aware both of his own needs and his anger that they are not being satisfied. The crisis occurs when, as the therapist said, this defence itself becomes the object of criticism; which of course occurs when *the demands from one area get into conflict with the demands from another*. Thus, in the present session, the boss complains that *his* demand for long-term projects is not being met because the patient is meeting the short-term demands *of customers*, and in the original crisis, the wife's demand that he should stay at home and meet *her need* for his company conflicts with the demand that he should *go to work*. When his wife now by implication criticizes the unsatisfactory way in which he had met the demands to maintain the upkeep of his home, the emotional boiler finally bursts in a colossal explosion.

In the heat of therapy no one can be expected to see all this as clearly as it has been formulated above, but it was seen clearly enough to get home to the patient. We may now give the essence of the rest of therapy largely in a series of quotations. The first is from Session 9: 'The patient said that the main thing is that he has come to feel that he has got to give up the attempt to meet all the demands at work. He will just have to explain that he has human limitations, and he will have to be given extra staff, or some work must be taken away from his department. He went on to talk about his growing awareness of the futility of trying to please everybody.'

In Session 11 the patient made the clearest possible statement of the discovery of constructive self-assertion: 'He said that the treatment must be having a good effect. He has become aware of feelings that he hadn't understood – of resentment – and he finds he is becoming indulgent towards himself and increasingly able to be angry when unreasonable demands are made on him. He has been spontaneously angry at work and has found that it achieves good results. It is not that he is making a deliberate attempt to be angry, but that it just seems to happen and only in retrospect does he see what he is doing.' He then made the rather strange statement that he felt angry about coming today – the anger is not with the therapist but is due to the fact that 'he has got what he wants from treatment and feels he needn't come any more'.

At this point the therapist drew his attention to the other area where changes were needed, namely the relationship with his wife. The patient agreed, and the main theme of the rest of the session consisted of his complaints about not getting enough from her, ending up with the feeling that he must make the best of it and seek satisfactions elsewhere – perhaps in his work. Now, with hindsight, one can see yet another strand that led to his outburst: his work had represented for him not only another demand, but a way of attaining alternative satisfaction, because he had been dissatisfied in his marriage. No wonder, therefore, that he exploded when his wife first 'demanded' that he should stay with her, and then by implication criticized what he had been doing at home. This was not really seen at the time, but nevertheless the therapist now made another major interpretation, making sense of the obscure communication about anger with therapy, and completing both triangles: 'I interpreted the similarity between his description of the marriage situation and his description of his childhood feelings (the O/P link) – that he must be grateful for what he has got, be uncomplaining, cut his losses, and look elsewhere for something to fill the gaps (defence) – the same happening here (O/P/T link), he must be grateful for what he has got from me and be uncomplaining about the very real dissatisfactions that still remain – his need to cut his losses and retreat, for fear (anxiety) that his demands, if they were to be expressed, would result in an aggressive, soiling attack (hidden feeling) upon the person to whom he feels gratitude.' (This interpretation of the 'making a mess' component in the aggressive feelings had been made on a number of occasions. There was never any direct response to it, and its significance remains uncertain.) The patient became very thoughtful, saying the therapist was right, but there wasn't anything he could do because his wife's capacity to give to him was limited. The therapist said that the patient himself contributed to the limited relation with his wife and the reason was his fear of his own demands.

In the next session (No. 12), the patient reported that when he got home after the last session he had had a showdown with his wife about her lack of enthusiasm for sex. She turned on him, saying 'there's more to marriage than sex', and the discussion degenerated into an argument. They were both left angry, and he felt the result had been a catastrophe. Two days later, however, she herself initiated love-making, and it was entirely satisfactory to both of them.

Thus the patient, in two separate areas, had discovered for himself the value of constructive self-assertion.

In Session 14, he announced his decision to stop coming.

'Koch's postulates' in psychodynamics

Here a further digression is worthwhile. One may ask, how is it possible to judge that a given explanation for a particular symptom is correct? The answer can be formulated in terms of four conditions, similar to 'Koch's postulates' by which one can judge whether a given disease is caused by a particular bacterium. These are as follows:

(1) That events in the patient's life, and particularly precipitating factors, suggest the nature of the conflict underlying the symptom.
(2) That a detailed mechanism can be clearly formulated whereby the symptom represents or expresses the conflict.
(3) That interpretation of this mechanism to the patient brings the conflict clearly into consciousness.

And finally, the most important:

(4) That this results in the disappearance of the symptom.

Now it is unfortunately true that often some, but not all, of these conditions are fulfilled. In the case of the Drama Student, for instance (see p. 34), the symptom of fear of travelling was precipitated by her husband's infidelity;

when the patient discovered this link she was able to talk the situation over with her husband, and the result was that the symptom disappeared; but the way in which fear of travelling resulted from her conflict never became clear. In other words, conditions (1), (3), and (4) were fulfilled, but condition (2) was not.

In the case of obsessional symptoms, and particularly obsessional rituals, it is often condition (4) that is not fulfilled – in other words everything becomes intelligible, and the patient becomes conscious of the conflict, but therapeutic results do not ensue. It is apparently true, for instance, that no authenticated case of an obsessional hand-washer being cured by psychoanalytic treatment has ever come to light. Correspondingly, as far as learning theory and behaviour therapy are concerned, condition (4) is often fulfilled, i.e. the symptom improves, but condition (2), namely the formulation of an adequate explanation for the symptom, is not. These facts would seem to imply that there is something missing from both approaches, and it is high time the two got together and tried to make a formulation that really *is* complete, instead of one that each likes to pretend is complete.

In the case of the Pesticide Chemist's compulsiveness and obsessional preoccupations, however, all four conditions were as nearly fulfilled as could reasonably be expected:

(1) The lack of a father in the patient's childhood, with the consequent implied demand that he should grow up without a father's support, is likely to have set up a conflict in him about whether he should express his anger and make demands on his own behalf, or control his anger and meet the demands of his environment.

(2) The particular solution of this conflict that he found provides an example of two defences: symbolic control in the form of perfectionism and obsessional tidiness, and over-compensation in the form of a compulsion to meet everyone else's demands. However, the 'return of the repressed' occurs both in the breakdown of the obsessional tidiness, and in the preoccupation with anxiety that his over-conscientiousness will fail and he will thus unwittingly do harm to the firm. In addition, this compulsive need to meet everyone's demands has three consequences: (a) he becomes increasingly angry that his own needs are not being met; (b) the demands of one area start conflicting with the demands of another; and (c) he is threatened with an eruption of accumulated anger when, as the therapist said in Session 5, his desperate attempts to meet everyone's demands themselves become the object of criticism. The final breakdown of all this explains his outburst of rage and its intensity.

(3) Interpretation of these mechanisms, though not put as clearly as hindsight now makes possible, leads to the patient's realization of the defence and the hidden feeling: that is he realizes 'the futility of trying to please everybody' (Session 9), and becomes aware of 'feelings that he hadn't understood, of resentment', and he now finds 'he is becoming increasingly indulgent towards himself and increasingly angry when unreasonable demands are made on him' (Session 11).

(4) Finally, not only do the hidden feelings emerge, but the obsessional symptoms disappear. This, which has not been mentioned so far, was shown at two-month follow-up: the quality and quantity of his work have

improved, he can shift from one job to another without obsessional worries, and his fear of making costly mistakes seems to be no more than normal. This position was maintained at a follow-up of nearly 4 years.

It should be added that the relation with his wife also improved at first, though there was later some degree of relapse.

The meaning of obsessional symptoms

The features that these two patients, the Maintenance Man and the Pesticide Chemist, have in common are as follows: (1) underlying problems of aggression giving rise to symptoms; (2) evidence that some of the unconscious aggressive impulses were concerned with making a mess; (3) the emergence of the aggressive feelings into consciousness; (4) the constructive use of aggressive feelings in the patient's outside life; and (5) the disappearance of the symptoms.

Of course these two examples only scratch the surface of problems of aggression and the various possible meanings of phobic and obsessional symptoms. In particular, I would not wish to give the narrow impression that obsessional symptoms are always a defence against aggressive feelings; or the even narrower impression that these aggressive feelings always contain a component of making a mess. I think the truth is that obsessional symptoms can be a defence against any kind of disturbing conflict – including sexual or Oedipal anxieties, and more primitive, psychotic anxieties.

In Chapter 8 I quoted the case of the Articled Accountant who became preoccupied with the fear of making small mistakes at work when a girl showed some interest in him. In this case the anxiety was almost certainly Oedipal in origin.

The following example, where the hidden feelings under control were sexual, is taken from the Magistrate's Daughter, a girl of 21 complaining of sexual inhibition, reported in greater detail in Malan (1976a) (see pp. 277–289).

In Session 5 (with a male therapist) she spoke of 'hating untidiness' and 'having to get everything done'. The therapist gave the standard interpretation of this kind of obsessional phenomenon as her need to *have everything under control*. He had inadvertently left the phone switched on in the room, and when it rang he moved quickly to switch it off. She said, 'You're jumpy too', and the therapist now interpreted the obsessional defence in the transference, speaking of her need to keep emotions between her and him tidy and controlled. At the end of the session she said that if her sexual feelings were liberated she'd be afraid that as she went out of the session she'd go to bed with any man she sees, thus entirely confirming her fear of loss of control.

One of the best ways of reaching insight into the inner mechanisms involved in neurotic symptoms occurs when such symptoms appear transitorily during the course of a therapeutic session. The following two examples are taken from the patient mentioned in Chapter 8 (see p. 63), who could not touch his mother to comfort her at his father's funeral. They illustrate the mobilization of obsessional defences when the therapist momentarily tries to go too fast.

In Session 2, the patient began speaking of another young man at work who was very competitive. The two of them were always competing with each other and 'thank God he was soon leaving the office'. It was difficult to have two such people in the same office – it just automatically led to a clash.

Here the theme of *getting rid of someone with whom the patient was in conflict and competition* was so clear that the (female) therapist tried to link this with the impulse to get rid of his father, with whom the patient had had a good deal of conflict in his 'teens. She said that to 'be an individual' meant to get into word battles with people, to get into fights with his father about having long hair, to get into competition at work, and it seemed that the solution to the disagreement was that *someone had to go*. The patient at first could not take this interpretation in, and when he did, he immediately veered off into saying *how pedantic* he was, and how he always *had to get everything right*.

In Session 4 he spoke about trying to make people, especially his GP, into father figures from whom he sought reassurance about his anxieties. The therapist reminded him of how he had said previously that he always developed very strong feelings towards people to whom he talked about his father, and she wondered whether he was worried about strong feelings he might develop towards her. Her account continues 'This led him into one of his roundabout discussions with himself about what he really felt about his GP. Was he really that special to him, would he really be upset if he died? Wasn't he really feeling the same things about his GP that he'd feel about anyone, etc., etc.? I said that it seemed to be difficult for him to get back to talking about the deep and very moving feelings that he had had at the end of the last session (where he had spoken of his intense wish to hug his father the night before he died). He said that the main reason was because he could feel an anxiety attack beginning ...'

In this first example the attempt to confront him with his wish to get rid of a rival, and to link this with the father, was obviously too much for him and mobilized a defence involving *being pedantic*. In the second example the confrontation with feelings about his woman therapist in the context of speaking about his father clearly brought anxiety to the surface. Subsequent events are then both exceedingly clear and extraordinarily interesting:

(1) He tries to control his anxiety by the defence of *obsessional rumination*.
(2) The content of his rumination consists of what he would feel about the death of his GP – here clearly representing his father – a subject which is obviously highly anxiety-laden.
(3) The rumination (which links with being pedantic) serves the purpose of *ironing out any spontaneous feeling* from the subject that he is considering – a kind of deliberate attempt not to see the wood for the trees (concentrating on the trees so as to prevent himself from seeing the wood).
(4) The therapist makes an interpretation that emphasizes the hidden feeling while hinting at the defence and the anxiety ('difficult for him to get back to the intense feelings', etc.).
(5) The patient's defence breaks down and he now admits to being on the brink of an anxiety attack.

It was in the next session that the patient finally spoke of his feelings about his mother at his father's funeral.

Thus in this patient, as in the Articled Accountant, obsessional phenomena were clearly being used as a defence against Oedipal conflicts.

In the next chapter we leave aside obsessional phenomena and consider further sources of aggression and further defences against it.

12

Three more linked themes: aggression arising from sibling rivalry; passivity and masochism; and the compulsion to repeat

In this chapter I consider four patients who are linked with each other in a somewhat complicated way. The first three suffered from *unconscious hostility towards siblings*, against which the second and third patients employed a number of passive *defences* resulting in their being ill-used and exploited. Thus these defences link with the obscure phenomenon of *masochism*, which is shown overtly by the third patient. Finally, the deliberate seeking of situations of suffering links with the even more obscure phenomenon of the *compulsion to repeat*, which is shown in the clearest possible way by the fourth patient. The evidence provided by the last three patients may possibly go some way towards making these two phenomena intelligible.

The descriptions of the first, third, and fourth of these patients have been taken from the much fuller accounts given in *Psychodynamics, training, and outcome* (Malan and Osimo, 1992).

Sibling rivalry

The book mentioned above consists largely of a description of the therapies of a series of patients treated with brief psychotherapy by trainees. Of these patients, nearly a quarter suffered from disturbances caused by guilt-laden jealousy and hostility directed towards a younger sibling – thus illustrating the importance of problems of this kind, which sometimes tends to be obscured by the importance of the relation with parents.

The Betrayed Son

This was a married man aged 25 whose main complaint consisted of phobic and hypochondriacal anxiety. He had one child, a boy, and his wife was now pregnant, near term, for the second time. The therapist was a male trainee psychologist.

In Session 3 the patient announced that the new baby had been born, but he entirely avoided expressing any feelings about this or even mentioning whether it was a boy or a girl. He went on to speak of intense competition over material things with a male colleague who had just lost a baby due at about the same time. The therapist suggested that rivalry might go deeper than material things, and that maybe he 'wanted to have a better baby than the other chap'. The patient responded with a highly positive unconscious communication to this acknowledgement of his feelings of rivalry with another man. He spoke of a long-standing fantasy of a house with two rooms, one of which was only for show while in the other he could really be himself. *He would only allow people into the second room when he knew them very well.* This was almost certainly a reference to warm feelings for the therapist, who had understood him.

Associating to the theme of rooms, the patient went on to speak of a time when he came back from holiday and *found his brother installed in his room* – an event likely to link back to the patient's childhood and his brother's birth when he was seven. The therapist reminded him of powerful competitive feelings for his colleague; and then made a tentative suggestion that he might have similar feelings about his brother, and also perhaps his father. Shortly afterwards it was the end of the session.

The patient arrived for the next session saying that he felt 'terrible', 'completely confused', and 'unable to concentrate'. This disturbance could not be traced to any event in the intervening period, and therefore it must presumably have been a reaction to the previous session. Since the patient had responded with relief to an interpretation pointing out his rivalry with another man in his *current* life (O), the cause of his anxiety must have lain in something that had occurred after this. In fact what had happened was that the therapist had also made the link with the lower corner of the triangle of person (P), namely his brother and his father. The question is, which of these was the more anxiety-provoking?

The evidence suggests that it was the brother. Later in this session the patient spoke of two fantasies, each involving the question of 'who gets the attention'. In the first he impressed people with his abilities and showed off his children, but his wife was never present (i.e. she didn't share in the attention); in the second he fulfilled all his artistic dreams, but he deliberately arranged things so that his *brother* took all the credit (a fairly obvious piece of over-compensation). The therapist (1) pointed out that the patient seemed to 'block his wife out' (defence) as he apparently blocked the new baby out; (2) suggested that this was because now both of them were the centre of attention; (3) linked this with the loss of attention in his childhood caused by his brother's birth (O/P link); and (4) suggested that he needed to protect (defence) his wife and the baby from his resentment (hidden feeling). In response the patient admitted that he had a block about the baby and at last revealed that it was a girl. He added that he did not like young babies – he found it very difficult to have the feelings of pride and satisfaction that one is supposed to have, and he had felt the same when his son was a baby, though not when he was older. Not long afterwards he began to speak of his brother. He said, on the one hand, that he got on very well with him and felt very close to him; but on the other hand he described how he had had to look after him when he was small, and how nowadays his brother excelled in various things and depreciated anything that the patient was good at. The therapist once more pointed out the need to protect people close to him from his hostility. The patient now responded with another positive unconscious communication – very similar to the one about the two rooms – namely that recently he had been more hopeful *because he had found a new friend with whom he could speak spontaneously and be himself.*

There is one aspect of the above sequence of events that requires an explanation, namely that the initial mention of competition with the brother caused considerable disturbance, whereas later work on the same issue produced relief. It is not certain why this was so; but we may note that initially the therapist mentioned only the hidden feeling (competitiveness); whereas later he spoke far more comprehensively, mentioning two defences ('blocking off' and the need to protect) and the link between the current situation and the past. This latter may well have relieved the patient's guilt about his current hostility to the new baby.

We may now turn to a female patient whose problems involved both a younger sister and a younger brother.

The Divorced Mother

This was a woman of 31 whose recent history was as follows: her husband had left her about 2 years ago, taking their son, Donald, with him, ostensibly for a holiday, and promising to let him come back. He had then broken this promise, leaving Donald with his own parents in the North of England – who were, however, people with whom Donald got on well. She had been unable to take effective action about this. She had then taken up with another man (Peter), who had left her 18 months ago. This had precipitated a state of depression.

Her background was that she was the second of five children. No obvious disturbance could be found in her childhood except that her father was in the Navy and her schooling was disrupted by frequent moves. Nevertheless she showed a neurotic character pattern that clearly lay at the root of her present trouble.

At the beginning of a relationship with a man she always presents herself as immature, helpless, and useless (the interviewing psychiatrist described her as appearing much younger than her years). This is followed by a stage of passive compliance which has resulted in her being exploited and ill-used. She is unable to assert herself to prevent such situations from developing, and on a number of occasions has failed to take action to escape from them. She was unable to take action against her husband over the custody of their child, and in the end has allowed *him* to divorce *her*, leaving the child with him.

It was clear that therapy would have to deal with this character pattern rather than the immediate depression, as otherwise she would just get herself into a similar situation again.

She was taken on for time-limited therapy at twice a week for 5 months. Her (male) therapist was an experienced psychiatrist and a sensitive and able man, but he was not fully trained in psychotherapy; and his tendency to rush into speculative interpretations, rather than using the step by step approach advocated throughout the present book, needed to be kept in check.

The compulsion to repeat

We may first prepare the ground by considering her possible psychopathology. The feature that is conspicuous in her story is the total absence of aggression of any kind. She has been exploited and ill-used by her husband, who has robbed her of their son, but she has neither been able to prevent this from happening nor to reverse it once it has happened, and indeed she seems even to *seek* such situations. This appears to be an example of the phenomenon named by Freud the *compulsion to repeat* (see Freud, 1914, 1920), in which the patient not merely *cannot avoid* certain neurotic patterns but actually seems to *select* people from the environment with whom such a pattern will inevitably develop (the Maintenance Man was probably another example – see p. 109). The explanation of this phenomenon, which will be discussed more fully below, is extremely obscure, but clinically this does not matter. What is needed in therapy is the same as in any other neurotic mechanism, namely to bring out the underlying feelings and trace them to their origin. It seems most probable that this particular patient is afraid of her natural aggressiveness and in some way is defending herself against it. The opening stages of therapy should therefore be concerned with identifying these defences and interpreting them.

The Divorced Mother (contd)

In the first session the therapist offered little instruction, support, or encouragement, deliberately raising her anxiety and precipitating her at once into a situation in which she was unable to employ her usual *defence* of finding out what the other person wanted and complying with it. She spoke of how she much preferred situations with set rules; and he said that *she was afraid of doing something that he would disapprove of*. Since the patient has already mentioned the *defence*, needing set rules – this interpretation of the *anxiety*, which also asks the patient's unconscious about the *hidden feeling*, and is couched in quite mild terms, is basically correct and appropriate. The patient then approached the hidden feeling by saying that she was *angry with herself* for being unable to act in the situation in which she found herself. Here he said that she was implying she was *angry with him* for putting her in this situation, and asked her whether it was not a pattern in her life that she got *angry with herself* instead of *with other people*. This interpretation of the defence of *turning anger against herself* was almost certainly absolutely correct and appropriate. However it was too fast for the patient, who simply said that she had no right to be angry with other people.

She then started speaking about her son, Donald, and eventually said that 'she would rather he did not exist in her thoughts' – presumably to save herself the pain of missing him. At this the therapist plunged into a speculative interpretation of a very disturbing hidden feeling, saying that 'she might even want him not to live'.

Here the ground had already been tested out when the patient had not responded to the previous relatively mild interpretation about aggressive feelings. It was a mark of the therapist's inexperience that he was not warned by this, and instead tried a much more disturbing interpretation. Not surprisingly, the patient simply denied it.

A fortiori, having received no response to this interpretation in the area of her *son*, he now tried a speculative link with the *father*, thus breaking one of the basic principles: that you do not make the link with a second area until you have properly clarified the triangle of conflict in the first area. What he did was to ask her what her feelings were when her father was absent at sea, to which, again not surprisingly, she answered simply that she didn't remember.

However, this talk of childhood now produced an important association in an entirely new area: that her younger sister, Janet, was very pretty, and she (the patient) *used to run away so as not to be compared with her*. Not only this, but she and her brother had thrown ink at one of her sister's dresses, in order to spoil her prettiness. Thus the hidden feelings of *jealousy* and *spite* emerged very strongly. The therapist, perhaps warned by her previous lack of response, did not mention jealousy itself, but spoke of how she halved her guilt with her brother. To this she said that she wasn't guilty, thus nullifying even this.

At the end of this first therapeutic session we may take stock. It is clear that the patient is very intolerant of her unacceptable hidden feelings, and the therapist will have to go carefully, concentrating on interpreting the defences. This therapist has been somewhat wild in his interpretation – it was probably this kind of activity that caused the patient to say at follow-up, 6 years later, that she thought in the early stages the therapist was 'poking around'. On the other hand, in spite of this, the patient has in fact come out with an almost open admission of *jealousy*, which is an indication of hope for the future.

However, in Session 2 the patient emphatically denied any feeling of anger or jealousy towards her sister, and said that in fact it was she rather than her sister who was preferred by her father. She also denied any jealousy towards her youngest brother (10 years younger), who had become the centre of attention for the whole family, saying that this was his due as the youngest. The only interpretation that she did agree with was – according to expectation – of a *defence*, namely that by keeping quiet and doing little she could deprive her therapist and other people of the means of criticizing her.

In Session 3 she said she did not like to speak because what she had to say *would be stupid*. The therapist, correctly, repeated the above defence interpretation, saying that by pointing out how stupid she was, she was forestalling his criticizing her, with which she now *emphatically agreed*. Thus, as might have been predicted, the first really clear response was to the interpretation of a defence. The patient went on to describe illogical things that she did, e.g. buying clothes she didn't want, and the therapist, again probably correctly, said that she was really trying to tell him not to be cross with her as she was '*such a lost chil*d who could not be taken seriously', i.e. another defence. She just responded to this as to an accusation.

Nevertheless, the work was bearing fruit. Towards the end of the session she spoke of feeling very bad about not writing to her son 'mainly because her reason for not doing so was selfish'. It was not clear what this meant, but the therapist correctly interpreted yet another defence, that she was again *forestalling his criticism by criticizing herself.*

In response to this the patient immediately spoke of the *hidden feelings* – the first that she explicitly admitted – namely that she did not write to her son *in order to make his father angry*. Towards the end of the session she admitted even more disturbing hidden feelings, namely that when her son was first born *she had hated him and refused to look at him.*

Session 4 was marked by further rapid progress in response to more interpretation of defences. She quickly became tense and silent, and the therapist made an excellent transference interpretation of a dilemma caused by two conflicting anxieties: if she kept silent she was afraid he might get angry with her, and if she spoke she might reveal things that he did not like. In response she spoke of refusing to have her picture taken at a photographer's until everyone else left the room, because she *was afraid that they might compare her and find her wanting*. The therapist again interpreted this in the transference, saying that she wanted to *run away* from him (defence) because he might find her wanting (anxiety), and linking this with her previous communication about the *past*, namely her running away for fear of being compared to her *sister*. The patient made an immediate response to this interpretation by speaking of a *hidden feeling*, though defensively disguised: that she could not bear to be compared, and she got very *angry* when people said *nice* things to her. The therapist immediately saw through this defence and said that she became angry when she was praised because then her anger was not completely justified (defence); and that she did this in order to forestall her real anger (hidden feeling) when disappointed, which she was really afraid of (anxiety). He went on to say that she employed all kinds of strategy (defence) so as not to become really angry, e.g. giving him implied instructions as to how to avoid making her angry. Her response to this was the clearest statement so far of the intensity of her hidden feeling: that when her husband had been angry with her she in her turn had just screamed with anger and literally banged her head against the wall.

I shall now jump ahead to Session 11, towards the end of which the therapist gave a major interpretation completing the two triangles. Previous features of the session had been (1) her cringing into her chair as if to hide; (2) her saying that she did not like to be seen in the light; (3) an account of how she had suspected her husband of being unfaithful; but (4) in the end he had persuaded her to commit adultery so that he could divorce *her*, promising to let her have Donald their son; (5) which promise he had then betrayed; (6) how she had fallen in love with the man, Peter, who had acted as co-respondent; but (7) how he had preferred his own outside interests to being with her; and finally (8) he had left her too.

In addition, in recent sessions, there had been a good deal of by-play over the 'engaged' sign on the door. On arrival the patient put it from 'vacant' to 'engaged' as if claiming exclusive right to her therapist, and then at the end putting it back to 'vacant', thus disclaiming her right and symbolically handing over to the next patient. We may now introduce another important general principle: although such actions might seem to be natural and trivial, they should always be carefully examined for hidden meanings. That they did in fact have a deeper significance seemed to be confirmed by subsequent events.

The therapist now said that she *did all sorts of things so as not to enter into competition*, i.e. she employed numerous defences. He cited many examples of this, such as appearing helpless, like a little girl; running away when compared to her sister; putting the 'vacant' sign on at the end of the session; not wanting to be seen in the light; being unable to compete with her husband for their son, or with Peter's other interests for his attention. He then added the *anxiety* and the *hidden feeling*: that if she competed in earnest she was afraid she would become angry and uncontrolled and lose the other person entirely. As the reader will see, this interpretation completes both triangles, since it mentions defence, anxiety, and hidden feeling on the one hand: and her sister (distant past), her husband and boy-friend (recent past), and the transference on the other.

Her response was to say rather cheerfully that she ought perhaps to start competing – somewhere else, of course, not here. The therapist then made explicit the competitive situation in the transference and her defence against it – that she wanted to make sure she did not compete with his next patient 'like the one born 4 years after her' i.e. her sister. This was thus an interpretation of the T/P link (where P stands for 'past'). Her only acknowledgement of these interpretations at the time was to say she now liked herself even less. This is an example of what one may call the depressive defence, emphasizing the guilt in order to hide the unacceptable feeling. At the end of the session she almost slammed the door and put the engaged sign off with some violence, thus indicating fairly clearly that her annoyance was not only with herself.

In the next session, however, when she was reminded of these themes, she came out with two crucial pieces of information: (1) that her mother had told her that she had tried to kill her brother soon after he was born; (2) that when she was 12 she had half tried to suffocate a baby by putting a pillow on him. During the rest of the session the therapist gradually reconstructed her fear (anxiety) of violent and even murderous impulses (hidden feeling) if she competed in earnest.

Almost certainly as a consequence of this work, in the next session there was a complete change of atmosphere. The therapist wrote that she no longer appeared as a little girl cringing back in her chair, but seemed to enjoy displaying herself as a positively beautiful woman. Perhaps the most important thing that she said was that she now knew what she had never known before, that she was a very jealous person.

Here I shall leave this therapy. The sexual transference was not far away, and had to be dealt with in the next phase. Her feelings about termination were of course a major issue. There were 30 sessions in all.

In fact this single course of therapy was not enough. She came back a few years later because of attacks of depression every time she saw her son, and had 18 months of group treatment. In accordance with our observation that patients who have had previous individual psychotherapy tend to do much better in Tavistock groups (see Malan *et al.*, 1976), she appeared to be able to use her group experience to good effect. She made clear at final follow-up that a long slow process of favourable change had been going on since her individual treatment 6 years before. She now had a stable and satisfactory relation with a man, knew what she wanted in life and seemed to have achieved it. Perhaps there was still some difficulty in standing up for her rights, but this seemed to be the only residual problem. In contrast to our patients in the above follow-up study of groups, who tended both to remember little about their experience in therapy and to speak unfavourably about what they did remember, she remembered her experience clearly. Of her individual treatment she said that the thing that had made a huge impression on her was that her therapist had told her *she did not like herself*; and she had also been amazed to find that she was extremely jealous of her sister, even though she herself and not her sister had been her father's favourite.

Passive defences against aggression and the link with masochism

This patient was remarkable for the variety of what we may call *passive defences against angry and jealous feelings*, and equally for the intensity and literalness of these feelings when they ultimately emerged. In this she strongly resembles the next patient to be described. Of her defences we may mention: appearing useless, helpless, stupid, and childlike; being compliant; trying to avoid being compared, even if she was the preferred one; appearing angry if people said nice things about her; and renouncing her claim to people she needed. She also showed two related defences in which aggression was turned against herself. In one, where she criticized herself in order to forestall criticism by others, or got angry with herself as a way of avoiding being angry with others, the aggression came from herself. This is related to depression, which is the main subject of Chapters 13 and 15. In the other, in which she allowed herself to be exploited, the aggression came from other people. This is related to masochism, which leads at once to a consideration of the next patient.

The Librarian who Sought Suffering

This 30-year-old married woman came to us complaining of recurrent depressions since puberty.

The important facts in the history of her childhood were that: (1) she was the eldest of a family of five; (2) all her happy memories were from before the age of 3, when her eldest brother was born; (3) after this time she received far less attention from her mother, and hardly any from her father, who tended to make fun of her; and (4) when she was 5 and in charge of her brother, then aged 2, he fell into a stream and was rescued by a neighbour – she does not know whether she pushed him in or not.

From her later history we may pick out the following: (1) she was almost entirely unaware of angry or jealous feelings; (2) she had a tendency to take up with men who ill-treated her or exercised power over her; (3) she found to her horror that she was excited when a man forced her to have sex with him; (4) some of her sexual fantasies involved being 'used' by a number of men whom she didn't know; (5) when her husband exposed her to situations of jealousy – which currently he was doing by having an affair with a woman called Denise – she would go out into the street with fantasies of being raped, murdered, or run over; and (6) she was actively promoting the relation between her husband and Denise, e.g. by suggesting that they should go out together.

The question of masochism

We may begin the discussion with a retrospect of the Divorced Mother, in whom we noted a number of passive behaviour patterns which had resulted in her being ill-used and exploited. Moreover there seemed to be a tendency not merely to fall into such relationships, but to seek them actively.

Such behaviour is often described as 'masochistic', but in her case this is rather a loose usage of the term; since, although she did appear to seek suffering, there was no evidence that she actually got pleasure or satisfaction from it.

In the case of the Librarian there were no such reservations: in addition to the tendency to seek out men who ill-treated her, she openly admitted that ill-treatment gave her sexual pleasure.

These phenomena are some of those belonging to a long list in the field of human psychology which contradict common sense. Biologically speaking, pain has obvious survival value, serving the function of warning the individual of situations to avoid, not to seek. This applies to mental pain as well as physical – the distress felt, and expressed, by a small child threatened with separation may persuade the mother to give up the idea of exposing the unprotected child to danger by leaving. Why should anyone develop the most un-biological tendency to seek mental or physical pain, let alone to derive pleasure from it?

These two patients, the Librarian and the Divorced Mother, may supply part of the answer, though it must be emphasized that the complete answer is probably much more complicated.

We may start with the Divorced Mother and ask the question, what emerged in her therapy that might shed any light on her psychopathology? Hers was an example of a therapy that can be largely summarized by a description of a few climactic moments. Here we may pick out the following sequence of three sessions: in the first the therapist interprets her defence against feeling jealous of his next patient (hidden feeling in the transference) and links this with her sister in the past (T/P link); in the second she admits that her jealousy of her younger siblings involved *murderous impulses*; and in the third session the consequence of this realization appeared to be immense relief expressed in a transformation of her whole personality – 'no longer a little girl cringing back in her chair, but a positively beautiful woman'. Moreover at follow-up her tendency to seek out men who ill-used her seems to have disappeared.

Could it be, then, that this seeking of suffering has something to do with violent, perhaps even murderous, impulses? We may bear this question in mind when considering the following climactic sequence from the therapy of the Librarian. The therapist was a woman social worker.

The Librarian (contd)

In Session 13 the patient said that she had been anxious to let her husband be free enough to have time with Denise, but he was tied to feeding some new puppies. The therapist said that this promoting of her husband's affair must be a way of expressing guilt about her anger at his rejecting her. The patient then told of a half-waking dream in which she found the puppies thin and dead, and her husband and Denise also dead in bed together, Denise having stabbed him and then taken an overdose. Here the hostile – indeed murderous – feelings towards the man, the woman, and rival children (represented by the puppies) were very thinly disguised indeed, which the therapist pointed out, making the link with the patient's father, mother, and siblings.

The therapist wrote in her account that at this point she began to feel a sense of withdrawal, expressed as sleepiness. This leads to a digression.

The use of 'counter-transference' in interpretation

'Counter-transference', as a term used to describe the therapist's reactions to a patient, is unsatisfactory, since these reactions may be entirely natural and not 'transferred' from anyone else; but I use it here because it has become common terminology. It may be remembered from the Imaginary Therapy that at one point (p. 93) the therapist made the mistake of expressing irritation with her patient, instead of understanding that what she was reacting to was a crucial pattern in the patient's relationships, which needed bringing into the open and tracing to its origin. Thus therapists need to be armed with enough self-knowledge and capacity for objectivity to examine their own reactions, and – without mentioning them overtly – to use them in the service of the patient.

The Librarian (contd)

The fact that the present therapist possessed these qualities led to a crucial moment in the therapy, in which transference feelings were brought out that otherwise might easily have been missed. The therapist recognized that she must be reacting with her own defences to something in the atmosphere between her and the patient; and she made the guess, which she incorporated into an interpretation, that the patient was expressing anger with her in some hidden way. The patient said immediately that this was true, and that it had to do with the therapist's small stature, which linked with the small stature of several other people in her life who were a cause of jealousy, in particular her younger sister. She added that her sister was preferred to her, and that she herself was humiliated by her father for growing into a 'big strapping girl'.

Bringing out these feelings caused the patient considerable distress, and she said, 'I feel you're stopping me from going forward. I came in here happy and now it's all gone.' The therapist then gave a major interpretation completing the triangle of person: 'I suggested that she saw me (T), as she saw her sister in the past (P), and now Denise (O), as coming between her and the man she wants – myself with her GP [with whom the patient was half in love], her sister with her father, and Denise with her husband – and that she feels guilty about her anger with all three of us.'

The day after this session the therapist received a phone call from the patient, of which the following is the therapist's description: 'She wanted to tell me that she was very angry with me yesterday for linking everything with her childhood. But suddenly things have fallen into place. She realizes that the guilt she feels towards Denise is in fact connected with her parents. She is afraid that Denise will die and that is what she felt about her parents – she was very fond of them in one way but hated their guts in another.'

The events described in this last paragraph represent an illustration of the phenomenon noted by Davanloo (1990) of 'unlocking the unconscious'. One of the situations in which this occurs is when a patient both *experiences and expresses anger* at a therapist's *correct* interventions. Here, anger at the link being made between the transference and the past led to the de-repression of crucial feelings throwing light on the origin of her problems.

The therapist's account continues: 'The patient opened the next session by saying that it was strange that she should feel so much better after realizing that her guilt about Denise was linked with her anger and guilt about her parents. She has come to realize that she has a *monster of violent anger* within her. She is glad that she no longer feels guilty about her anger towards Denise for wanting her husband. She realizes that she wasn't allowed to express even small amounts of anger to her parents, which made her anxious about her aggression and afraid that they would die.'

At 6-year follow-up both her tendency to depression and the masochistic phenomena had disappeared. She had divorced her husband. She now spoke with distaste of her husband's need to exercise power over her, and her subsequent relations with men were warm and gentle. Of her therapy she spoke as follows: 'When I was only offered 30 sessions I was very angry, but I feel that I worked through a tremendous amount in that time. I was able to have feelings which I regarded as wicked, but it didn't make me into a wicked person, so that I learned not to be afraid of them. Talking with my therapist enabled me to disentangle what belonged to my father and what belonged to my husband.'

Comparison of these two patients

This story and that of the Divorced Mother are extraordinarily similar: (1) in both there was ample cause for jealousy in childhood; (2) both showed a long-standing tendency to seek situations which caused them to suffer and be exploited; (3) at the height of therapy both came to realize intensely aggressive, guilt-laden feelings, in both cases involving murderous impulses; (4) in both this resulted in immense relief and a major transformation of their personality; and finally (5) both were found at follow-up to have lost their tendency to seek suffering, and to have replaced it by the ability to establish warm and close relations with the opposite sex.

Discussion of the issue of masochism: the 'superego'.

These two patients do not *prove* anything about the mechanisms underlying the phenomenon of masochism. The evidence is not strong enough. It would be stronger if we knew that masochistic tendencies began to disappear at the very point at which the patients became aware of their violently aggressive feelings, but unfortunately this observation was not made in either case. However, Davanloo – with his immensely powerful technique of unlocking the unconscious – has indeed made this observation in one patient after another, and the connection between masochism and violence must be regarded as established. Thus the two patients described here *illustrate* this connection, though they do not prove it. It is important to add that the violent feelings do not always involve jealousy, still less jealousy of siblings, but may result from any cause.

The question is now, what are the mechanisms involved? It seems that these are twofold. On the one hand patients defend themselves against the realization of their own outwardly directed violence by turning it against themselves; and on the other hand this serves the purpose of expressing their guilt about their violence through *self-punishment*. As will be touched on in the case of the Nurse in Mourning (p. 144), this is an example of the operation of a pathological conscience containing some of the patient's own aggression, for which Freud coined the term *Oberich* or 'superego' – a concept that will be discussed more fully in Chapter 15 (see the Irishwoman with the Cats, p. 174).

Mechanisms in the compulsion to repeat

Three patients, the Maintenance Man and the two just described, showed phenomena that come under the heading of the 'compulsion to repeat'. The first married a woman resembling his mother, who was dominating and disgusted by sex. This act, at first sight quite unintelligible, becomes intelligible if we understand it as the expression of a defence, with the aim of keeping his guilt-laden sexual impulses under control, possibly combined with self-punishment for these same impulses. The two women patients repeatedly formed relationships with men who ill-treated them. This in turn can be understood if we formulate it in a similar way, as a fusion of (1) a defence against outwardly directed and highly guilt-laden unconscious violent impulses, and (2) an expression of guilt through self-punishment.

If we can understand such repetitive acts as expressing these powerful forces of defence and guilt within the psyche, then it would seem that no further explanation is required. But it may be asked, is such an explanation always valid or complete? The answer may be considered in connection with the following patient.

The Victimized Telephonist

This single woman of 34 came to therapy after some sensitive work by an osteopath. She consulted him about pain in her back, but he detected the depression and emotional strain in her and referred her for a psychotherapeutic opinion.

The essence of her story was that she had been involved for 7 years with a much older married man named Andreas. He was extremely generous to her in a materialistic sense, but emotionally everything had to be on his terms; and he had broken with her when for the first time she began to make demands on him. This was one year ago.

She described a childhood largely empty of affection. It was clear that she had dealt with this by a pattern of bending over backwards to please, which she had continued in her relation with Andreas.

She was assigned to brief therapy with a male trainee psychiatrist, which unfortunately was limited to only 12 sessions by his departure for his home country. The main theme of his interventions was to point out repeatedly her pattern of trying to please and her inability to make demands on her own behalf, linking this with her upbringing. Short as her therapy was, she quickly began to show remarkable improvements, discovering the capacity for constructive self-assertion in a number of situations.

We had great hopes for her, but at final follow-up (nearly 4 years) she revealed a catastrophic situation:

She had fallen in love with a man named Stefan on a visit to Poland and eventually they had agreed to get married. This would serve the additional purpose of enabling him to get out of Poland and come to Britain. She said two highly significant things about him: first, that he resembled Andreas in several ways; and second, that she wanted to help him. When she was asked what she wanted to help him with, she said, 'How can I explain? I suppose with life.'

However, when she visited him a second time the situation had changed in a disastrous way, and yet she had gone through with the marriage just the same.

The story is best told through condensed extracts from the follow-up interview:

PT: When he met me at the airport, instead of kissing me he didn't take any interest in me. This horrible feeling came over me. I was just trapped.

TH: Why were you trapped? Surely you could have left?

PT: I couldn't. I was illegally in his house. There was no way I could go.

TH: What would have happened if you had taken the first plane for London?

PT: I couldn't. When you are there and all his relatives are there, how could I get out? I suppose I didn't want to hurt, to create a big scene.

TH: I think we can agree that you weren't materially forced to remain there. So what was the feeling that pushed you to marry him anyway?

PT: Because I was in his house, with all his relatives. I think basically I am not ruthless enough.

TH: In spite of your awareness of always putting yourself in the victim position, you still do it. Why can that be?

PT: I think it belongs to my childhood. My parents – I was taking responsibility for them.

TH: Why?

PT: My mother needs to be looked after and I have never really communicated with my father.

TH: What I am impressed with is that these two characteristics – needing help, and not communicating – are present in your relation with Stefan.

PT: Now that you say that, it's funny, but he reminded me of my father.

TH: In what way?

PT: Father was often shouting. When I was with Stefan he couldn't talk to me as I am doing to you. He would raise his voice and shout. And the other thing is that he didn't seem to be interested in me as a woman or as a person, the same as my father towards my mother.

Discussion

This tragic story is perhaps the least accessible to common sense of all those in this book. How can we understand someone wanting to marry a man who resembled her father in that he shouted instead of communicating, and wasn't interested in her as a person or as a woman?

First of all, there is evidence that this patient sought relationships that caused her suffering in the same way as the two previous patients described above. Thus she had fallen from the frying pan into the fire, having been deserted by her self-centred man-friend, only to marry a man who resembled him and who neglected her. So, although there is no direct evidence in her case for guilt about angry feelings, it might seem reasonable to assume that they were there and the same mechanisms were at work. Also, it might be possible that in taking up with these unsatisfactory men she was expressing a hidden attachment to her father. Yet, although both these factors may have been present, they somehow do not feel as if they provide a complete or adequate explanation in this and similar cases.

Freud came up against the same problem of repetitive psychic phenomena that caused suffering when he considered recurrent dreams of traumatic events, particularly in patients suffering from war neuroses (see *Beyond the pleasure principle*, 1921). Here we could use an even more modern example, namely concentration camp victims: when they were in the camp they dreamed of a life outside, but after they were released many dreamed they were back in the camp. This kind of phenomenon forced him to abandon the position that dreams were always an expression of a (conscious or unconscious) *wish* – the wish is obvious in the former dreams, but is unthinkable in the latter. Again, we can express Freud's ideas with the aid of knowledge that has accumulated since his time, by considering the stage of *intrusive thoughts* of a traumatic event, which many people who have suffered such an event have to pass through (see Horowitz's book, *Stress response syndromes*, 1976). These thoughts can probably be explained as follows: At the time of the trauma the individual is faced with stimuli that threaten to be overwhelming, and an automatic protective mechanism is set up preventing the full emotional reaction from occurring. The victim feels stunned, numb, incredulous. The intrusive thoughts represent the beginning of the delayed emotional reaction; and if all goes well the event and the reaction to it can be *assimilated* gradually without permanent damage. But if the reaction is still too great to bear, even in small doses, then the individual may never get beyond this stage, and the intrusive thoughts just continue without resolution. This is thus an example of the 'compulsion to repeat', here to repeat thoughts of a traumatic event. Freud postulated that the compulsion to repeat traumatic relationships was in part driven by the same mechanism – the feelings involved had never been properly experienced, and they were pressing for expression so that they could be assimilated, or, as he put it 'mastered'.

Yet it seems to me that even this does not complete the possible explanations, and that a clue to an additional factor may have been provided by this patient herself. The dialogue given above was broken off at the point where she described two resemblances between Stefan and her father, one being that her father used to shout and the other that he was not interested in her mother as a person or a woman. At this point the therapist asked a question:

TH: So why should you look for such a man?
PT: I really don't know why. Security, familiarity ...?

Could it be, then, that a further reason why people may seek a relationship of this kind is that they feel more secure in it because it is familiar? Perhaps the Telephonist wouldn't have known how to deal with a loving man because such a relationship was beyond her experience, and she unconsciously preferred to employ patterns that had been established and ingrained since her childhood. But this speculation about her possible reaction to a loving man leads back to 'assimilation' or 'mastery': if she was full of pent-up unconscious feelings about her neglectful father, how could she express them and get rid of them with a man who cared about her? This would explain why people may actually *need* the types of relationship that gave them pain in the past – but of course it doesn't work: what happens is that they simply get caught up in the same maladaptive patterns as they employed in the past, which solve nothing, with the result that the repetition becomes endless. In fact this is surely the driving force behind the transference, and leads to the basic principle of most dynamic psychotherapy: no matter what the therapist is like, patients perceive him (or her) as some person in the past who has caused them conflict, and react in the same maladaptive way; and it is because the therapist can perceive this, bring it to the surface, and trace it to its origin, that the maladaptive patterns can be broken.

Finally, it is worth noting that all three of the women patients described here suffered from *depression*, a vast subject which will begin to be considered in the next chapter.

13

An introduction to depression

It is almost impossible to give a number of clinical examples without coming across a patient suffering from perhaps the commonest of all neurotic symptoms, namely depression. Several such patients have already been mentioned and will be used in the following discussion. As will be seen, although the basic concepts in the psychopathology of depression are extremely simple, the subject is one of the most complex in this whole field.

One of the complexities, of course, starts before we enter the field of psychopathology at all, and consists of the still unanswered question of whether there is a fundamental difference between 'neurotic' and 'endogenous' depression, and whether the latter is fundamentally biochemical rather than psychogenic. I do not intend to get involved in this question, but will simply adopt the standpoint that some depressions have an emotional basis – with which few workers in this field would disagree.

The best starting point is a patient of a kind represented by the following:

Depression and miscarried grief – the Nurse in Mourning

The patient was an unmarried woman of 32, a qualified nurse working as matron in a mixed boarding school. Her initial interview, which was carried out by a (woman) psychologist, may be used as not only an introduction to the psychopathology of depression, but also to continue illustrating some of the principles of psychotherapeutic consultation.

The Nurse in Mourning, initial assessment interview

When asked where she would like to begin, the patient said that she was suffering from depression which she had had for about 18 months, 'but perhaps the new tablets prescribed by her doctor might help her' – thus revealing at once her resistance to the idea of a psychotherapeutic approach.

Now the patient had already shown, by a questionnaire filled out before the consultation, that there was ample apparent cause in her history for psychogenic depression, and therefore that her pinning of hopes on anti-depressants almost certainly represented a defence against facing painful feelings. Such a patient needs to be brought into therapy by partial interpretations, which must be carefully adjusted so that, without raising too much anxiety, they convey the message that she is understood and can be helped.

Here I am going too fast. As I always teach, it is quite unjustified for anyone to make interpretations until he knows what kind of patient he is talking to. For all we know, in spite of the patient's dating her depressions from 18 months ago, she has suffered from cyclic depressions alternating with manic attacks for years, or alternatively she is seriously suicidal and needs to be handled with the utmost care (see Chapter 19, especially pp. 246ff., for a full discussion of these issues).

The psychologist therefore at once went carefully into the quality and severity of the depression. This consisted mainly of the feeling that life was not worth living, and at one time had been bad enough for the patient to take 5 weeks off work; but there were no 'endogenous' features such as early waking, and she denied suicidal ideas. There was no evidence for any diagnosis other than depression, the patient had been apparently well until 18 months ago, and the psychologist now felt it safe to go into the whole story.

The patient went on with a direct statement of her resistance to examining her feelings, saying that *4 years ago her fiancé had died*, but 'it was all such a long time ago'. Since then she had filled her life with many activities, and 'she couldn't go on for ever hanging onto the past'.

The psychologist gradually coaxed her to tell the story in detail. She had met her fiancé while working in the North of England. He had been severely injured in an explosion at the chemical factory where he worked, and had died in hospital, in her presence, a few days later. She had felt terrible, but *had not cried*, and very quickly had begun throwing herself into hectic activity – going to wild parties, drinking too much, and working out of hours.

The reader who has familiarized himself with the concepts put forward in the foregoing pages will see at once, first, that this is a highly abnormal reaction to such an event, and second that it is clearly an example of a *defence of over-activity* against shock and grief. It almost certainly bears a relation to the phenomena of mania and hypomania, and is loosely referred to as the 'manic defence'.

Thus, although this is an abnormal reaction, it is entirely understandable that she should have needed to defend herself in this way, and one might think that there is no need to look any further into the causes of her depression. But there is very little simplicity in the field of psychodynamics, and one does need to ask the question of why this patient in particular found it so difficult to face her grief. The psychologist therefore asked her why she had to rush away from the pain so quickly, to which she replied that she thought that what she had done was the best way of coping.

Now the psychologist knew from the patient's written material that in fact the story was much more complicated than this, and therefore offered the simple comment that 'there had been too many deaths, and she couldn't cope with another'.

This brought out an account of two previous traumatic occurrences. When the patient was 16 her mother had been killed while out shopping by a lorry that had run out of control. Then, when the patient was 28, her father had developed headaches, treated by her GP with aspirin, and finally, after an acute exacerbation, had been admitted to hospital, where he had died of an intracranial tumour. It is important that her reaction to these two earlier events had been quite different from her recent reaction. After hearing of her mother's death, for instance, she had sat at home all afternoon disbelieving it, and had followed this by crying a great deal. Thus she illustrates once more the principle that traumatic events often owe their damaging effects to the fact that they are a repetition of something similar that has happened in the past.

The patient herself made clear that she understood this by saying, 'When it happened once more, I just couldn't go through it again.' The psychologist then offered an interpretation linking this series of events with the depression, saying that the fiancé's death must have aroused not only feelings about that event itself, but those left over from the two previous deaths, and that all these feelings must be there *but instead of being aware of them she was depressed.*

At this point the patient showed the beginning of her therapeutic alliance by putting her finger on one of the unanswered questions of her whole history: her fiancé's death had occurred 4 years ago, but she had not become depressed until about 18 months ago, and she herself now asked, 'Why so much later?'. To this the psychologist responded by suggesting that she should look at events since she came back to London about 2 years ago. From this it emerged that, first, she had formed a relation with a man but had broken it off, quite consciously aware of this as a *defence* against the *anxiety* of being hurt again if she became too involved; that she had again filled up her life with activity by working all the summer holidays; and finally that she had become depressed on returning to school in the autumn – 'perhaps it was the fact that now she had been given extra responsibility.' The psychologist said that this didn't seem to be sufficient reason, and it now emerged that soon after the beginning of term one of the girls had come to her *depressed because she had just lost her mother.* This had clearly threatened to reactivate the patient's own grief, and thus the whole series of events was explained.

The fundamental principle that this patient illustrates with the utmost clarity is that one of the important roots of depression is concerned with feelings of loss, and *particularly with grief that has in some way miscarried and has never been worked through.*

The treatment of responses to traumatic events

This patient also illustrates, with equal clarity, both a 'normal' way and one of the maladaptive ways of reacting to a traumatic event, in this case the sudden and unexpected loss of a loved person. As described in the previous chapter, the normal reaction often begins with a protective phase of shock or denial, lasting for hours or days; which is followed by a phase in which the grief begins to come to the surface and needs to be expressed over and over, until every aspect of the loss has finally been worked through and life can begin again. This is exactly the reaction that the patient showed to the death of her mother. (As an aside, it is worth mentioning that an initial period of numbness does not necessarily follow *unpleasant* events – how often has one seen someone being interviewed after some major achievement, saying 'Well, it hasn't sunk in yet'? Presumably this initial failure to respond operates as a protection against too great stimulation of any kind, including joy or triumph.)

Returning to grief, the process may go wrong in two main ways: there can be *too much* reaction or *too little*. When there is too much reaction, the person's feelings threaten to become overwhelming; when there is too little, the phase of denial and numbness continues and the grieving is never properly begun; and moreover these two phases may occur alternately in the same person. There is also the phenomenon, described in the previous chapter, of *intrusive thoughts*, in which the denial begins to break down and images of the event or the lost person keep presenting themselves unbidden, but without sufficient feeling to enable the grief to be worked through.

As Horowitz (1976) has made clear, treatment differs according to the phase in which the patient is seen. The aim is always to enable the process of grieving to occur at the right pace, namely the pace – however painful it may be – that is bearable. If the reaction threatens to be overwhelming, then it needs to be reduced; and such measures as moving the patient away from places associated with the lost person, and/or support, rest, and sedation are appropriate. If denial goes on too long, or the patient is suffering from intrusive thoughts unaccompanied by appropriate feeling, then the therapist must try to bring on the grieving process and help the patient to pass through it.

The therapist's role in acute grief

Obviously the Nurse's reaction to her fiancé's death came into the category of 'too little' grief rather than 'too much'. Here it is worth imagining that she had consulted a psychotherapist immediately after the death of her fiancé. How should she be handled? The answer is very simple: she must be helped to face her grief, and in the first place must be helped to cry – the therapist must try gently to bring on the healing tears. This utterly elementary principle is often very difficult to grasp and even more difficult to put into practice. There are too many conventional ideas standing in the way – we admire people who are 'being very brave' and 'carrying on just the same', without realizing the price they may be paying; we feel compelled to offer comfort, when often no comfort can be given; and the resulting feeling of total helplessness is very difficult to bear. All this is compounded if we have not entirely faced our feelings about similar experiences ourselves – as I tried to illustrate in the Imaginary Therapy described in Chapter 10 (p. 96). Yet the truth is that we are *not* helpless, and the greatest service we can give to people in these circumstances is to stay with them and simply *share their grief.*

The Nurse in Mourning, motivation

The principles of treating this patient, even after a gap of four years since the precipitating event, are exactly the same. But before this can be carried out it is necessary to make sure that the patient has the *motivation* to face her painful feelings, which in this case was by no means certain. In fact the patient showed very marked reluctance, still trying to pin her hopes on medication, but to cut a long story short she eventually realized that this was not going to work, and she started therapy with a female therapist, with a time limit of about thirty sessions at once a week. (For further discussion of the important question of motivation, see p. 238).

The Nurse in Mourning, therapy

In the first session she continued to show her ambivalent motivation with the utmost clarity. She started utterly passive and resistant, with many silences, repeatedly saying that her mind was blank. Yet towards the end she made the following statements: (1) that the things that were going through her mind were not worth saying; (2) that by concentrating on trivialities she used to stop herself from thinking painful thoughts; and (3) that it no longer worked and this was why she was depressed. She thus showed spontaneous insight into one of her defences and how it was breaking down, and indeed at this point in the session she began to become tearful. This mixture of passive resistance and therapeutic alliance characterized the whole of her therapy.

At the beginning of Session 2 she said that she almost didn't come today because she had felt terrible all the last week – the moment she had got out of the previous session she had been in floods of tears and hadn't been able to stop herself crying all that evening. Thus, even though very little had been mentioned in that session about the cause of her depression, the process of helping her to mourn had already begun. Yet here we need to be careful, because these tears both were, and were not, the healing tears that we are looking for – in answer to a question from the therapist she said she had been 'crying about nothing'; and even in the next session, where she reported that the process had continued, she said that she had been crying for 'no apparent reason'. This is the first example of many subtle defensive manoeuvres found in depression – 'depressive tears', which seem to be mourning, and yet are not really in touch with what the mourning is about. Nevertheless, in this patient, who had been unable to cry at all, they are to be welcomed.

For reasons of space I cannot go into too much detail, but I wish to use this therapy to illustrate certain important themes, some of which have already been touched on in the Imaginary Therapy.

The first is the part played by coincidence in psychopathology and psychotherapy, and the second is the difficulty the therapist may have to contend with in facing the patient's feelings. In Session 5 the patient reported a major coincidence: that the fiancé of a girl-friend of hers had been severely injured in an accident and was now in an intensive care unit. This brought memories of waiting at the hospital at the time of her own fiancé's injury and death. Some quotations from the therapist's account of the session are as follows: 'There was a desolate look on her face and I felt half guilty about pressing her and half alarmed that I might precipitate some strong reaction ... I was struggling with the material and felt I couldn't think ... though trying to provide interpretations I was telling myself that these were silly ...' There was in fact too much interpretation and too little of simply trying to share the patient's feelings, and the session never really came to life.

The third theme arose when the patient said in Session 2 that the reason why she was depressed was that she could no longer commit herself to a relation with a man because she was afraid she would lose him. She thus introduced the idea of *loss of hope*, or *despair*, which is such a feature of some states of depression, and yet despair which in truth is self-imposed because of the patient's inability to face her real feelings. Another example of this was shown by the Director's Daughter (see p. 49), who described her feeling of despair at self-imposed isolation from men, which in turn was due to Oedipal guilt. This emphasis on despair on depression can itself be used defensively, as I shall describe later (see p. 144).

The issue of ambivalence in depression

The next theme is the most important, and indeed is fundamental to the whole issue of the psychopathology of depression. It may be introduced through a rhetorical question: is it ever possible to meet depression that results simply from being unable to face grief and is uncomplicated by mixed feelings ('ambivalence') about the person who has been lost? I think the answer must be yes, and that this is in fact met particularly in short-lasting depressions that occur in the initial stages of a relatively normal mourning process – where, as mentioned above, the first duty of the therapist, or friend, is to help the bereaved person to cry. Be that as it may, the commonest reason for miscarried grief is this very complication – anger, hostility, resentment, which is often already guilt-laden, but is made enormously more so if the other person dies. The therapist needs to exercise constant self-discipline to remember this and look for it, and to lead the patient *gently* towards it – all of which of course is not easy; it is difficult enough to face the grief without forcing the patient's unwilling attention upon such an unacceptable kind of feeling. It is of course considerably easier if the cause of the loss is not death, but rejection or desertion, where anger is part of the natural response to the situation.

The question of ambivalence was central to the present therapy. It is obviously true that this patient, with two previous sudden deaths in her history, would seem to have ample cause to be unable to face her feelings about a third. Once again, by the principle of economy of hypothesis, there should be no need to look any further. Yet, as this therapy unfolded in my brief psychotherapy unit, the question was always present in our minds whether the patient's grief might have been complicated by previous quarrels with any of the three people who died. In fact in Session 2 the therapist questioned her closely about this. No trace of any such problem was ever elicited in relation to her fiancé, but she did admit that in her teens there had been quarrels with her mother, who would not let her go out in the evenings on weekdays.

Very little more direct evidence on this question was elicited throughout the whole of therapy, and yet indirect evidence was considerable. On at least three occasions the patient reported improvement after therapeutic work directly or indirectly concerning anger. One of the climaxes of therapy occurred in Session 12 when the patient reported two nightmares. In one her current (platonic) boy-friend, Derek, betrayed her and then told her off for crying; in another she was looking for her cat and found instead many cats sitting and staring at her, while Derek appeared, but it wasn't Derek and he had a horrible leper face. He went downstairs and then began to come up again, and she awoke terrified as steps approached her door. The most terrifying thing of all was that in the dream she had woken up from a dream within a dream, and thus when all these things happened she thought they were real.

What can we make of these disturbed, somewhat persecutory dreams, that seem in this apparently very normal woman to have emerged from a deeper, paranoid layer of her psyche? This introduces the whole question of the meaning of paranoid feelings, which needs to be considered now, but will be considered more fully in Chapter 16 (pp. 201 ff).

The meaning of paranoid feelings

The most familiar paranoid delusion is the patient's feeling that people are talking about him or plotting against him. It has always seemed to me that whereas phobias can in a sense be understood as an exaggeration of everyday fears, and even compulsions as an exaggeration of superstitions, paranoid feelings are in some way more mysterious. The feature that paranoid feelings have in common is the sense of sinister, hostile forces in the environment, directed against the individual. What can be the source of this? The answer cannot be reached by common sense, even by someone familiar with psychodynamics, and can only be reached empirically. It is found in fact that in the right circumstances paranoid feelings can be caused to disappear by the interpretation that they really represent hostile feelings in the individual, which, by some primitive and little understood mechanism of 'projection', he perceives as being located in the environment rather than in himself.

With the help of this basic concept, we can approach this patient's dream. In them Derek first betrays her, then becomes unsympathetic, and then turns into someone terrifying; equally her cat, a loved creature, turns into many cats, who in turn become sinister. Here we may be reminded of the intuitive insight of a previous patient, the Director's Daughter, who said of her father 'First I *hate* him, and then I think he's *horrible*, and then I'm *afraid* of him', thus describing an inner mechanism by which hate turns into fear. The part about the cats can also be understood better if we use an association that the patient revealed in a later session, namely that she had come home from university on one occasion to find that her cat had been put to sleep by her parents, i.e. of course killed. All this would seem to add up to the possible interpretation that the patient is terrified of elements of hostility in her own feelings towards people close to her. It would of course have been going much too far to have said this to her, and the therapist, quite correctly, only interpreted that she was frightened of something inside her that was very upsetting and horrible to look at. The account of the session continues: 'She anxiously replied, what is it then? I repeated my comment about the persecutory, frightening quality of whatever it was, and ended the session there.'

In spite of the fact that the underlying feelings were only hinted at, the patient reported in Session 15 that she had been feeling better ever since the session in which these nightmares had been reported. At the same time she had once more become extremely resistant, and in Session 16 the therapist made interpretations about anger in the transference, basing this on her own feeling that the patient was deliberately trying to irritate her by being obstructive. The patient utterly denied this, but nevertheless, in the next session (No. 17) she said she had been trying to remember occasions on which she had been angry, and reported three episodes of *being let down* by people, including a previous boy-friend who, she discovered, had been going out with many other girls as well as her. No such feeling could be elicited about her fiancé. Nevertheless, after telling of these instances of anger, she once more reported that she had recently been feeling better.

In Session 18 the therapist therefore returned to searching for hostility against the patient's *mother*, and brought out some more details of the conflict with her mother in her teens. This led in Session 19 to another of the climaxes of therapy. The patient now allowed her therapeutic alliance to over-ride her resistance by spontaneously writing down her dreams and bringing them to the session. In one of these a woman called Anne had been murdered – Anne is the patient's second name and also that of her *grandmother* – and a man was following the patient and her grandmother, possibly intending to murder them. This was followed by the association that she sometimes gets so irritated with her grandmother – who is very old and whom she regularly visits – that she *wishes she would die,* and then she feels terribly *guilty,* with the thought that she had not done enough for her.

Thus the patient introduced the theme of *guilt,* which is such a prominent feature of many depressions, though it had not been manifest in hers. This is of course closely linked with the theme of ambivalence, because the guilt is most frequently due to buried hostility against someone who is also loved. Guilt is also related to depressive self-reproaches, which will be considered below (see pp. 149ff.). Like so many features of depression, the guilt itself can in turn be over-emphasized – together with the consequent despair – and then used defensively to mask the hostility which is the most painful and furthest from consciousness of all the feelings involved. In the therapy of most deeply depressed people, it is this *conflict between love and hate* that needs to be reached (the 'depressive position', see Chapters 15 and 16), and when it is reached it can afford the most profound relief – with the result that the *despair* and *utter deadness* of depression become converted into *hope* and *life.* This was illustrated by the patient described here when, in the same session as that in which she had reported the nightmares, she also reported a 'healing dream', in which *the ice of an Arctic landscape became green and was transformed into grass.*

In Session 21 she reported an incident in which, shaking with anger, she had sworn at a bus conductress who had behaved with utter callousness to an old lady. This incident may be used to introduce yet another important mechanism in psychopathology: as we have just seen, this patient, who clearly genuinely loved her grandmother, also felt irritated with her and sometimes had the feeling that she wished she would die, about which she felt guilty. Thus there were two halves of her, one in conflict with the other. It is almost certainly true that in fact the patient would do anything rather than allow actual harm to come to her grandmother, or to behave in any way unkindly to her. What does she feel, then, when someone else (the bus conductress) behaves unkindly to an old lady? Naturally she is outraged, but her rage may be complicated and intensified by the fact that she sees in the conductress an aspect of herself – in other words there may be in her rage an element of *self-hatred.* This in turn links with depressive self-reproaches and with suicide, and it also leads towards very mysterious and primitive mechanisms, in which the primitive conscience, or what Freud called *superego,* seems to take on a persecuting quality, which is apparently in some way derived from the individual's own primitive aggressiveness. This will be considered in Chapter 15 (see the Irishwoman with the Cats, pp. 172ff.).

In Session 24 the patient told of an incident in which her friend, Derek, had failed to arrive to meet her, and she had been afraid that something terrible had happened to him. 'It's always the same thing. I'm worried that something is going to happen to people I'm fond of.' 'And', said the therapist 'with whom you've had a disagreement and expressed some irritation to.' This was a very clever guess, for it was immediately confirmed when the patient said that she had nearly quarrelled with Derek the day before.

Once more, in the next session she was extremely silent and resistant; but in the next (No. 26) she admitted that recently she had been much more aggressive. In the example she gave, of a girl at school who had answered her back, the anger seemed to be quite uncomplicated and straightforward, unlike that in the incident with the bus conductress.

In Session 27 she opened by saying that perhaps the therapist wouldn't believe it, but she had spent the morning trying to convince a friend who was depressed that she should see a psychiatrist, because she herself had been helped so much. She went on to tell of having burst into tears because she had been let down by another friend who had invited her and then cancelled. She reported this as a temporary relapse, but from the point of view of the therapy it marked an extremely important advance: for now her tears were in touch with their cause, which her depressive tears had not been before. Thus, having previously reached uncomplicated anger, she was now able to reach uncomplicated grief. Of course it was not entirely uncomplicated, because it was out of proportion to the immediate cause, and carried with it the fear that this friend was going out of her life. The therapist made the link with the past, and the patient then told of two further nightmares, both about ghosts. The therapists gave her some deeply thought out interpretations, explaining that often the belief that people will come back as ghosts, if they haven't been properly buried, is really about the psychology of the survivors, who haven't dealt with all their memories and feelings about the people who have died.

The patient continued to the end her mixture of extreme resistance and therapeutic alliance. It seems clear that what she was doing was determinedly going at her own pace and never allowing the therapist to take her beyond what she could bear. Thus the last few sessions contained long silences and little communication. In particular, interpretations about feelings of loss at termination produced no response whatsoever.

In the final session, however, she listed a number of changes that seemed to go well beyond the mere lifting of her depression: she said she felt *different* – she could now tell when she was upset, whereas previously she had never been conscious of sadness or unhappiness. Recently a seriously bereaved girl had come to her and the two of them had cried together, and she had felt she was crying for herself as well as for the girl. The other members of staff could see she had been crying but it no longer mattered.

As the reader will see, much of the therapeutic work was indirect. There was really no direct recovery of either grief or ambivalent feelings about any of the three people whom she had lost. Ambivalent feelings and guilt appeared in relation to the *grandmother*; and she became able both to grieve and to be angry about *events in the present*.

This patient illustrates with the utmost clarity the long and complex process of unravelling some aspects of depression, which we may summarize as follows:

The first step, which occurred before she came to us and was a necessary condition to her seeking help, was the conversion of the *manic defence* into *depression* itself; which was followed by the conversion of the deadness and emptiness of depression into *depressive tears*; then the reaching of *ambivalence*, and *guilt*; then *anger*, complicated by *self-hatred*; then *straightforward anger*; and finally the conversion of depressive tears, which are not in touch with their origin, into *healing tears*, which are; in summary, the conversion of depression, which leads nowhere, into *grief*, which leads to *hope* and the possibility of a new life in the future.

This was completely confirmed at 5-year follow-up, which fulfilled all our hopes. The patient had taken the conscious decision to allow herself to become emotionally involved with a man again. She had now been married for two years, and the relation with her husband was loving and full of shared feeling and companionship. She was able to be effectively aggressive when the situation required it. And finally, she was able to be upset at situations as they occurred, with the result that there had never been any recurrence of her depression. (For further details see Malan and Osimo, 1992, pp. 3–6 and 59–65.)

Retrospect of depressive patients

In the light of this therapy, which illustrates so many features of depression and their meaning – and yet, as will be seen, still only scratches the surface – we may look back at some of the patients already described in whom depressive symptoms have been found.

The central feature in this patient was *miscarried grief*; but there was also indirect cumulative evidence that a complicating factor consisted of *ambivalent feelings* towards people close to her, which in turn gave rise to guilt. Because the evidence was so indirect, it is as well to take as our next example a patient in whom this kind of evidence was unequivocal, namely the Daughter with a Stroke (see p. 38). This patient certainly suffered from depression, but the most prominent feature of her illness consisted of severe anxiety attacks in which everything went red before her eyes. It became clear that the precipitating factor had been the death from a stroke of her difficult and dominating mother two years before; and that the central problem was her guilt about her hostility towards her mother, with consequent inability to work through her feelings about her death. There was no doubt about the *hostility*, which was expressed in a dream in which she told her mother she shouldn't be there because she was dead. The *guilt* became manifest from what were essentially two interpretations during the initial interview: the first was the link between the 'redding out' and the patient's fantasy of what it was like to have a stroke, from which it emerged that a recent attack had occurred on the second anniversary of her mother's death; and the second was the suggestion that her fear of *falling into something* expressed her feeling that she ought to be with her mother in the grave, at which she broke down and wept uncontrollably. The attacks of 'redding out' clearly illustrate a mechanism that was described above in connection with Sifneos's Phobic Patient with Dyspnea, namely *taking the other person's illness on oneself*, by some process of guilt-laden identification.

This patient raises a number of further questions: to what extent did she fear *self-punishment*, and to what extent did she fear punishment by some fantasied external agency, a more appropriate term for which would be *retribution*? Equally, if it was self-punishment that she feared, to what extent was this due simply to *guilt* about hating someone close to her, and to what extent was it due to hate conflicting with *love*, which leads more in the direction of *concern, protectiveness, reparation,* and *remorse*? Then, to what extent was her hostility to her mother the product of her mother's controlling and restricting personality, and to what extent was it a reaction to what she felt to be *failure of love and care* on her mother's part? Finally, although there was clearly reason enough for hostile feelings in the direct relation with her mother, to what extent was hostility also complicated by *Oedipal jealousy* in the triangular relation that included her father?

These questions cannot be answered on the evidence available, but they are not idle speculation, as they are given point by such cases as those described in the following paragraphs.

Oedipal depression in women

Depression was the main symptom in the first patient of all, the Economics Student, who as her exams approached began to suffer from attacks in which she felt she was *worthless*; then, just before her exams, she suffered from an uncontrollable fit of weeping brought on by a feeling of *loneliness*; and finally, some two years later, she had a depressive attack, accompanied by a feeling of self-hatred, brought on by a situation of jealousy. There was considerable evidence from her story that her basic problem was *guilt* arising from Oedipal feelings, which was expressed in depressive self-reproaches. The guilt led to the feeling that she could never form a relation with a man, which in turn led to *despair*.

Here we may ask yet another question: to what extent was her guilt simply caused intrinsically by the incestuous element in her feelings about her father, and to what extent was it guilt in relation to her mother? Again this question cannot be answered, but it is given point by a patient already described, the Director's Daughter (see Chapter 7).

In this latter patient the main presenting symptom was anxiety, which during therapy was relieved dramatically on a number of occasions by the expression of hostile feelings against men. This in turn was almost certainly derived from her disappointment in her relation with her father, and there was no evidence that it was accompanied by guilt or remorse, so that it did not contribute directly to her depression. Part of this latter was clearly the result of *despair* consequent upon her inability to form a relation with a man – 'and it seems as if life consists of nothing but washing up and making jam'. But part was the result of her Oedipal strivings conflicting with her deep and genuine love for her mother. During therapy she had the irrational thought that if her mother died she could have her male therapist to herself, which she described in her own words as being accompanied by strong feelings of *remorse*. Equally, she felt that if she went away with a man she would be abandoning her mother to loneliness. Her situation was thus one in which if she formed a relation with a man – which of course was not only what she wanted more than anything in the world but indeed was necessary to her happiness and mental health – she did this at her mother's expense, whom she loved more than anyone in the world. This is one of the central issues in depression, *the individual's need to express instinctual impulses, but only at the expense of someone deeply loved*, an insoluble dilemma from which really the only way out is suicide. This is one of the deepest and most painful of all the conflicts that human beings have inherited, which we shall meet time and again in the following pages.

Oedipal depression in men

Whereas the main psychiatric symptom in Oedipal problems in both sexes is *anxiety*, these last two patients illustrate very clearly the syndrome which may be labelled 'Oedipal depression'. An exactly corresponding syndrome exists in men. The depressive element arises particularly when in addition to the Oedipal rivalry there is a strong element of love for the father (see p. 62 for an example already given). It also arises when love for the father is frustrated and disappointed, which may appear even if the picture of the father is of someone utterly unsympathetic and unpleasant, as in the following example.

The Depressed Tailor

The patient, a married man aged 33, was complaining of attacks of depression about once a year for the past 14 years, in which he had intense feelings of inferiority, found himself unable to converse with people, and lost his capacity to remember things. His father had dominated the whole household, was often out in the evenings, and the patient remembered little contact with him in childhood. Precipitating events for the attacks of depression included: (1) *conflict* with his father while working for him in the family business; (2) *success*: at the age of 25 – as a result of the conflict with his father – he started his own business, did extremely well in the first year, and repaid a large loan, and it was at this point that he became depressed; (3) *being let down by men*: (a) a younger man who worked for him but left, promised to come back, and then let him down; and (b) an older man who had previously worked for him and with whom he had been extremely friendly, who promised to relieve him during a holiday period, let him down at the last moment, and then died (this was the precipitating event for the attack that caused him to seek help).

It is possible to recognize in this story the combination of Oedipal and depressive features. In therapy a constantly recurring theme consisted of asking for guidance and teaching from his male therapist. This was almost certainly a plea that the therapist should make up to him for what he felt his father had never given him. The correct treatment was to make no attempt to give him what he was asking for, but to interpret that the plea for guidance was a defence: an attempt to avoid confronting the therapist with the anger (hidden feeling) which was aroused when he was failed by men, as he had been failed by his father (T/P link). Only by working through the anger in the transference in this way and making the link with the past, was it possible to arm him against future depressive breakdowns. This line of therapy was entirely successful, as was shown by a follow-up several years later.

The Son in Mourning (contd)

A very similar basic conflict was shown by the Son in Mourning (see pp. 71ff. and 80ff.). Here the psychiatric picture in a young man consisted of anxiety and hypochondriasis. The anxiety had first arisen 8 years ago, when he thought he had made a girl pregnant and was terrified of his father's reaction. The hypochondriasis had arisen 3 years ago shortly after his father's death from a heart attack – the patient had become increasingly worried about his health, with the fear that he would die, like his father, 'in the prime of life'. Here the theme was very clear of taking upon himself his father's illness and death – the fear of self-imposed retribution, exactly as found in the Daughter with a Stroke. Oedipal themes concerned with rebellion against his father's authority, and conflict over taking his father's place, became prominent in therapy. In addition, however, there emerged intense frustrated love and mourning for his father, conflicting with Oedipal hostility and anger about being rejected, which revealed that a major component of his illness was depressive in nature.

Depression and rejected love

The complexity of this whole subject is illustrated by the fact that it has been possible to get so far into the present chapter and only now begin to discuss depressive patients in whom *rejected love* lay at the heart of the problem – a situation to which *mourning complicated by anger* is intrinsic, and which therefore can be seen *a priori* to be a likely potent source of depression.

An example was provided by the Farmer's Daughter (p. 37), whose depression was eventually traced to the fact that her current man-friend, with whom she had taken up after dreadful experiences with her psychopathic husband, had first raised her hopes of marriage and had then disappointed them. From what we already know, there is ample reason why this should have given rise to depression, and we would expect to find despair, weeping, and possibly suicidal feelings, all of which were in fact present. But, as has so often been observed, little goes exactly as expected in psychodynamics – which is what makes it both so fascinating and so difficult a subject – and no one would predict that the main manifestation of her depression would be *severe self-reproaches* about the fact that (under pressure from her husband) she had given away her two children.

Depressive self-reproaches

Here we may ask, what on earth is the connection between this symptom and her recent disappointment? This raises the whole difficult problem of the origin of depressive self-reproaches, a problem which has been touched on already and now needs to be considered in more detail.

This question was first considered from a psychodynamic point of view by Freud in one of his most famous papers, Mourning and Melancholia (1917) – a paper which, like most of Freud's writings, shows his strengths of brilliant and profound insight and clarity of expression, together with such weaknesses as clinging to mechanical models of the psyche and offering generalizations without a trace of published evidence.

The passage relevant to depressive self-reproaches is as follows:

> If one listens patiently to the many and various self-accusations of the melancholiac, one cannot in the end avoid the impression that often the most violent of them are hardly at all applicable to the patient himself, but that with insignificant modifications they do fit someone else, some person whom

the patient loves, has loved or ought to love. This conjecture is confirmed every time one examines the facts. So we get the key to the clinical picture – by perceiving that the self-reproaches are reproaches against a loved object which have been shifted on to the patient's own ego.

There is no need to be greatly surprised that among those (self-reproaches) … some genuine self-reproaches are mingled: they are allowed to obtrude themselves since they help to mask others and make recognition of the true state of affairs impossible …

From this and similar statements has grown the generalization, so often heard, that 'depression is aggression turned against the self'. Is it true?

I hope that enough has been said hitherto concerning the complexities of depression to make clear that at best this is a facile statement which can only be a fraction of the truth. It is also important to note, first, that Freud was writing about 'melancholia' i.e., what we would now call psychotic or severe endogenous depression, and therefore that he was probably referring to the kinds of persecutory self-accusation that approach or attain the quality of delusions; second, that *neurotic* self-accusations may not be the same thing, and third that Freud quite specifically says that not *all* self-accusations, even in melancholics, necessarily fit the pattern that he is postulating.

Now I have no evidence to offer from this kind of very severe depression; but it is often true that milder or more transitory symptoms give clues about the meaning of symptoms that have become severe enough to have really taken the patient over, as in psychoses or severe neuroses. It is therefore worth while to examine some examples of self-accusations in depressive patients, with Freud's hypothesis in mind.

An example of a patient suffering from self-criticism has already been met in the Divorced Mother. Towards the beginning of Session 1, for instance, she spoke about being *angry with herself* for her inability to function in therapy, and the therapist made a direct interpretation of the hidden feeling, saying that she must be *angry with him* for putting her in this situation. To this she made no response. In Session 3 she spoke of feeling very bad about not writing to her son, and followed this with the self-criticism that her reason for not doing so was selfish. The therapist said that she was criticizing herself in order to *forestall his criticism of her*; and she then admitted that she didn't write *in order to make her ex-husband angry*, i.e. it was an aggressive act, expressing her own anger with him for robbing her of her son. In Session 6 the therapist gave her the interpretation that she might be angry if she were not the preferred one, and that this would then be one of her reasons for forestalling criticism, by criticizing herself. Her reply was to say that this might be right, that this made her a horrible person, and that *because she could not be what she really wanted she disliked herself*. There was of course abundant evidence during the course of this therapy that underneath her helpless exterior she was an extremely angry and jealous person.

A second example is from a young woman who had been put on the waiting list for psychotherapy but asked for an urgent appointment because she had suddenly become depressed. It emerged at interview that the precipitating cause for her depression had been her anger and jealousy at her flatmate and the latter's boy-friend, who had been making love together all week-end in the flat, while she herself was left alone. Each time she spoke of this her stream of talk quickly passed over into saying what a horrible person she was for thinking like this.

A third example is as follows:

A male patient who fulfilled all the criteria for brief psychotherapy had been set a time limit of 6 months, had worked extremely hard at his therapy, had made remarkable progress, and had been discharged as planned, apparently grateful for the help he had received. Some months later he returned in a state of quite severe depression. One of the things that he said to his male therapist was, 'You must be very disappointed in me'. It was not difficult to give him the interpretation that surely what he really meant was that *he was very disappointed in his therapist and his therapy*. This led almost at once to the overtly expressed feeling that he had been discharged prematurely, that he did not like having the length of therapy controlled by the therapist, nor the rigid way in which the therapist had stuck to his time limit, and that if he were to return to therapy he wanted the discharge to be in his own control. The theme of therapy had been entirely concerned with the patient's relation with his father, including, repeatedly, the T/P link. Now shortly after the above work, it emerged very clearly how the patient felt considerably deprived at the hands of his *mother*, which gave the opportunity for another T/P link. The depression lifted at once.

This sequence of events fulfils all of the 'Koch's postulates' formulated above (see p. 118): the symptom is understandable in terms of known mechanisms, these are put to the patient in the form of an interpretation, the hidden feeling emerges overtly, and there is an immediate therapeutic effect.

The foregoing examples show a number of distinct but related mechanisms. In all of them the hidden feeling is *anger* in conflict with *guilt*, and in all of them the guilt is emphasized at the expense of the anger, with the aim of either avoiding anger altogether or at least avoiding the expression of it. In other words the guilt, which represents one side of the conflict, is used as a *defence*. Moreover in the third example the self-accusation – as in Freud's hypothesis – exactly fits the hidden accusation against the other person. This is thus an example of the 'return of the repressed', in which the manifest symptom, originally intended purely as a defence, so to speak, takes on the hidden expression of the feeling it is intended to avoid. According to this formulation, the depressive self-reproaches can be seen to represent a *fusion between anger and guilt* – the guilt is manifest, and the anger is expressed against the self. If this is true, then it may well be that suicide at least sometimes represents this mechanism taken to its ultimate conclusion.

It does seem, therefore, as if Freud's hypothesis sometimes fits the milder self-accusations found in neurotic depression. With the help of these observations we may now return to the Farmer's Daughter (see pp. 37ff.). Here the content of her self-accusations was intense preoccupation with guilt about giving away her two children, and the precipitating factor was disappointment at the hands of her man-friend, Len. If we now change the words 'giving away' to 'abandoning' we suddenly see that her self-accusation *might* in fact fit her hidden accusation against Len, though this interpretation was never thought of until I began to write the present chapter, and no direct confirmation was ever obtained in therapy. (For two more, clearer, examples, see the Mother of Four, p. 169, and the Fostered Irish Girl, p. 252.)

No systematic evidence has ever been collected on the subject of how often self-accusations fit Freud's hypothesis and how often they do not; still less on how often suicidal impulses represent aggressive feelings against another person turned against the self. These are examples yet again of the uncritical acceptance of psychoanalytic theory as laid down by the founder.

Suicide

However this may be, the subject of self-accusations may be used to introduce a fundamental principle in the therapy of almost every case of depression, particularly when suicide is an issue: that what the therapist needs to reach, by every means in his power, is *hidden anger against someone whom the patient needs or loves* – or in Freud's words, *has* loved or *ought* to love. Moreover, in psychotherapy of any depth, this is likely to be reached in the first place through the *transference* (for an example see the Man with School Phobia, p. 226). As has been mentioned above, this mixture of love and hate for the same person is one of the deepest and most painful conflicts that human beings suffer from, and depressive patients will do everything in their power to avoid it.

The forces in the individual opposing the acknowledgement of this anger or hate are of many different kinds. There is first of all simply the *pain of conflict*; there is *guilt*, already mentioned many times; and there are all the offshoots of love, which include *sadness* and *grief, concern, tenderness, remorse, protectiveness, compassion*, and the *need for reparation*; and in the end these may lead to the ultimate sacrifice, the feeling that one will kill oneself rather than acknowledge, or bear the pain of, or give expression to, the impulse to harm the other person.

Defensive use of genuine feelings in depression: A Man of Sorrows

As I have foreshadowed several times already, one of the important features of depression is that these *genuine* feelings such as grief and concern can be over-emphasized and used defensively in order to hide the anger underneath. And yet, although these feelings are genuine, because they are not in touch with the anger they are also false, and until they can be integrated with the anger they are of no use therapeutically.

In the first session of his analysis a male patient broke down as there came into his mind the line from Omar Khayyam:

Nor all thy *tears* wash out a word of it.

and it later emerged that many similar quotations had a special significance for him:

We need never be ashamed of our *tears*, for they are rain upon the blinding dust of earth, overlying our hard hearts.

(which moment of poetry in prose comes from *Great Expectations*).

During his analysis it became clear that this had to do not only with his own tears, but with his profound compassion for his mother's tears after the death of his father. Yet the de-repression of such feelings had only a limited therapeutic effect. A clue about why this might be was given by another theme that crept into these quotations; for instance the last line of Schubert's song, *Am Meer* (By the Sea), from a poem by Heine,

vergiftet mit ihren Tränen

which means (freely translated in the context), poisoned by her tears; and still more, by the English song, *Henry my son*, perhaps the bitterest folk song ever written, in which a lover tells his mother of being poisoned by his mistress, and the refrain beginning *Oh make my bed* takes on a shattering new meaning in the last verse:

How shall I make your bed, Henry my son?
How shall I make your bed, my beloved one?
Long, deep and narrow, long, deep and narrow.
  Oh make my bed, I am sick to the heart,
  And I fain would lie down.

This now put in context something that occurred during the course of his analysis, when, by some unexplained rearrangement of internal forces, he quite suddenly became aware that he was spoiling his whole life out of resentment about the permanent loss of closeness with his mother caused by his father's death; and for a few hours he felt free from this, and experienced an intense inner clarity of thought and feeling which transformed the whole world for him. The effect was temporary and was never recaptured.

The helping profession syndrome

A particularly common example of the use of these genuine feelings for a defensive purpose occurs in what I call the *helping profession syndrome*, whereby the individual devotes his life to giving to others the care and concern he would like to have for himself. He then frequently comes to treatment when he breaks down into depression, accompanied by conscious resentment about the demands being made on him. This theme will be taken up in the next chapter (see p. 161).

14

Regression and long-term therapy

So far the major clinical examples have mostly been taken from once-a-week, time-limited therapy, in which patient and therapist sit face to face. In this kind of therapy the patient rarely needs to be given any instructions, but simply understands that he is asked to talk. Patients assigned to brief psychotherapy are very carefully selected, and, as the reader will have seen, they yield nothing to any other kind of patient in intensity of interaction, particularly in the transference, and depth of feeling. They can thus be used to illustrate almost all the phenomena of dynamic psychotherapy. What is the difference, then, between this type of therapy and long-term therapy, in which the patient is seen several times a week over a period of years, lies on the couch, and is given the 'fundamental rule' of psychoanalysis, namely to say everything that comes into his mind? Perhaps the reader might consider the following three clinical examples from this point of view.

The Mental Welfare Officer

This was a male social worker aged 30, in treatment with a female therapist. The following two sessions were taken from towards the end of the first year of three-times-a-week therapy.

In recent months there had been repeated quarrels with his wife, the theme of which had always been an exactly symmetrical conflict: the urgency of *his* needs, which are guilt-laden, conflicting with *hers*, which are resented and felt as unreasonable *demands*, though in turn he feels he ought to meet them. With roles reversed, she of course feels exactly the same; and a vicious circle of resentment and guilt has been set up between them, which is in turn affecting the two children. Taking note of his occupation, the reader should immediately recognize an example of the *helping profession syndrome* mentioned at the end of the previous chapter.

At this stage of therapy, the two other corners of the triangle of person must be taken into account: first, it had recently emerged that the patient felt his *mother* to have been dissatisfied with her life and to have laid the burden of her needs onto her relation with the children – which obviously would account for his present conflict with his wife – and second, almost certainly another factor in the situation is the patient's *dissatisfaction in his relation with the therapist*, which of course he cannot reasonably express, so that his resentment

154

has been displaced onto his wife, exacerbating the tension between them. It is thus an example both of *acting out* and of *transference*.

Here it needs to be said that in fact this kind of tension had been present between the patient and his wife long before he ever came to therapy; and at this point anyone inexperienced in psychotherapy, quite reasonably applying the principle of economy of hypothesis, might ask what is the evidence that there is anything to do with transference in the present situation whatsoever? As I have said above many times, however, in psychotherapy one must not be deceived by this excellent scientific principle. Long and salutary experience has shown generations of psychotherapists that if this kind of situation is missed – and it is very easy to miss, as I myself have reason to know – the consequences may well be intensification of the acting out to the point at which it becomes uncontrollable, and deadlock in the therapy, with the result that relations outside and the therapy itself are put in serious jeopardy. In this particular case the evidence for the importance of transference came from later events, and as will be seen was overwhelming.

In the session with which we are here concerned, the patient gave a now familiar account of quarrels with his wife, in which the above theme appeared over and over again. When he had finished, the therapist gave him the required O/T interpretation, spelling out the nature of the defence, implying the anxiety, and specifically mentioning the hidden feeling, that he was expressing towards his wife the *resentment that he could not express towards his therapist*, which was about his not getting the attention he wanted from her, as shown for instance by the coming summer break and the fact that one day treatment would end.

This deepened rapport, immediately freed the patient from his rather repetitive account of external events, and enabled him to give far more than a simple confirmation of the interpretation. He said, '*The ending I feel most is the ending of each session.*' He went on to say that on every occasion he feels in a daze and needs time to recover, and that his feeling is twofold: (1) a feeling of *relief*, because by the end of the session he feels he has *given as much as he can*; and (2) a feeling of *hurt* because his therapist is sending him off and as much as saying 'that's enough now, off you go'. He goes on to elaborate on (1), and the therapist, spotting that this is an example of the defence of emphasizing the easier half of the conflict in order to hide the more difficult half, in her turn emphasizes the hurt about being dismissed, which he can't express so easily. To this he says that it's not reasonable to express such feelings, because the therapeutic relation is one that has been set up especially for him, so how can he complain? He then himself spontaneously makes the T/P link, saying that this reminds him of how his mother gave him the feeling that she existed only for his sake – so how could he protest, after all that she had done for him? In a previous session he had described his view of his mother as an isolated, friendless person, who didn't get enough from her husband and turned to the children for compensation.

In the next session the therapist began by saying that after the coming holiday break she would have to change the regular time of one of the sessions, and offered two alternative times. She explains that this is because of someone else's timetable, which she has to fit in with.

In reply to this the patient mentions work commitments which would make both alternative times difficult for him, and goes on to describe a difficult interview with a young man who had ended up in tears because his father wouldn't have him home for Christmas – our patient had a sense of being 'crowded' and 'jostled', and this had been intensified by being literally jostled in a small busy shop.

Here the therapist interpreted that the patient felt jostled and pushed by her request for a change of time, on top of all the other demands he had to meet; and, in an attempt to get at angry feelings, said that perhaps he wanted to hit back when he was pushed in this way. This the patient denied, but he went on to say that he couldn't protest if there was someone else who had to be given his time, he just had to accept it.

At this point the therapist, who had known how the patient would react and felt very badly about having to change the time, acknowledged openly to him that she had had to explain the reason for it because of how she felt.

The patient now said how difficult the alternative times were for him; but he reiterated that he couldn't protest, adding the important new detail that if he did so, he felt that it would only result in her 'preferring the other person even more'. This is an example of the way in which intense transference feelings, essentially derived from childhood, get drawn into what would otherwise be a relatively simple piece of reality. (The reason for the change of time was in fact that the therapist had to fit in with the time of a clinical meeting, and it was a particular colleague whom she was considering rather than another patient.)

The therapist, correctly, intensified the language of childhood by saying that as he felt, 'if she loved him at all she would do what he wants and needs her to do.' This interpretation was entirely confirmed – the patient says that it's an all or nothing thing and he does feel unloved, but powerless to do anything about it.

The therapist then pointed out that he hadn't considered another way of proceeding, namely that he should put forward some times of his own and see if she could fit in with them. This, he says, he couldn't possibly do, because she is *giving* the sessions to him, and anyhow the only time he can think of would be an evening time, and he isn't sure that he himself wants to give up this time, let alone ask it of *her*. He comes back to this several times and eventually says that he is aware of trying to push her into offering that time to see if she is willing to make a sacrifice for him, when he is not at all sure that if she did offer it he would want to accept it. The therapist, again trying to get at angry feelings, suggests that his proposal of this time was really a way of equalizing things between him and her, rather than actually asking for something he wanted. He agreed with this, and now responded by coming closer to the possibility of angry feelings, saying that if she had offered him the evening time he might well have said that he didn't want it anyway. He then himself made an important link to one of his life problems going back to childhood, namely his habit of sulking – which of course often consists of rejecting the other person after being rejected oneself – rather than expressing his anger directly.

He went on to say that if he did come at another time he would probably arrive late and not talk about how he really felt, as a kind of 'passive resistance'. The therapist said that on the contrary, this would be a pretty active way of making her and the treatment unimportant; and, having now clarified the conflict in the transference, she apparently correctly proceeded to make the T/O/P link, namely the comparison with how he currently behaved with his *wife* and how he used to behave with his *mother*. The patient, however, showed that there was still unfinished business in the transference, saying it had crossed his mind that the therapist really had set the whole thing up in order to test him, and would then go on to tell him that the treatment had finished. He then said an extraordinary thing, that he feels 'demolished and childlike', and 'if the two of them stood up now he would just about come up to her knee.'

Towards the end of the session he began employing one of the many depressive defences mentioned in the previous chapter, reproaching *himself* for his selfishness, rather than reproaching *her*, which the therapist interpreted. He ended up by saying another extraordinary thing: he was afraid to refuse to change the session time because if he did he would have won a victory and then *she* would be utterly dependent on *him* – he would have made her into some sort of slave and this would mean *he* would have to take all the decisions, and this frightened him. This was the end of the session.

The Carpenter's Daughter (contd)

The patient may be remembered from Chapter 9 (see p. 79), where she was used in illustration of the use of transference interpretation to remove a block to communication in the early stages of therapy. This previous session was taken from a course of once a week psychotherapy with a time limit of about 30 sessions; but this plan had proved unrealistic, and she was later assigned to long-term therapy at three times a week with a second therapist, also female. The following is an account of the 46th session of the second course of therapy.

In fact the patient had shown repeated evidence that her life consisted largely of a struggle between her attempts to get some *satisfaction* for herself on the one hand, and the exhaustion consequent upon the need to meet the *demands* that seemed to come from every quarter on the other – demands simply to get up and get dressed, to look after herself, to get to work, and to cope with a job which as far as 'objective' reality was concerned, was far below her capacity and could not be seen as being demanding at all. One can formulate such a struggle as being concerned essentially with the 'emotional balance of payments'. One of the very few satisfactions in her very isolated life was provided by her therapy, and at the same time even this could become a demand, as was illustrated very clearly by the next passage.

The present session was the first after the patient's return from a visit to her parents in the North of England, a previous session having been cancelled by the therapist. The patient opened with a distressed account of how she had been trying to work out her feelings about her parents, but this had all got lost in the last two days because of the heat, to which she is very sensitive. This was an example of one of the major features of her current life, namely her tremendous struggle to keep going at all.

The therapist clarified the struggle and linked it with the transference, saying that the heat and the feelings about her family are *demanding* a lot of her, and to have missed the previous session must have made it all the more difficult.

This interpretation was immediately effective, as the patient became calmer and remained quiet for about 5 minutes. However, it was only partly effective, for when she resumed, the theme was the same: the difficulty of adjusting back to life in London – everyone else seemed to manage, but she is by now nearly exhausted – she wants to think about her family but the heat gets in the way, she can hardly stand, she gets panicky feelings, and her skin feels as if it is burning.

Here the therapist, realizing that what was left out in the previous interpretation was that *even therapy was felt to be too much of a demand*, said that she thought the patient was speaking about her need to be able to make use of lying on the couch to take some rest here in the session.

At this the patient visibly relaxes and remains quiet and apparently resting for about ten minutes. Now when she speaks, having had the satisfaction of being properly understood, her associations turn from 'bad' to 'good'. She speaks of how she now realizes that her visit to home had really gone very well – it must be to do with coming here. Her relations with her father and siblings had been surprisingly satisfactory. On the other hand, she feels confused about the relation with her mother, to whom she feels close in one way yet somehow in a different world in another.

The therapist now linked this once more with the transference (P/T interpretation), saying that the patient was speculating about what relation she already has and might have in the future both with her actual mother and with her therapeutic mother, and part of the confusion is the contrast between the image that she has in her mind, on the one hand, and her actual experience, on the other.

Again there is a long pause, after which the patient starts speaking in a quietly anxious way of her uncertainty about her summer holiday – she is not going home for any length of time, she won't be coming here, and she feels 'empty' about it.

The therapist here emphasizes the patient's feelings about missing therapy, when she, the therapist goes on holiday. The patient agrees, but says there's more to it than that: she has the problem of fitting in both with the demands of work and with visits of other relatives at home – she must see to it that she doesn't burden her mother too much.

The therapist emphasizes the patient's problem of competing with the needs of other people, that she must feel 'squeezed out' by the other relatives at home and must have similar feelings when the therapist goes on holiday, and even when the latter cancels a session, though of course she is in further conflict because of her need not to burden the therapist any more than her mother.

The patient says, 'That's just it', and is silent for the last few minutes of the session.

The Cricketer

This was a married man in his late thirties being treated by a male therapist at five times a week. The sessions are taken from the fifth year of treatment.

In the first session the patient opened with some denunciations of the lack of generosity of private banks in giving money to charity. The therapist interpreted this as referring to himself, saying that the patient felt that what was given to him in therapy was given unwillingly, which aroused his fury and made it very difficult to receive anything. There were in this clear implications, which both patient and therapist knew without having to spell them out, of the therapist's being seen as a 'bad mother'. Shortly after this the patient went to sleep on the couch.

The phenomenon of going to sleep during the sessions had been a prominent feature for many months. It usually seemed to happen when the patient felt he had been understood.

Another phenomenon, which also happened now, was for the patient to wake up briefly, mutter something, and immediately go to sleep again. On this occasion he said something about somebody 'having him round the middle'. When he eventually woke up, some ten minutes later, the therapist asked him about this. He said that he had been dreaming of being tackled at rugby football.

Since this was concerned with a symbolic fight between two men, the therapist made a tentative interpretation about himself and the patient being rivals. The patient then greatly intensified the implications, giving an association to the idea of *poison being poured into someone's ear*, which in his somewhat fuddled state he momentarily thought was a reference to *Macbeth* rather than *Hamlet*.

It is worthwhile examining the implications of this concentrated communication. The patient has had a dream about a struggle between two men. The therapist has introduced the idea of *rivalry*, which the patient – having received many such interpretations before – knows perfectly well is leading towards Oedipal conflicts. He has just been *asleep*, and his next association is to something from Hamlet, where the King is murdered while *asleep*, which in turn he mistakes for Macbeth. The link between Hamlet and Macbeth is of course that in both plays a 'good' king is murdered in his sleep. Moreover, since the patient had a serious conflict with his own father, he is essentially identified with the son against the father, and hence, by association, with the murderer in both plays. Yet his own father was always represented as a 'bad figure', and in this case the association is to the murder of a 'good figure'. Moreover, the dream occurred in the setting of his having been understood by the male therapist. We may therefore suppose that a major issue is the patient's *guilt* about hostile feelings towards the therapist, which persist in spite of the therapist's adopting the role of helper. Finally, in the dream the patient is the potential *victim*, and moreover it is the *patient* who has been asleep, so that the fear is of himself being murdered in his sleep, apparently in retaliation or retribution for his hostile feelings against the therapist, who here seems to represent *both a good and a bad father*.

There are two phenomena here which Freud wrote about in the early days of psychoanalysis. The first is that mistakes like slips of the tongue – here muddling up two different Shakespeare plays – are often not just chance occurrences, but are the resultant of identifiable forces, as they obviously are in this particular case. The second is the extraordinary wealth of significance that can be concentrated into a single communication. It has taken me about 20 lines of typescript to elucidate a communication that took less than three lines to describe. As already mentioned (see p. 10), this phenomenon was named by Freud *condensation*.

The therapist therefore interpreted that when the patient fell asleep, he (the therapist) was first seen as a *good mother* who had understood him; but that then the patient had to deal with his perception of the therapist as a *rival man* who might murder him in his sleep.

In further associations the patient now compared his sleep to that of a baby or a cat, just curled up enjoying itself, i.e. with the implication of the therapist being seen once more as a *good mother*. Later he spoke of having fallen asleep with his head on the shoulder of a girl-friend, and another girl-friend who had fallen asleep with her head on his. Thus, his anxieties having been interpreted, sleep had become no longer something dangerous but something to do with love, trust and fulfilment.

Next day the therapist reminded him of the events of the previous session: how he had had to cope with the fear of being murdered by the therapist while asleep, but that later he seemed to be considering the possibility that going to sleep might not be dangerous but might express a warm and loving relationship. Within a moment the patient was asleep once more.

This time he was suddenly woken up as the telephone rang in the room. He wondered aloud what sort of things the therapist thought of while he, the patient, was sleeping. The therapist's account of the session continues as follows: 'I suggested that the question in his mind was whether my attention was still on him, or whether I wandered off into my own thoughts. I then reminded him of how he often wakes up and makes some odd remark and goes to sleep again as soon as I reply. I suggested that this was to make sure I was still there and still available for him. He smiled and said that, when he was small, people (his mother or a nanny) used to sit with him after he went to bed, but would try and tiptoe out when they thought he was asleep.'

Discussion

Once-a-week, time-limited, psychotherapy on the one hand, and long-term therapy at several times a week on the other, really represent a continuum, and there is little or nothing in these sessions that distinguishes absolutely between the two. Nevertheless there are a number of phenomena whose intensity makes it likely that these sessions are taken from intensive long-term therapy and nothing else.

These phenomena, and other issues into which they lead, are discussed below.

Regression and dependence

As will have become evident from practically all the examples already given in this book, most current conflicts are found to have roots in childhood, and the link with the past is an essential part of psychotherapy. Moreover, attachment to the therapist, and dependence on him (or her) develops rapidly in many patients, and is thus often a major feature even of brief psychotherapy. But the intensity and quality of the dependence in these three examples, and the way in which the patients were temporarily but utterly taken over by it, are characteristic features of the long-term therapy of a particular kind of patient, namely those who have suffered a greater or lesser degree of childhood deprivation. This is an aspect of the phenomenon known as 'regression'.

Thus the Mental Welfare Officer showed some of the 'normal', 'adult', reactions to the proposed change of time, such as protesting and bargaining, but in addition he said he felt 'demolished' and 'childlike' and that he would 'just about come up to the therapist's knee'; and he interpreted the whole situation in extraordinarily black-and-white terms, saying that if he refused he would 'make his therapist into a slave', utterly dependent on him. The Carpenter's Daughter was in a state of such regression that she had to rest and be symbolically mothered before she could even express herself to her therapist. And the Cricketer did not merely *rest* but actually fell *asleep* during the session, later very clearly and explicitly linking this with his need to have someone sit with him while he was asleep, when he was a little boy.

These considerations lead into the next section, which represents an example of a particular kind of conflict frequently encountered in regressed patients; and this in turn will lead to an important question that applies to long-term therapy in particular, namely the meaning of the term 'corrective emotional experience'.

'Needs' and 'demands'

A new-born child is a mass of needs – to be fed and held and kept warm and kept clean – is entirely dependent on the people in his environment to see that these needs are met, and (as far as we know) is not equipped even to perceive the needs of others, let alone to meet them. The most important thing he can give is the satisfaction of being seen to respond to the care that he is *given* – a satisfactory state of affairs indeed. On the other hand, when he is grown up, a substantial portion of his life will consists of putting aside his own needs and impulses and taking responsibility for those of others. How is the transition effected? The answer seems to be that there are two essential requirements. He must first be *given enough* – his *needs* must be met sufficiently. The second is that he must then be initiated gently, firmly, and at the correct rate, into the realization that not all his *demands* can be met at once, if at all, and that other people have needs as well as him. He in turn will experience this second requirement as a *demand*, which of course it is.

If the second requirement is carried out too slowly, or ineffectively, or not at all, he is likely to become spoiled and selfish, and unable to tolerate frustration. If the first requirement is not met, and/or if the second is carried out too quickly or brutally, he will be genuinely deprived, will be full of unsatisfied *needs*, and intolerant of *demands*. This conflict between *needs* and *demands* is likely to play a major part, one way or another, in his later life, and will of course become a major issue in psychotherapy.

One type of situation that this conflict leads to is what I both humorously and seriously call the *helping profession syndrome* (see also p. 153), which is a derivative of Bowlby's 'compulsive care-giving' (see Bowlby, 1977). Here the individual defends himself against the conflict by a form of over-compensation, i.e. he compulsively gives to others what he would like to have for himself, which of course leads to a severe deficit in the emotional balance of payments. Other people's *needs* then begin to be felt as *demands*, and the individual is likely to break down into guilt-laden resentment, leading to depression. When two such people come together, the consequences may well be a perpetual struggle about whose needs are going to be met by the other, as in the first of the above examples, the Mental Welfare Officer. As mentioned above, this is a constantly recurring theme in psychotherapy, and the more intensive and longer term the therapy is, the more intensely it will be manifested in the transference. This is shown both by the Mental Welfare Officer and by the second example, the Carpenter's Daughter. In the first, a change of time leads to the issue of whose needs are going to be met, which is described in the most extraordinarily intense and black-and-white terms; in the second, the patient at first has nothing left over even to *speak* to the therapist, which is felt as an impossible demand from which she must withdraw. The therapist recognizes this need, and sits sharing the silence until the patient is ready to speak again. When she does so, the theme of what she says has changed from *complaint* to *satisfaction*. This symbolic mothering, and its effects, lead at once into the next heading.

The 'corrective emotional experience'

This is a term introduced by Alexander and French (1946), in the following words:

> ... reexperiencing the old, unsettled conflict *but with a new ending* is the secret of every penetrating therapeutic result. Only the actual experience of a new solution in the transference situation or in his everyday life gives the patient the conviction that a new solution is *possible* and induces him to give up the old neurotic patterns.

Ever since this passage was written it has been the subject of misinterpretation and controversy. Almost certainly what the authors meant can be illustrated by the example of the Mental Welfare Officer. Here the patient had married a woman suffering from problems similar to his own, and the result was a relentless *vicious circle* of quarrels about needs and demands, from which – without therapeutic help – it was difficult to see any escape other than separation. When such a patient comes into therapy the same issues arise with the utmost intensity in the transference relationship. Obviously, if the therapist reacts in the same way as the wife, another vicious circle will be set up, and the whole situation will perpetuate itself. However, because the therapist is not involved with the patient in the same way as his wife is, and because she has (one hopes) at least partly overcome any similar problems she may have had, she *reacts in a way that breaks the vicious circle* and enables the patient's problem to be understood and worked through. This is almost certainly what Alexander and French meant by the phrase 'with a new ending'.

The question is now whether they also meant more than this. Here let us reverse the sexes but retain the difference between therapist and patient so that 'he' and 'she' distinguish the two. The above phrase has often been interpreted as meaning that the therapist must actively *give* something to the patient, must go out of his way to be kind to her, must mother her, or father her, to make up for what she has missed. Is this true?

This is a very controversial question, and its history needs to be considered in some depth. Freud's original dictum, written in 1915, was that 'The treatment must be carried through in a state of abstinence', by which he meant that the patient must be given unconditional acceptance and understanding, and *nothing else*.

Now this means, of course, that although the therapist's actual interventions consist of nothing but making interpretations, he is usually giving a great deal of warmth and support; and moreover, unconditional acceptance and deep understanding are both very potent gifts which the patient is most unlikely to have ever experienced before. Therefore in a sense the therapist is in reality making-up to the patient for things that she has missed in the past. But although this is true, there is a great deal that the therapist does not give – in particular he resolutely refuses to yield to demands for such things as advice, interventions in her life, and of course any active expression of love, neither verbal nor – above all – physical.

What, then, is the aim of therapy in patients of this kind? The answer seems to be very similar to the aim in patients suffering from depression due to miscarried grief, such as the Nurse in Mourning described in Chapter 13. It may be recalled that this patient had suffered three traumatic losses, culminating in the recent death of her fiancé in an accident. Here there are two important things to note: first, no one can bring her fiancé back; and second, at present no one can make up to her for the loss of her fiancé, because she is in no fit state to accept anyone who tries – again it may be recalled that she had deliberately broken off a relation with a man for fear that history might repeat itself once more. How then can she get well? The answer is that she has to be helped to experience and work through her feelings about the loss. Only then can she overcome what she has suffered and be receptive to any opportunities that her life may offer in the future.

Almost exactly the same two statements can be made about the majority of patients whose childhood has been unsatisfactory. First, quite possibly no one – and certainly not the therapist – can make up to them for what they have missed; and second, even if opportunities are offered for some kind of recompense, the patients are in no state to make use of them – like the patient in the Imaginary Therapy described in Chapter 10 they are liable to spoil them in some way. That, of course, is the basic reason why they have come for help. It might be thought, therefore, that there is nothing that can be done, but – in many cases at any rate – this is not true. What can be done is the same as in such patients as the Nurse in Mourning: their grief and (above all) their anger about past deprivations need to be experienced and worked through. It is then found empirically that they can be brought to the point of accepting those satisfactions that life can offer, even though these may often be nowhere near the recompense that they would like. Put briefly, *the aim of therapy is not to make up to patients for the love that they have missed, but to help them work through their feelings about not having it.*

There is also a feature here that was not present overtly in the Nurse in Mourning, namely that the person in relation to whom this grief and anger are worked through is the therapist. It used to be one of Winnicott's striking and paradoxical epigrams that the function of the therapist was not to *succeed* but to *fail*. This is a profound truth dressed up to sound absurd. Of course it does not mean that he must fail as a *therapist*, but as a *substitute parent*. The therapist can never make up to his patient for what they have suffered in the past, but what he *can* do is to repeat the failure to love them enough – which, after all, is intrinsic in the therapeutic situation – and then share with them and help them work through their feelings about his failure. This is perhaps the most important aspect of the 'new ending'.

When this goes well there occurs a change that in some ways consists merely of a change in emphasis, but in reality is a striking and dramatic transformation, heralding the beginning of a crucial therapeutic process: the patient, instead of perceiving only the 'bad' aspects of the therapeutic situation, e.g. the frustration and deprivation of the therapist's professional objectivity, becomes aware of, and able to make use of, the true satisfactions that she is offered, namely the therapist's unconditional acceptance and understanding. These now begin to represent the experience of being loved, and are felt to enrich her and to provide her with resources that she can use throughout her life in the future. This phenomenon is intimately linked with the 'depressive position', which will be a central theme of Chapters 15 and 16 (see pp. 153ff., 198–9, 202–4).

Let us return to Freud's dictum about abstinence. It needs to be remembered that psychoanalysis was originally developed as a treatment by male therapists for female patients suffering from hysteria. Here a basic problem usually consisted of intense, guilt-laden, unfulfilled sexual feelings, with an incestuous component, which were often crystallized in a real or imaginary childhood seduction by an adult. These feelings arose rapidly in the transference, and were expressed in powerful sexual fantasies and hidden or overt demands that the male therapist should respond. Thus (as already mentioned – see p. 74) the first patient of all, Anna O, developed an intense attachment to her therapist, Breuer, which he himself found difficult to resist; had a phantom pregnancy of which Breuer was clearly the phantom father; began to come between Breuer and his marriage; and finally embraced him and caused him such alarm that he threw up this work altogether and never returned to it. Freud had the courage, like Odysseus faced with the Sirens, to tie himself to the mast (there being no one else to do it for him); and to go on to accept, work through, trace to their origin, and never to respond to, his patients' intense demands for direct love and physical contact; and when he did so he found he could resolve the situation. Once more, this is an example of a 'new ending', though very different from that imagined or consciously desired by the patient.

Of course, where the patient's feelings are sexual, it is quite wrong and indeed dangerous to yield to them in any way, even symbolically. But when the patient is in a temporary state of regression, it can be a crucial part of therapy to give a parent's care in ways that are essentially symbolic, do not step beyond the bounds of the therapeutic situation, and yet are something more than just making interpretations. This is shown in two of the above examples: in the Carpenter's Daughter the therapist made an interpretation that in effect gave the patient permission to rest; while the Cricketer was actually allowed to sleep. In both cases the 'fundamental rule' of free association was temporarily abandoned; and in both cases the therapist did far more than just stop making interpretations, on the contrary creating an atmosphere in which she (or he) *watched over* the patient like a mother with a child.

Transference and the transference neurosis

After choosing these three sessions and summarizing them I discovered that they show yet another characteristic feature, which may be verified by the interested reader, namely that every single intervention by the therapist contains a reference to the transference. This is neither a necessary nor a sufficient condition for identifying long-term therapy – much non-transference work can continue in long-term therapy, and there may be periods of short-term therapy that concentrate entirely upon the transference – but nevertheless it is mainly in long-term therapy that this phenomenon occurs. As has been illustrated particularly in Chapter 9, transference feelings may develop the moment a psychotherapeutic situation is set up, but once intensive therapy has continued for some time, transference often becomes intensified to the point that every communication in the therapy, and indeed many significant actions outside it, possess a transference component. In other words, much of the patient's life is taken up with working over his relation with the therapist. This is what Freud referred to as the *transference neurosis*.

There is of course nothing absolute about this phenomenon – it forms a continuum with the kind of transference illustrated in previous chapters; there is no definite point at which it is possible to say that 'transference' ends and 'transference neurosis' begins; and in many sessions of long-term therapy the central point of feeling is concerned not with transference but with one of the other two corners of the triangle of person. Nevertheless its existence does mean that the therapist needs to be even more on his guard than ever not to miss the transference component in the patient's communications or behaviour. This applies particularly, even in the early stages of therapy, where some new behaviour appears in the patient's life outside, or some old behaviour is intensified, both of which may represent instances of *acting out*. Characteristic examples are when a young female patient, early in her treatment with a male therapist, starts an affair with a much older man; or when a patient, while showing exaggerated high regard for the therapist or the therapy, starts quarrelling with some person outside. This latter is likely to be an example of 'splitting' of the transference, 'good' feelings appearing manifestly in therapy, while 'bad' feelings, which also are aroused by the therapist, are directed elsewhere.

As has already been mentioned, it is absolutely essential that the transference component in this kind of phenomenon should be brought out by interpretation as soon as possible. If it is not, on the one hand therapy will reach deadlock, and on the other the patient may get more and more caught up in inappropriate behaviour in his life outside which may damage himself, other people, or both. Inexperienced therapists may find this difficult since the transference component is often not at all obvious, and they may feel they are flying in the face of common sense – after all, why shouldn't a female patient become attracted by an older man, or a male patient quarrel with a wife whose behaviour has always been unreasonable anyhow? Therapists who feel like this can be helped by remembering both that such phenomena are not absolute – of course some older men are likely to be attractive and wives infuriating in their own right – and also that most interpretations are essentially experiments and can be given in the form of direct or implied questions: 'I wonder if part of what is happening is that your relation with me is stirring up sexual feelings in you, which contribute to your attraction for this man', and so on. The result of such interpretations is likely sooner or later to be, first, the gradual emergence into consciousness of the hidden feelings, and second a reduction in the compulsiveness of the acting out and therefore in its damaging consequences.

Acting out of this kind is likely to be encountered particularly when the patient is *dependent* and the therapist is *unavailable*, i.e. during gaps in treatment, or when the therapist is going to become unavailable, which applies both to future gaps in treatment and especially to the prospect of termination. These issues form the subject of Chapter 17.

15

Deeper layers of depression

Maternal deprivation

In Chapter 13 I introduced the subject of depression with a patient in whom
the main problem was *loss* and *miscarried grief*, though with hints of ambivalent
feelings towards the loved people who had died. From this I went on to review
other patients in whom the element of ambivalence was more prominent. The
most striking of these was the Daughter with a Stroke, who clearly could not
face the tangled emotions of love, grief, hate, relief, and guilt, surrounding the
death of her dominating and controlling mother. This led on to patients such
as the Divorced Mother and the Farmer's Daughter, where the loss was not
through *death*, but through *rejection* by a lover, a situation to which ambivalence
is intrinsic. All these examples still leave out of account another kind of *loss*
or *rejection*, which is almost certainly the most important single root cause of
depression, namely maternal deprivation.

When one takes the history of such patients it is often difficult to decide
where loss ends and rejection begins. Rejection inevitably implies loss; early
loss of the mother may be followed by rejection on the part of the father or
other relatives; and loss may itself be irrationally seen as rejection. Most
commonly, therefore, there is a mixture of the two.

Much of the rest of the clinical parts of this book will be concerned with
the consequences of maternal deprivation. The subject may best be introduced
by reference to the story of Roberta in Hospital, which I described in Chapter
2 (see p. 12). Here the little girl, abandoned in hospital, reacted by rejecting
her mother when she visited; and I pointed out that this may well have served
both a defensive and an expressive function, the expressive part being probably
concerned with *anger*. This, of course, is simply an anecdotal observation, but
the evidence is overwhelming – both in humans and other primates – that
aggressive behaviour or feelings form part of the response to separation and
other forms of maternal deprivation (see Bowlby, 1973).

The depressive position

The whole subject of human aggression is both one of the most crucial to the
future of the world and one of the most obscure, complex and controversial.
I shall discuss it further below (see pp. 212ff.). Here I shall content myself

with the purely clinical statement that in deeply depressive and borderline patients therapeutic effects follow from reaching and working through what Melanie Klein and Winnicott have called the *depressive position*: that is, the full realization that *love and hate are directed towards the same person*. This person is essentially the mother, who is at one and the same time the person who has met the patient's needs and has failed to meet them. In depressive patients it is usually the 'positive' feelings that appear on the surface, and the therapist needs to reach the aggression. In borderline patients it is usually the other way round. Thus the key to depression – and also, it is worth noting, to suicide – is usually aggression. This is the theme of the following examples.

The Ghanaian Girl

The patient was a young black woman of 28 suffering from depression for 4 years. This had been of acute onset and had been severe enough to have kept her off work for the first 6 months. She would not admit to any precipitating cause, and her GP had treated her with anti-depressants without much effect. Finally she had come to him in great distress and had admitted under some pressure that the precipitating cause had been her hearing the news that her mother had been murdered with an axe in Ghana, by the man she had been living with.

She spent much of two psychiatric interviews in silence, with her eyes cast down and tears running down her cheeks. The psychiatrist managed to piece together the following story: that she was a member of a fairly large family living in Accra. Her father left the home when she was 5, and the patient was sent to live with her grandmother in the country, though her mother visited fairly frequently. The mother had a number of children by other men. Finally, when the patient was 20 her mother began living with yet another man and the patient moved in with them. This man was extremely violent, and the patient took upon herself to be her mother's protector – 'he would never touch her while I was there'. The patient did her best to persuade her mother to leave, but she wouldn't, and this resulted in many quarrels between the two of them. Finally the patient got a chance to come to England. Some years later the event occurred which precipitated her depression.

During the course of the interviews the patient said, 'I feel it's my fault'. This was, of course, an example of depressive guilt; but at the same time there was some logic in it, in the sense that if she had remained in Ghana she might well have saved her mother's life.

We may pause at this point and review the many features of the pathology of depressive illness that the patient illustrates: there is the background of considerable early *maternal deprivation*, in the form certainly of *loss* and possibly of *rejection*; there is the later actual *loss* of the mother through her death; there is *protective love*; there is direct evidence for *resentment* in the quarrels; and finally there are the depressive manifestations in the form of *lack of spontaneity*, *depressive tears*, and the emphasis on *guilt*.

Although, like the origins of human aggression, the causes of depression constitute a vast, complex, and obscure subject, some of the inner mechanisms involved are supported by overwhelming clinical evidence. The early loss or rejection sets up aggressive feelings against the mother, which conflict with the need for her and love for her; the aggressive feelings are then balanced and held in check by the 'positive' feelings of *guilt, grief, concern*, and *protectiveness*. One of the universal depressive mechanisms is then that these positive elements become emphasized but detached from their origin. As in this case, the patient presents with guilt, grief and protectiveness, which become used defensively to hide the fact that they partly have their origin in aggressive feelings.

The *lack of spontaneity* is perhaps more difficult to explain, but it almost certainly has something to do with the patient's *inability to express one side of her true feelings*, namely the aggressiveness: put in other words, the patient cannot be *real* because part of the real feelings cannot be expressed. Finally, as mentioned in Chapter 13 (see p. 147), the element of *hopelessness* or *despair* arises because the *only way of becoming real involves admitting aggressive feelings towards someone loved*, which is the one thing that must be avoided at all costs. It needs to be emphasized throughout all this that the love is as genuine as the aggression; but at the same time it is *not* genuine if it is expressed *without* the aggression, and the only way of making it genuine is for the two opposite feelings to be expressed together.

Therefore, the way of handling such a patient therapeutically is to put her in touch with the aggression, which is usually very difficult and must be done with tact and no faster than the patient can bear. With the present patient this is what the psychiatrist tried to do; and towards the end of the second interview the patient eventually came out with the remark, 'I always felt she disliked me'. Thus the evidence for *rejection* as well as *loss* became conclusive. At this point she went into an impenetrable depressive silence, and she failed to attend for the next appointment. Gentle as he was, the psychiatrist had tried to go too fast.

In this patient the element of anger, though capable of being clearly inferred, never became manifest. In the rest of the examples, the anger broke through the depressive defences unmistakably.

The Mother of Four (contd)

This patient has already been described in Chapter 9 (p. 77) for the purpose of illustrating transference. Here the originating situation had been the fact that her own mother, who almost certainly had a deprived childhood herself, had difficulty in giving genuine care and affection, used material things as substitutes, and expected gratitude in return. Presumably at least partly as a consequence of this there was considerable disturbance in all her four children. In the patient, the main disturbances consisted of a problem over *giving and receiving*. First of all, she showed a lifelong pattern of over-emphasis on giving – even after her therapy she could hardly conceive of any spare time activity that did not involve giving things to others, which indeed she enjoyed and did very well. All the evidence suggests that this was one of the typical depressive defences, already mentioned many times, in which the quite genuine wish to give is over-emphasized, in order to keep at bay resentment about having to give without receiving enough. This defence has a tendency to break down suddenly when the individual's emotional balance of payments gets into serious deficit. In her, this had occurred in an acute and dramatic fashion once before: she had been working as a *nurse* ('helping profession syndrome'), and she had had an *outburst of rage* in which she smashed a number of things in her room, the cause of which was that her boy-friend wanted sex from her without loving her enough. In the present situation the breakdown of her defence had recurred in a different form and was what had led her to seek treatment: she had become depressed 18 months after the birth of her fourth child, with the feeling that *everything was getting on top of her and she couldn't cope*; at its worst she felt she *couldn't look after the household,* and she once had to *retire to bed for three days*; she felt tearful and at times suicidal, and *reproached herself for not being a good enough wife and mother.*

The reader will see how almost every manifestation of disturbance in this patient fits into the formulation already given, which can be summarized as follows: *inadequate mothering* leads to *resentment*; resentment leads to *guilt*; the guilt is held at bay by *compulsive giving*; the giving leads to a deficit in the emotional balance of payments, which leads to more resentment and a vicious circle; on one occasion the resentment breaks through in a manifest attack of rage; on a later occasion the defence breaks down without the emergence of resentment, but instead the illness at times takes the form of actually *preventing her from giving any more* – which, if it had appeared with deliberate intent, could have been correctly labelled as *going on strike*, and is thus an example of the *return of the repressed*; and all this results in an intensification of the *guilt*, which is the main surface manifestation of her depressive illness. Once more the depressive defence takes the form of emphasizing the 'positive' feeling of guilt in order to hide the negative feeling of resentment. It is also very interesting that not only do her depressive self-reproaches – that she is not a good enough wife and mother – have some justification if the above formulation is correct, but in addition they fit (in Freud's words) 'someone whom the patient loves, has loved, or ought to love', namely her own mother.

Many authors write, following such thinkers as Karl Popper, that psychoanalytic formulations are incapable of being tested and are therefore unscientific. In doing so they entirely ignore the way in which these formulations are made operational and are then tested daily in our clinical work, and could be tested systematically if only some of us would undertake the task. The test consists of *making interpretations* and *observing responses*. Moreover, especially where the interpretation involves the *transference*, the whole process is concerned with *observables* which can be put on videotape and thus recorded objectively. In this particular case (which was unfortunately not even audio-recorded), the process was as follows:

Although in the early stages of consultation the patient gave a great deal of useful information, she conveyed a feeling of sullenness and defiance throughout, and communication eventually came to a halt with her silence, followed by the remark: 'I think you're playing some sort of game with me, expecting me to say something.' The interviewer then put together in his mind a number of pieces of information leading in the direction of a formulation like that given above, i.e. he made a *hypothesis*. He then *tested this hypothesis* by putting it to the patient in the form of an interpretation that included the transference, with the implied *prediction* that this would resolve the situation: namely that she was resentful because she felt he wanted to get a lot of things out of her without giving anything back. As already described in Chapter 9, this interpretation had the most dramatic effect, the patient first crumbling into tears and then becoming fully cooperative for the rest of the interview. In other words, not only was the implied prediction fulfilled, but evidence was obtained confirming – for this case – the formulation of the depressive psychopathology.

Therapy was very brief, consisting of pointing out and working through this pathology during the course of seven contacts in all. The result was relief of the depression, together with considerable improvements in relations within her current and original family. However, the over-all pattern of giving too much and not taking enough for herself was not resolved, and there were several crises during the course of the next few years. Some of these were handled by persuading her to take more time off from the children and fulfil her need to have her husband to herself.

The Convent Girl

This was a young woman of 23 referred because of an attack of mild depression and irritability of a few weeks' duration. In accordance with one of the basic principles of psychiatric consultation (see pp. 33ff.), the (male) interviewer started by concentrating on the precipitating factor. This emerged clearly as the fact that the patient had been *transferred*, in her job as secretary, to a new office in which there was an *unsympathetic woman boss*. Asked to give an example of something that made her irritable, she told of an incident in which one of her two flatmates, who was ill, had asked her other flatmate to go out and buy her some cigarettes, and the latter *had refused*. The patient had been furious but had said nothing and had gone out and bought them herself. The interviewer asked if she had been depressed before, from which it emerged that 5 years ago she had had an attack of 'migraine' lasting a fortnight. This had occurred while she was working as assistant cook in a *hostel for old people*, where there was an *unsympathetic matron* who did not understand that the old people were not *getting enough food*, and sometimes the head cook and the patient used to supplement this out of their own wages. The headache disappeared as soon as she gave in her notice.

It is not difficult to recognize in this story a similar pattern to that found in the Mother of Four: the recurrent themes of caring for people, on the part of the patient, and failing to care on the part of other people, almost certainly giving rise to hidden resentment. Any experienced clinician who studied this story would predict that maternal deprivation, in one form or another, would be found in the patient's background; and would say that, like the previous patient, this girl was using her wish to *give* as an over-compensating defence against her own resentment about not being given enough.

The source of resentment was hardly very far to seek, as emerged from the following story: The patient was the eldest of three children, and although her early life seemed to be free from disturbance, her father – whom she had loved very much – had gone away to the war when she was 5. He returned when the patient was 10, was then found to be going around with another woman, and left the home. The mother was very distressed and confided her troubles to the patient, who felt she was expected to take her father's place. The mother then got seriously depressed and was unable to cope with the children. At the age of 14 the patient was told she was going into hospital to have her tonsils out, but when she got there she discovered that she and her brother and sister had been sent to a residential convent school. She remained in institutions, being *transferred* several times, until she got her first job.

This young woman has thus been *both* betrayed and abandoned, *both* by her father and by her mother. It is hardly difficult to postulate her conflict as being between love and grief on the one hand, and intense resentment on the other; the whole complicated by *guilt*, because her mother was so much the injured party. What then appears on the surface is the reparative urge of looking after other people, which breaks down into symptoms when the causes for resentment get too much to bear. In the story it is *women* who appear as the villains; but it is also worth noting that the patient had entirely kept away from men, never having had a boy-friend.

The dialogue between patient and interviewer then went as follows: The interviewer pointed out the *defence*, saying that she seemed to spend her life doing things for others – what was there in it for her? To this she said that all the *responsibility* of her childhood had made her a very serious person, and something seemed to stop her going out and enjoying herself – she just didn't seem to be able to make the effort. The interviewer re-emphasized the defence, linking it with her mother, saying that as a child she had had to take *responsibility for her mother's troubles*, and since then she seemed to have a need to look after others and an inability to take things for herself. This produced a long brooding silence, which the interviewer broke by asking her what she was thinking. In response she told a story, the essence of which was that she had had to put off doing something for one person because of the needs of another – she hated disappointing people. Encouraged by this word, the interviewer decided to introduce the *hidden feeling* and the *anxiety*, saying that most probably she herself felt *disappointed*, was *angry* about it, and *guilty* about the anger, and it was the guilt that stopped her taking things for herself. Once more there was a trance-like silence, longer than before, which the interviewer had to break. She said that she was thinking about all the things she could join, such as youth clubs; and later she said that if she once started going out she felt it would hardly be possible to keep her at home. Thus, in imagination, the stranglehold of her guilt was broken.

This patient was only seen for consultation, since she declined an offer of treatment saying that she wanted to manage her problems on her own – an action that repeated her pattern of refusing things for herself. When she was followed up four years later, there were remarkable changes. She no longer seemed to suffer from any compulsion to look after other people, was able to enjoy herself, and could even deal with difficult women bosses. On the other hand, a relation with a young man had come to nothing, and she said quite openly that men didn't really interest her. Many years later, however, we heard that she had got married. The patient was one of a series who had only been interviewed, not 'treated', and there was considerable statistical evidence that the single interviews were partly responsible for therapeutic effects – see Malan *et al.* (1975).

The theme of feeding

This story shows many features similar to those of the Mother of Four – maternal deprivation, compulsive giving, emphasis on the positive to hide the negative feelings, and the breakdown into symptoms when the defences are over-burdened. However, I would like to emphasize one further aspect, namely the theme of *feeding*, which appears in the story of the old people who did not get enough food. Obviously feeding is part of maternal care for children of all ages, but particularly for babies. In the analysis of deeply depressive and borderline patients in particular, themes that relate to feeding appear with great frequency, and as the analysis deepens these become more and more literal and concerned with mouths and teeth and the mother's breast. These issues will become of increasing importance in subsequent case histories.

The Irishwoman with the Cats: an internal persecutor

This was a woman of 50 living alone. Her two children were grown up and had left home, and her English husband had left her a year ago. Her complaint was the feeling that she is 'possessed' by her mother – she wishes that she could have an operation to remove her mother from inside her. Careful questioning made clear that these feelings were figurative and not delusional.

The psychiatric enquiry also revealed that she suffers from two different kinds of depression. One is reactive, is usually set off by feelings connected with loss, and consists of becoming preoccupied with all the terrible things that have happened to her, accompanied by the feeling that she cannot cope. Although the idea of suicide does cross her mind, she described herself as 'greedy for life', and conveyed the impression that suicide was not a serious risk. When depressed she suffers very seriously from early waking, getting to sleep 'like a baby' but waking sometimes as early as 12.30 a.m. and being unable to get to sleep again. The second type of depression is more 'endogenous', coming on and disappearing suddenly for no apparent reason. Its main manifestation is that everything appears grey and lifeless.

In view of her complaint, we may ask what was her actual relation to her mother? The answer is that she feels her mother hated her from birth, and she had the idea – for which there is some evidence – that the reason for this is that she is not the child of the man her mother married. From the beginning her mother constantly criticized her and she could do nothing right. This is apparently not a distorted memory, since it has been confirmed by other relatives.

The feelings to do with her mother inside her are as follows: she is persecuted by feelings of guilt, and she hears her mother's voice inside her constantly criticizing her, just as actually happened in real life. When she looks in a mirror she sees her mother's face and becomes terrified. She once saw a photograph of the murderess, Marie Bernhardt, who poisoned all her family with arsenic – the eyes were her mother's eyes. It is when she feels most identified with her mother that she is most likely to *become violent*, and she was in fact referred by her (woman) therapist, a psychoanalyst and social worker, for a psychiatric opinion as to whether she might really be a danger to people.

When a psychiatrist is asked for such an opinion, what can he do? How is he to know? The answer, obviously, is that he can't, but what he can do is to ask for details of incidents in which she has become violent, and assess the atmosphere and quality of these, the amount of damage she has actually done, and her capacity for impulse control.

Two types of incident were as follows. On one occasion she had hit her husband on the shoulder with a rolling pin while he was in bed. In fact she had not done him any serious harm. Although she has been fully aware of murderous impulses, this was an isolated instance of violence actually directed towards a person. On other occasions she has expressed her violence by throwing things at the bedroom door, which now bears many scars.

A second type of incident concerns her three cats. Again, she has frequently felt like killing the cats, but she has actually never laid a finger on them. They have learnt to keep away from her when she is in one of her moods – they get frightened because she screams. She described a typical incident: in her anger she moves quickly and they disappear into the next room; she then carefully shuts the door between them and her, and waits till her anger has subsided; then she lets them in and makes it up to them by cuddling them.

There was thus tremendous warmth in this woman side by side with tremendous violence. The impulse to *give* was further illustrated by her fantasy that if one of her parents died she could go back to Ireland and look after the other. She mentioned this to them but all her father answered was that if her mother died he would go to a 'proper place for old people'.

The psychiatrist later offered his opinion, for what it was worth, that since in her fantasies and actions she had shown not only this degree of warmth but a very clear ability to limit her violence, there did not seem to be danger of her doing serious harm.

When she was asked what might set off these feelings of violence she answered, first, that the incident with her husband had been set off because he had the time to go to the pub and get drunk but said he didn't have time to put up a shelf for her. As far as the cats were concerned, she said that a typical precipitating factor might be, '*if I have just fed them and they come and ask for more*'.

The theme of *needs and demands* is obviously very prominent in these two types of incident, and at least with the cats there are strong hints of mother – child relations, with the element of *feeding* appearing once again. She is clearly enraged when the cats seem to be *greedy* and make excessive demands on her; but we also know that she is a guilt-laden person, she has described *herself* as 'greedy for life', and it is only too likely that her anger is complicated by self-hatred, which would contribute greatly to its intensity (compare the incident with the bus conductress in the Nurse in Mourning, p. 144).

If this is so, what are we to make of her feeling that her mother's voice is constantly inside her, criticizing her, that when she looks in the mirror she sees her mother's face, that she compares her mother to a murderess, and that when she feels most identified with her mother she is most likely to become violent?

The first answer, of course, is that the mechanisms involved are very obscure indeed, and that no one really understands them with any certainty. It seems likely, for instance, that there is some mechanism present akin to that in brain-washing, whereby the victim's resistance is finally broken down and she becomes more or less permanently identified with her persecutor. This is referred to as 'identification with the aggressor', and is presumably at least partly *a defence* against the pain, fear, and effort of constantly keeping up resistance.

But even if such a mechanism is at work, it may not be the whole story. We may ask the question whether this internal image of her mother may not also play some part in expressing some of the inner feelings of the patient herself.

Now we already know that the patient is packed full of violent anger and murderous impulses, and that a standard feature of depressive illness is *guilt about aggressive feelings*. Certainly it seems probable that this internal persecuting mother allies itself with the patient's conscience, constantly dealing out some kind of internal punishment.

Yet this is also a very strange kind of conscience, possessing as it does downright persecutory qualities, even one might say, the quality of *cruelty*. What could be the source of this? Well, the patient's mother was undoubtedly cruel, and perhaps we need to look no further. Indeed it is not at all improbable that she wanted to get rid of her daughter, so that the patient had some reason to perceive her in spirit as a *murderess* as well. Yet we know that the patient herself has murderous impulses, and the therapist even feared she might be a danger to people. Moreover, the times when she feels most identified with her mother are the times when she is most likely to be violent. There thus seems to be some fusion between the *mother's* aggression and that of the *patient*. We can therefore ask another question: could it be that some of the patient's own violent – even cruel – aggression is locked up in this internal persecuting mother/conscience and turned against herself?

These questions cannot be answered with any certainty, but they need to be taken seriously. As we shall see in the next chapter, psychoanalysis has revealed powerful evidence for very strange, totally unexpected, and disturbing primitive phenomena in human beings. In the analysis of borderline and psychotic patients, it does seem as if the primitive human conscience deals in something very different from the everyday feelings of *guilt* and *concern* as we know them, and deals far more in the principle of ruthless and cruel retribution, like the primitive justice of many human societies. Moreover, the 'operational' evidence is that bringing out the extent of the violence, directed against the therapist in the transference, mitigates the severity of the conscience. This now allows a new identification with a benign authority in the shape of the therapist, and leads to the emergence of concern, and tolerance of the patient's own impulses, rather than the drive towards pitiless self-punishment.

This concept of the primitive conscience which contains some of the patient's own aggression is one with which every psychotherapist needs to be familiar. It was partly phenomena of this kind that led Freud to coin a special term, *'Oberich'* or *'superego'*, instead of using the word 'conscience', which, in its everyday use, does not convey this aspect of the psyche in its true complexity.

Yet, as I have written in this book so many times before, the complexities never seem to end. We may now ask the question whether the mother was really as bad as the patient perceived her. If the patient had never been given any love, how did she acquire the capacity to give so much love herself? This question cannot be answered in this particular patient, but there is an immensely important observation that is repeatedly made: that when the full extent of the hatred is experienced in the transference, side by side with the love – in other words, the *depressive position* is reached – there emerge a number of related transformations, amongst which is the *recall of some good memories from childhood* which had hitherto been totally ignored or forgotten. Thus, in the present patient, the internal persecuting mother may play a part in the patient's aggression in another way, as the object of angry denigration and depreciation.

In fact this speculation was fully confirmed. The patient was seen once a week for a total of 6 years. At termination her violence had been considerably mitigated. However, the most important information was that she had invited her mother to visit her from Ireland and there had been a major reconciliation between the two of them – thus indeed suggesting that the reality of her mother was not as bad as the patient's hate-ridden memories had painted her.

An even more striking example of this kind of transformation is given in the next case history, which consists of an account of a therapy in which depressive mechanisms were dealt with in great depth.

The Personnel Manager: the depressive position

In the first two patients described in this chapter, depressive mechanisms were interpreted and this resulted in some response at the time. In the present patient they were not merely *interpreted* but *worked through*, at length and in depth. I am convinced that this at least partly accounts for a feature that sets her apart from most other therapeutic results described in this book, namely the *depth of feeling* which she showed at follow-up. This was in marked contrast to her somewhat intellectual defensiveness which was observed at consultation.

The patient was an unmarried woman of 40 who came to therapy because she had developed a severe *phobia of driving* after recently buying a car for the first time. Four clues to the meaning of this phobia, which emerged at consultation, were as follows: (1) an incident contributing to the precipitation of her anxiety was that her driving instructor had told her that *she did not have herself under proper control* – this had worried her because she had always had a reputation for great calmness; (2) she said that, in previous group therapy, she had come to realize that she was an *unwanted child* and her mother must have resented having her; and (3) that to cope with the consequent insecurity she had become determined to *have everything under control*, and 'to go ahead along a narrow path without paying any attention to what there might be on either side'; and (4) she said that in her driving she was afraid of *getting into a difficult situation and not being able to cope with it*.

Now since this woman was both in a highly responsible job and emanated a strong air of competence and efficiency, there was clearly at first sight something paradoxical in her story of panic attacks merely at the thought of driving a car. However, simple application of the principles that run throughout this book resolves the paradox without difficulty. It looks as if her efficiency is a mask (defence) hiding a deep sense of insecurity (hidden feeling, here also an anxiety). She is thus one of those people who can be described in Winnicott's graphic phrase as possessing a *false self*, which is a kind of defence that can be massive and all-pervading. In her, this defence serves the purpose of *keeping everything under control*, and she breaks down into severe anxiety when her control is threatened. Therefore, although there was never any evidence that she was obsessional, her defence has clear affinities with the obsessional defence described in Chapter 11 (see pp. 113ff.). This similarity was strongly confirmed when she revealed the obsessional's *fear of change* because it introduces the *unfamiliar*. She said that she felt she would experience the same panic as she had when driving, at any major change in her life, such as forming a relation with a man (something she had never succeeded in doing), or being sent abroad in connection with her work. The inner mechanism involved here is almost certainly that the patient hopes to meet only familiar stimuli, to which she can respond with pre-programmed responses, thus making sure that no feeling is surprised out of her which might be more than she wants to face. This whole defence is threatened if she meets a situation that is unfamiliar or unforeseen.

During the consultation the interviewer dimly saw the psychopathology implied by her description of her feelings, but when he tried to lead her towards this he drew a blank. When she made the remark about 'going ahead along a narrow path without paying any attention to what there might be on either side' he pointed out the possible connection with the car phobia, namely that when one was driving this was exactly what one couldn't do. She agreed with this but could not make use of it. Thus her need to have everything under control and not to be faced with the unfamiliar seemed to include her attitude to new insights about herself. Similarly her insight about being an unwanted child, which she had acquired during her previous group therapy, and her response to this, seemed to be largely of an intellectual kind. This has an important bearing on the climax of her individual therapy, described below.

The patient was assessed in Balint's Workshop, and although the above pathology was seen, she was assigned to therapy (with a male therapist at once a week) with the aim of trying to deal with a quite different problem, namely supposed masculine identification hiding resentment against men. However, as is now clear, this was not an appropriate focus, and in addition her therapist was strongly oriented towards dealing with problems in the early relation with the mother. The result was that, between them, patient and therapist very rapidly changed direction. In Session 3, for instance, the patient said she had come to realize that she felt anxious in many situations where she was *away from home*; she later said that she distrusted her *mother* and felt that her mother had '*destroyed an essential part of her*'; and she then recalled an incident as a child in which she had got lost at a railway station and a kind stranger had helped her find her family again, and she had been *surprised that tears could bring help and comfort*. Thus this patient, though brought up in a home where she was fed and clothed adequately, is giving clear evidence of hidden but severe emotional deprivation – she had earlier said that she was *unwanted*, and now she is implying that her mother did not understand that a child who cries is asking for comfort, and we have no reason to doubt her word for this.

The treatment of maternal deprivation; internal spoiling

So, once more we are up against the problem of maternal deprivation. The question is now, what can be done about this in psychotherapy?

The answer must depend on the extent of the deprivation. There may well be some severely deprived patients – e.g. those showing severe sociopathic behaviour – who have missed something that is so essential to normal development that nothing can be done whatsoever. There may be others with whom it is necessary to help them *regress* to a childhood state, and then really to try and give them some of what they have missed – the schizophrenic girl described in Sechehaye's book *Symbolic realization* (1951) is an example. Equally, Winnicott (1958) developed a technique known as the 'Winnicott regression', in which such patients are kept at home, are absolved from all adult responsibilities, and are cared for while – within limits – they are allowed to express what they like, including all the anger about what they have missed. Obviously this desperate measure requires very special home conditions and is usually impracticable. Fortunately, also, it is often not necessary.

One thing is certain, however, namely that *just* giving what the patient has missed is not enough. A dramatic everyday example of this was given in Chapter 2 under the heading Roberta in Hospital (see p. 6). Here the little girl, who felt abandoned and neglected in hospital, was offered her mother's presence again at visiting time. Her reaction was to refuse it. Almost certainly this refusal served the usual twin defensive and expressive functions – by refusing contact with her mother she both saved herself the pain of potential further abandonment and expressed against her mother her angry feelings about being abandoned. Only when these feelings were brought out could she accept her mother again.

The story, also from Chapter 2, of the Social Worker and her Father, illustrates a further stage in this kind of process, here directed at the father rather than the mother. Not only did she reject her father, but in talking of the incident later she said she now realized that she didn't love him, she disliked him. This statement was patently untrue – without question she loved him more than anyone else in the world. She was in fact expressing her anger about all the abandonment and neglect in the past not merely by rejecting him but by *depreciating*, or *spoiling*, or *destroying* the image of him. Carried to the limit, this mechanism spreads not merely to the image of the other person now, but to everything to do with him, present and past, with the result that the whole memory of him is spoiled.

This *spoiling of memories* or of *previous experience* leads into very deep issues indeed. Here one may ask a question which at first sight seems rather abstract and philosophical: what, psychically, do we consist of? Again, it may seem rather facile to answer 'all we have experienced'; and in any case this is clearly only partially true, since it leaves out of account what we bring to what we have experienced, and how this in turn has interacted with our experience. Yet such a description does seem to have a surprising degree of practical relevance. Much clinical evidence suggests that part of the normal growth of self-confidence and self-regard depends on receiving enough *good experience*, which is felt to be *taken in* and *held inside*. Deprivation tends to lead to a disturbance of self-regard in two ways: first, there is insufficient good experience; and second, what good experience there has been is in some way angrily *spoiled* or *destroyed*.

The result is a feeling of being empty, worthless, or dead inside; or worse, rotten and contaminated. Moreover new good experience, which is offered, may be of no use because it in turn is depreciated, spoiled or destroyed, and the result is a state of despair. The reader may recognize in the above description, when taken to the limit, some of the manifestations of what one may call 'in-patient' depression, in which the despair is total; or in which these feelings take on a literal quality and appear as delusions – that the inside of the patient's body is empty, or full of rubbish or faeces, or poisoned, or that she (or he) has destroyed the whole world.

However, it is these very self-destructive mechanisms that in fact lead to the possibility of therapeutic help. If the only factor were that the patient has not received enough, then it would seem probable that nothing could be done short of giving them what they have missed, which, as mentioned above, is usually impracticable (see p. 177). But if the patient is spoiling memories of the past and destroying what she might otherwise receive in the present, then perhaps this can be brought out, worked through, and ultimately neutralized and reversed.

What, therefore, is the therapist's function in patients of this kind? The answer is an aspect of the 'corrective emotional experience' mentioned in the previous chapter. We may mention once more Winnicott's epigram that the function of the therapist is 'not to succeed but to fail'. What the therapist must do first is to *offer symbolic care* – which he does in any case by the mere fact of listening and trying to understand. He must then *fail to give enough* – which is hardly difficult, as it is absolutely intrinsic to the therapeutic situation. He must then accept, tolerate, and understand the patient's rejection of him; and then he must bring out, accept and tolerate all the anger and destructiveness directed at him for what is felt as his neglect. When this goes well, what happens next is unexpected and dramatic, as is illustrated by the present patient, to whom we may now return.

The Personnel Manager (contd)

In Session 5 she was already beginning to show signs of depression. The therapist made an interpretation about her conflict between a need for her mother and her wish for independence. In the next session she was clearly reluctant to become involved, and she said that she felt *sick* at the thought of coming. The therapist said that she felt he was forcing her back to re-experience the painful conflicts associated with her childhood.

In Session 7 she spoke of her feeling of being *left out* in her childhood, feeling an outsider with *no rights* of her own. She had to master her rebellion and anger at having to settle down to an apparent conformity. The result had been the feeling that she had to manage on her own – it was no use relying on anyone else. The therapist linked this communication with her feelings about him, and she began to become aware of her resentment against him for leaving her to manage on her own between sessions.

Session 8 illustrated with great clarity that events occurring outside therapy (see previous examples of this in the Imaginary Therapy, p. 97, and the Mental Welfare Officer, p. 155), may possess an important transference component. She told of how, at the week-end, her car had stalled and the starter had become jammed. Although this had happened before and she knew the technique of dealing with it, she had felt panic-stricken and had had to call in a mechanic. This, however, had only led to her becoming more agitated. She had then tried to drive but had allowed the car to become out of control and had mounted the pavement. This led to her becoming extremely distressed at her own incompetence and then having a further panic attack. She had felt desperately in need of talking to the therapist about it and had poured it all out to people at the office but had felt she had no right to ask for an earlier appointment.

One can see in these events a number of different themes. First, there is the clear breakdown of her defence of *managing on her own*, being competent, and *having everything under control*. When this breakdown occurs she reveals extreme anxiety, an inability to cope on her own, and a desperate need for help. The meaning of the car begins to become much clearer: as a symbol of independence that she cannot really cope with, and which reveals the need for help underneath. Thus, the competent person who knows how to deal with the situation is swept aside and she has to call in the mechanic. The transference implications of this are inescapable; and these are confirmed by her quite conscious need for the therapist, together with the feeling that she *has no right* to ask for him – a clear echo of her childhood. She has to use the people in the office as substitutes.

This much is obvious. What is less obvious, but clearly hinted at, is the possibility that her lifelong resentment against her parents for being made to cope on her own, of which she has become quite conscious, is now being transferred to the therapist; and therefore, that among her feelings over the week-end – when the therapist was not available – was resentment against him, and that her inability to cope was a sort of living reproach to him for abandoning her and forcing her into the situation of having to manage without him. Yet he is the one person in her life offering help and understanding, so that the relation with him at all costs must be preserved. This conflict, of being deeply angry with someone deeply loved and needed is – as mentioned before (see pp. 167ff.) so often the basic dilemma in depressive patients.

Thus, in this session, the therapist wrote of his interpretations in the following words: 'I also sought to make her aware that the panic was related to her anger, and that I was quite prepared to recognize this anger and to help her to do the same.'

In the next few sessions the patient appeared much more depressed, while perhaps as a consequence of this the importance of the car seemed to have receded. She felt the therapist *offered her nothing of value*; she was defeated and helpless; there was no point in going on; the things that she wanted were no longer available. At the same time she experienced each session as a relief and at the end was reluctant to leave.

Transference aspects became even clearer in Session 12. She said that on two or three occasions during the early part of the week she had forgotten about her coming session and found herself arranging other appointments at that time. The therapist interpreted that she *hated him* for not being more freely available. In response to this she told of having unexpectedly seen her former group therapist at a railway station, being taken aback, and having involuntarily *turned away from him*. The therapist said that the same applied to himself – she *turned away from him in hate and anger* during the week's interval between sessions, which was felt to be too long. She then told a dream in which three kittens were *left for a week*, after which one had disappeared, one was dead, and one was alive. Some of the details of this dream were certainly obscure, but she herself linked the *week* with the interval between sessions, and said that she felt the therapist *gave* her things during the sessions in the form of his interpretations but did not give her enough time. She went on to recall that she had difficulties over *feeding* when she was a child, in which she *hated the food* that she was given and had to be forcibly fed.

Here we meet the deep issues that have been discussed earlier in this chapter. Some of the implications of what the patient has said are very clear: without question she sees the therapist as *giving* to her, she is not *given* enough, and the weekly interval is too long. If we now turn to the dream, then we may say that kittens – like human babies – need to be looked after and *fed* if they are to be kept alive, and the message about whether or not they remain alive after being left for a week appears to be somewhat ambiguous. However, there is more to it than this, for it seems that she is implying not only that she is *not given enough* to keep her alive but that she *hates what she is offered* and wants to refuse it. This the therapist interpreted to her, and he wrote that towards the end of the session she appeared far less worried and more relaxed.

As has been described above, corresponding to this hatred directed outwards towards what she is offered, there is often found a hatred directed *inwards* towards what she has already received, so that everything inside becomes spoiled. In many therapies this is manifested as follows: the patient goes away feeling she has received something of great value from her therapist, but as time passes this feeling evaporates and she feels as bad as ever. Thus in the next session the patient reported that she had left the previous session with a great sense of peace and inner calm. She longed to make this state more permanent, but on the contrary, as the time for coming approached, she had experienced a mounting sense of panic and inner turmoil. The therapist interpreted that she wanted to preserve him inside herself as something 'good', but feelings of hate began to supervene the longer she was away from him; and thus the image of him inside her became spoiled. In response to this work her true mixed feelings came much closer to the surface, and she became aware both of glimpses of resentment and protest on the one hand, and love and friendliness on the other.

In the next session (No. 14) the ambivalence came even nearer with an intensification of language. She spoke of how she had been aware of great tension during the week – in fact it was like *living near a volcano*. This the therapist interpreted as her inner turmoil, spelling it out as consisting of very powerful love and hate towards him. She told a dream in which she found herself having a fantasy of being in the Clinic, but instead of her therapist there was a figure like a statue.

The meaning of the statue became absolutely clear in the next session. She linked her dread of coming to therapy with her early experiences with her mother, in which she felt intense need but found her mother *failing to respond*. The therapist interpreted her fear that she would repeat the same experience with him, thus acknowledging that he repeated the deprivation; but he then added her own reaction, that this would result in her *turning away from him in hate and anger* and being *plunged into a state of despair* – a very clear statement of part of the dynamics of her depression.

Throughout all this there had been an emphasis on interpretation of the *hidden feelings*, and if I had been supervising this therapy I would perhaps have made the criticism that not enough work had been directed towards underlining her two main *defences* of competence and efficiency on the one hand and keeping everything under control on the other. For instance, the therapist had a clear opportunity to do this in the 'volcano' session, in which she had spoken of having two contrasting experiences of herself: at work she was competent, decisive, and prepared to take responsibility; whereas in her relation to therapy she could only feel intense dependence and anxiety. In Session 21, however, he did make use of such an opportunity: she spoke of having been given a new job at work which would mean being isolated, working on her own. She would very much like to cry about it, but another part of her forbids her to. At this point the therapist emphasized the defence: *how much she needed to keep herself under complete control.* In the next session she said that she had been thinking of this all the week, and she realized how true it was. The theme of much of the rest of the session was how she had never been allowed to *be herself* at home, and at this point the therapist *emphasized the positive aspects of therapy*: that here she could allow herself to be her true self and find out what she was really like beneath her defences.

I think this understanding of her defences had important consequences, as in the next session (No. 23) she told of a dream in two parts, the second being a dream of hope: in the first a small girl of about 8 was in very great distress, needing help, but very afraid of a woman who would compel her to do her will. In the second, the patient was busy in the attic of a house, planning the lay-out for a new occupation. She saw herself sitting by a large window, looking out on the world, with a feeling of great pleasure and peace. She realized that the woman in the house below was beautiful – she associated her with her elder sister.

This is a crucial moment, the first time her view of the world has allowed the existence of any kind of 'good mother'. Yet it is still not quite the point to which the patient needs to be brought, the true *depressive position*, in which the 'good' and the 'bad' person – usually the mother – are the same. This was reached by the following therapeutic work, in which the gap of three weeks in therapy caused by the Easter break played a prominent part:

The last session before the break was largely taken up with her quite conscious anger at being left alone for such a long time. She felt utterly discarded, pushed out on her own, *persecuted* by all the demands of reality, and left with a sense of *inner emptiness and despair.*

Anyone who has worked with psychotic patients will recognize here two feelings which, if greatly exaggerated, appear in the· form of delusions in paranoid and depressive patients respectively. As already described, the depressive delusion is that the patient's body is empty, or full of rubbish or faeces; the paranoid delusion is that the patient is being persecuted by some outside agency, which of course may be organized into some systematic conspiracy.

Such delusions not only appear totally meaningless to common sense, but also are usually utterly refractory to any form of psychotherapeutic intervention, and certainly to rational argument. However, when they appear in the much milder form of transitory feelings in neurotic patients, particularly – as here – in the context of identifiable feelings in the transference, their meaning becomes at least partly intelligible.

In fact in such circumstances they admit of absolutely standard interpretations, which have been reached by generations of empirical work, and which need to be known by every psychotherapist. The chief contributors to our knowledge in this area have been Melanie Klein and Winnicott.

There are two elements in the patient's feelings: *inside* is the depressive feeling of emptiness, *outside* is the paranoid feeling of persecution. The interpretation of these feelings which is found to produce a response is concerned with the patient's own primitive aggressive feelings, which are felt to destroy everything *inside* her, and (as mentioned in connection with the Nurse in Mourning, Chapter 13) can also be in some way felt to be coming back at her from *outside*, resulting in a feeling of persecution. Both the inner feeling of emptiness and the outer feeling of persecution will be relieved if the patient can be brought to acknowledge their origin in *destructive feelings within herself*, which in turn owe their origin to a sense of deprivation, and in the present context are directed both towards the therapist and towards everything that he gives her now or has given her in the past. This was the theme of the therapist's contribution in this session: 'I made interpretations of her anger and resentment towards me and the internal attacks resulting in my destruction and annihilation; and of her utter helplessness and despair at her predicament.'

Climax of therapy: reaching the depressive position

When she returned from the 3-week break (Session 30), she both reported that she had been very depressed, and spoke of *not wanting a relation* with a woman whom she had met during this time. The therapist interpreted her *defence* as being a withdrawal from the relation with him.

In the next session she said that she had never felt so depressed and *rotten* as she had during last night and this morning – a word by which she may or may not have implied feelings of inner destruction and contamination. She went on to describe one incident after another during the course of her life in which she had been left with the responsibility, lonely and isolated. Here, once more, what she needs is not only compassionate understanding of her very real deprivation, but also a sympathetic but ruthless interpretation of the way her reaction to it has set up a vicious circle of isolation – in the previous session she had spoken of not wanting a relation with a particular woman, and in her history it needs to be remembered that she had never had a relation with a man. This the therapist did, emphasizing her deep need of him; saying how she had been re-experiencing in her relationship with him the same feeling of being left with the responsibility, of being unwanted and unloved; and how her reaction has always been to turn away from people in hate and anger, thus putting herself outside relationships and intensifying her loneliness.

It is to be noted that this interpretation mentions both the 'positive' feelings (the deep need) and the 'negative' feelings (turning away in hate and anger) together; and that both these feelings are *directed towards the same person* – the person needed is the *person also hated*. It is the integration of these two opposite feelings, the *depressive position*, that is the point towards which the whole therapy has been leading.

The consequences of this intense session may be told in the therapist's own words:

'Last week on leaving here she felt very unsettled and disturbed. This feeling increased as she approached her office, and having arrived there she realized that she wanted to talk to me. It seemed terribly important to be able to do this, though the things she wanted to say were very much the same as what she had told me in the session. She then realized that all this had to do with feeling herself to be UNWANTED. She thought about this for a while and felt very disturbed, but this was followed by a feeling of great peace and content. Since then this feeling has persisted. She described it as if a great load had been lifted off her mind.'

At first sight this reaction of peace and content to reaching a feeling of being *unwanted* may seem both puzzling and paradoxical. It is *puzzling* because the patient has spoken of being unwanted many times before – indeed she mentioned it in the consultation. Why should it have such a dramatic effect now? The answer is almost certainly that she had *said* it before but had not fully *experienced* it – it had been *said* by her false self but was now *experienced* by her real self. Part of the anxiety that had almost overwhelmed her before had been due to the fear of this experience, which now, as always, turned out not to be so terrifying as had been feared.

However, it is also *paradoxical*, because being unwanted is an extremely unpleasant feeling: why therefore should it have led to a feeling of peace and content? The answer is quite simple, namely that it is almost always a relief to experience one's true feelings, however unpleasant they may be – it is better to feel the grief of being unwanted than to maintain false competence and efficiency; it is better to be torn apart by love and hate than to exclude oneself from all relationships, so that one can never receive anything of real value; it is better to feel one's childhood as a mixture of happiness and despair than to paint it entirely black.

For now something happened that is intrinsic to the experience of the depressive position: first, the realization that the past has not been so uniformly desolate as one's retrospective anger has made out; and second, the turning to the present with hope and the possibility of allowing oneself to be enriched in the future.

The patient now said she realized that there *had* been happy experiences with her mother, though she had been made to pay a high price for them in terms of being required to conform and submit; and she ended by saying that *she had received something very precious and important from her therapist.* This may be contrasted with her previous remark that he offered her nothing of value.

Termination

Of course one must not hope that such a moment will mark the end of therapy. In fact the experience has to be worked through over and over again before it can be consolidated; and since the patient's problem was essentially to do with *loss*, it will inevitably be reactivated by the prospect of *termination*, and this will have to be worked through in its turn. The patient was given 30 more sessions. The therapist wrote that he confronted her again and again with her need for him and her resentment arising out of its lack of fulfilment, particularly because of termination; and – once more carefully emphasizing the positive – he spoke of the possibility of her emerging out of this experience with an increased ability to deal with life. Therapy occupied 62 sessions over the course of 18 months.

Follow-up

When the patient was followed up nearly 7 years later, not only was she entirely free from her phobia, but she also showed a new-found and most exceptional depth of feeling, and a capacity to use her feelings in her life to get, and give, satisfaction [for further details see Malan (1976a), pp. 192–7]. One remark that sums up the therapeutic process, and especially the climax described above, was: 'I have realized the value of letting your feelings overwhelm you, so that you know what they are.'

An important word of caution

Although the *content* of this therapy is typical of the process of working through the depressive position in a non-borderline patient, there are many other features that are not typical at all. The *form* of the therapy, at once a week and face to face, and the *duration*, only 62 sessions spread over 18 months, are highly unusual for work of such intensity and depth. In general it would not be realistic to attempt to do this at less than three times a week, and the expected duration would be considerably longer. Moreover, with many types of patient, any attempt to do such work might well result in uncontrollable regression and dependence and considerable danger of suicide – which gives point to the necessity for extremely careful initial assessment (see Chapters 18–23). And even further, with certain therapists the work might become nothing other than sadistic. Therapy of this kind should not be attempted by anyone who has not had intensive training and personal psychotherapy, unless he is under close supervision. This applies *a fortiori* to patients such as those described in the next chapter (see the Refugee Musician and Foster Son), where the danger is not only *suicide* but *homicide*. It needs to be noted that in the case of the Personnel Manager the therapist was an analyst of many years' experience.

The patient herself was also exceptional. She clearly possessed exceptional strength and capacity to bear her feelings. Moreover, she had already had 2½ years' group treatment, which had cleared a number of subsidiary problems out of the way. To repeat, all this emphasizes the importance of assessing the potential dangers of dynamic psychotherapy at the very beginning.

16
Primitive phenomena

Psychodynamics and the failure of common sense

In the early chapters of this book I was able to illustrate all the basic principles of psychodynamics by the use of everyday examples or simple case histories, which involved such ordinary human feelings as jealousy, anger, resentment, guilt, and grief. I could show how such feelings are kept at bay by various simple defence mechanisms, and how when these mechanisms break down the feelings may return in a disguised or displaced form. These examples thus illustrated the basic psychodynamic principles of defence, anxiety, hidden feeling, and the return of the repressed, all of which were relatively easily accessible to honest introspection.

Yet even in the first example of all, the Economics Student, there were important details that I delayed until Chapter 7, because they were most certainly not accessible to everyday introspection. The reasons for this were of two kinds: in the case of the patient's sexual feelings for her father the *feelings themselves* were of a nature that we do not readily acknowledge; and in the case of the nightmares before her exams, what was obscure was the *connection* between the sexual feelings for her father on the one hand and the examination anxiety on the other. This led into the whole question of Oedipal feelings in women, which is a difficult and obscure area, and then to the even darker area of Oedipal feelings in men.

In subsequent examples this kind of obscurity has alternated with far more accessible material. There seems little difficulty, for instance, in thinking oneself into the Daughter with a Stroke, who was faced with tremendously conflicting feelings after the death of her dominating and controlling mother, and apparently so feared retribution that she developed anxiety attacks in which she suffered the same as what she imagined her mother had experienced. Clearly this involves some kind of 'identification'. So does the phenomenon shown by the Irishwoman with the Cats (p. 172), who saw her brutal mother's face when she looked in the mirror, yet the inner mechanisms here are far less obvious.

We can use a parallel from the development of physics, in which from the beginning of the twentieth century onwards there began to accumulate a series of observations that could not be explained by classical ideas. The result has been the growth of systems of knowledge very far from common sense, such as relativity and quantum theory. Yet it must be remembered that these systems of knowledge are firmly based on empirical observations, which, being different from what would be predicted by common sense, require explanations that appear to contradict common sense.

Over much the same period something very similar has been happening in the understanding of human beings. In exactly the same way, the observations contradict common sense, and the explanations must therefore do the same. This will be the theme of the present chapter, beginning with the following example – which, though it may appear very complex at first, is in fact utterly simple.

'Fed upon his mother's tears' – an experience under LSD

A doctor in his thirties, whose long analysis appeared to have reached an impasse, began to try to reach deeper layers of his psyche by the use of LSD. This was in the days when LSD was manufactured officially and could simply be bought on prescription. Strangely enough, his early experiences with the drug were of heightened superficiality. Then, on perhaps the fourth occasion, the following occurred:

He sank into a dream-like state, and the image presented itself of his body being connected to that of his mother by a sort of U-tube, in such a way that – as would happen in reality by the laws of hydrostatics – the fluid contents of the two bodies would find their own level, equal in the two. There was then the feeling that *there was not enough to go round*, and both bodies were deprived and depleted, so that in the end both were just *skin and bones*.

He then became preoccupied with a photograph that he had taken a year or two before, of his girl-friend sitting by a fence in lush country, with a mountain in the background. The bare wooden fence reminded him of bones; and it therefore seemed to him that this photograph symbolized a profound truth about his inner feelings, namely that somewhere within the experience of the beautiful girl in the sunlit and verdant countryside, which seemed to offer so much in the way of mutual satisfaction and enrichment, there lay the opposite experience – an interaction in which both partners were depleted, and reduced to a feeling of skin and bones.

Before continuing with what happened on this particular occasion, we may underline this experience with something that happened under LSD a few weeks later. Here, the patient's unconscious constructed two contrasting neologisms, worthy of a creative schizophrenic or of Lewis Carroll. The first was 'beautuquent', a kind of fusion of 'beautiful' with some word suggesting 'liquidness', which was associated with the way in which a cooked sausage is tense and full of goodness, ready to eat, but also almost as if it had *come to life*. The second – utterly opposite – was 'threevled', possibly with associations to 'threadbare' and 'shrivelled', which somehow eloquently expresses the concept that it represents, namely the feeling of one's mouth being full of dust and cobwebs. This was associated in his mind with a patient whose student he had been in a surgical ward, who had suffered from inoperable cancer of the tongue. The surgeon, in an impulsively heroic act, had removed the whole of the patient's tongue, leaving him with little more than a layer of skin as the floor of his mouth. The image was of this man, desperately – and clearly hopelessly – clinging to life, trying to drink, with nothing left by which he might swallow, or even by which he might speak to the nurses looking after him.

What on earth could all this mean? The doctor seemed to know some inner experience of starvation, and yet if anything was certain it was that, brought up as he was in a loving and prosperous middle-class home, he had never experienced anything of the kind.

The LSD experience continued. He now began to recollect a French cartoon film that he had seen, with his mother, in his teens, and which had made – for reasons unknown – a haunting and indelible impression on him.

In it there is a sick – perhaps dying – child with her young widowed mother, living in poverty in a single room. It seems that the child feels that there is one thing that will restore her to health, and she cries out for it, 'Mummy, I want an orange, a big round juicy orange.' The truth is that her mother has no money to buy her an orange. The only way she can earn enough to keep them alive is by making furry toys, and as she bends over to hide her weeping, her tears drip onto the teddy bear that she is making.

Here, magic begins to happen. The tears soak into the teddy bear's body and he *comes to life*; and after the mother has gone to bed, he gets up and goes out of the house. The rest of the film is about his adventures, which end in his managing to steal an orange from a stall; and he brings it back and stands on the end of the child's cot, and peels it and throws her the segments one by one; and, well, of course, the implication is that the child recovers. And, as the patient recollected this story, he was overcome by wave after wave of sobbing.

This led to another recollection of his work in hospitals. Shortly after he became qualified he worked for a time as houseman in the children's ward. One of his patients was a 4-month-old baby boy suffering from some condition leading to severe dehydration, who was on a glucose/saline intravenous drip. One Sunday, when there was no one but himself in charge, the baby – in spite of the drip – was obviously fast deteriorating, appearing grey and shrivelled ('threevled'?), and it seemed clear that unless he could be given exactly the right combination of salts he would die within hours. But how was anyone to know what to give? The hospital's laboratory was not at that time equipped to carry out the necessary analysis, and in any case, being a Sunday, it was closed. It so happened, however, that there was a registrar in the hospital on that day, who was doing some research on the analysis of salts in the body by flame photometry. The houseman went and asked him if he could help, receiving a mildly irritable answer, that the registrar had his own work to do and was not there to do routine laboratory procedures. The houseman persisted – 'but the baby is dying' – and unwillingly the registrar (the reluctant caregiver who yet did enough) consented and took a blood sample. An hour later he came back and said, 'I would give him a mixture of so much sodium and so much potassium. Start by giving him six fluid ounces.' This the houseman did. The effect was miraculous, the baby turning from grey and shrivelled to pink and healthy-looking. And, as should happen in a fairy story, the child survived. At the time when this story was recollected this one-time baby must have been about 15, and the doctor wondered what memory of this experience there might be, locked away in the young man's unconscious.

Again we may jump forward to something that happened later in the doctor's analysis, namely that there kept coming into his mind the story of the Woman of Samaria in St John's Gospel, condensed quotations from which are as below (the version used is from *The Bible Designed to be Read as Literature*, London: Heinemann):

Jesus therefore, being wearied with his journey, sat thus on the well. There cometh a woman of Samaria to draw water: Jesus saith unto her, 'Give me to drink'.

Then saith the woman of Samaria unto him, 'How is it that thou, being a Jew, askest drink of me, which am a woman of Samaria?' For the Jews have no dealings with the Samaritans.

Jesus answered and said unto her, 'If thou knewest who it is that saith to thee, "Give me to drink"; thou wouldest have asked of him, and he would have given thee living water. Whosoever drinketh of this water shall thirst again; but whosoever drinketh of the water that I shall give him shall never thirst.'

The woman saith unto him, 'Sir, give me this water, that I thirst not, neither come hither to draw.'

As the patient said, it always seemed to him – if only one could see beyond the fog of religion – that this story revealed Jesus in a most unsympathetic light, playing cruel verbal games with a simple woman who could not possibly understand what he was talking about. Again, the combination of compassion for the woman, the beauty of the prose, and the theme of water and thirst, produced in him wave after wave of tears.

It is now high time that this long exposition led to some elucidation. The central event of this patient's later childhood had been the sudden death of his father when he was seven; which had produced in his mother a state of distracted grief, followed by numbness, leading in turn to inaccessibility, in face of which her seven-year-old son could only sit helpless, having lost not only his father but his mother also. Much of his feeling could be summed up in his desperate need to bring her back to life, without of course having any means of doing so. Sometimes however she would come to life of her own accord, and this was usually when she could cry – see the theme of healing tears in Chapter 13 – and thus tears could be said to be life-bringing for both of them. This must have something to do with the material given above.

Yet it cannot account for more than part. What about the experiences of starvation and life-threatening thirst, which are depicted in such literal terms in the experience of skin-and-bones, or the fairy story of the dying child, or the true stories of the dying man and the nearly dying baby in hospital?

One may answer, of course, that under the influence of this immensely powerful drug, the mind produces all sorts of distorted and deranged phenomena, including apparent memories that cannot possibly be memories. I am very sceptical, for instance, about people under LSD who appear to remember the process of their birth – one patient reported the feeling 'It's high time that big red-bearded doctor came and got me out of here'! Nevertheless it must be remembered that although the experience reported above started with an exceedingly obscure and highly symbolic vision, the rest consisted of memories of real events, and what the drug did was simply to highlight the connection between them by releasing the feelings associated with them. Moreover, if, as with dreams, associations give an apparent meaning to the whole, perhaps this should at least be seriously considered. The final association of this particular patient – still under LSD – was to the following incident:

When he was perhaps 4, the embarrassing moment came that most parents dread – and certainly parents dreaded in the 1920s – namely that he asked the question how he was born. He was of course told 'another time, dear', which was not unreasonable, seeing that he and his mother were in company at the time. Some days later his mother gathered her courage together and told him part of the truth; but what she emphasized was how she had *dutifully* breast-fed him till he was 6 months old, and *how much it had hurt her*, so much that *it used to make her cry*. He recollected a kind of *déjà vu* feeling, that she was telling him about something very familiar that he had forgotten, accompanied by the wish that he had never asked.

We are now in a position to discuss all this complex material in depth, under a number of headings.

First, some important words of caution. It must always be remembered that these experiences were occurring in an adult, and that any inferences that may be made about the distant past are in danger of what may be called 'psychological anachronism', i.e. attributing to an infant phenomena that really belong to a much later and more sophisticated stage of development. Moreover, any phenomena that may be inferred can only be the result of extrapolation and reconstruction, and no one can speak with any certainty about their significance in terms of human development, and behind this, of human evolution. Finally, of course, there are many details that are unique to this particular patient, as there inevitably are in most patients' stories.

Nevertheless there are phenomena in this material that are encountered time and again in routine analyses; and the inferences made from them – though often stated with far too great certainty – are based on very considerable cumulative evidence.

Having said all this, we may start with the central fact that everything in this long chain of symbolic visions, memories, and associations, is seen in what we may call 'nutritional' or 'homeostatic' terms, which the final association links firmly with *feeding at the breast*. It may be recalled that, in the previous chapter on deeply depressive phenomena, the theme of *feeding* kept recurring in a somewhat similar way. This is a phenomenon so commonly observed in the analysis of patients with any depth of disturbance, and so regularly invested with such colossal emotional significance, that it must be regarded as a major issue in the psychic development of human beings.

What, then, was the core experience apparently being recollected in this series of memories and associations? Surely the evidence suggests that this consisted of trying to get enough nourishment, in face of the fact that any attempt to feed himself caused his mother, the reluctant care-giver, pain. The inference must be that at least sometimes he failed to do so, and in consequence had some kind of experience of starvation. When a baby is small a few hundred millilitres of the right mixture of electrolytes will make all the difference between life and death. This would account for the quite desperate quality with which the whole theme is invested – the baby in hospital and the ill child in the French cartoon, for both of whom death was averted at the last moment, and the man without a tongue, for whom death was inevitable.

It is common psychoanalytical jargon to say that all this is connected with the 'oral' phase of development, since the theme of hunger and thirst, eating and drinking, runs through the whole of the material, and the part of the body that mainly mediates these feelings and the relationship with another human being – the mother – is of course the mouth. This is in contrast to the much later phase in which a relationship of equal importance and intensity is principally mediated by the male and female *genitals* – the 'genital' phase. But in this particular material the word 'oral' to some extent misses the point, because the basic feeling is really about the *inside of the whole body*. This again is an issue that is invested with colossal emotional significance, and which occurs so frequently in analysis that it must be assumed to be universal. Here the contrast is between the feeling of being empty, shrivelled, and at the point of death, on the one hand, and being turgid and full of life on the other. What this example does not illustrate so clearly is the contrast between being 'full of good things' on the one hand and 'full of bad or poisonous things' on the other, which figures very frequently in depressive and paranoid patients, and was considered in connection with the Personnel Manager (p. 177) and will be considered in Chapter 19 (see pp. 254 and 255). The feeling of being 'full of bad things' seems to be associated with *destructive feelings* and *guilt*. In this particular example these feelings appear to be absent, but instead we find two quite different phenomena which will need to be discussed separately. One is the feeling about the inside of his *mother's* body, and the other consists of *concern* and *compassion*.

The first is represented by the most obscure part of the whole experience, the feeling that the patient's body and his mother's were connected, 'there was not enough to go round', and that *both* were merely skin-and-bones. No one can be sure of the significance of this – and any reference to an umbilical cord cannot be anything other than psychological anachronism – but it is an example of something repeatedly encountered in psychotic patients, and in regressed patients in analysis, namely that what is 'inside' and what is 'outside' appear to be the same. A plausible inference is that there is an early stage of development when a human infant cannot distinguish between inside and outside and automatically attributes the same properties to both. In psychotic patients this breakdown of the boundaries of the self appears to be represented by such phenomena as delusions of influence and thought transference; and, as will be discussed later, it can be used defensively in the form of 'paranoid projection'.

In this particular patient, however, there was no suggestion of such phenomena, but on the other hand the overwhelming feeling was one of sadness for his own predicament and compassion for his mother's. The question is now, what phase of development does this belong to? Was this something that arose only when his mother tried to tell him the facts of life, when he was 4, or after his father's death when he was 7, and was then projected back into his infancy, or did he really have such feelings for his mother when he was feeding at her breast? Who can tell?

Here one must say the following: that part of what we observe in regressed patients consists of what we may call the *embryology* of human instincts, emotions, and relations. Compassion and concern are two aspects of human relationships. There must be a time when they first arise. The question is, when? The answer seems to be that, as far as we can reconstruct the process from the analysis of adults and from direct observation, a human infant begins to become aware of his mother as a separate person somewhere around the age of 4–6 months. It is thought that the element of *concern* arises at the same time, and – as has been mentioned before – this represents the *depressive position*, the point at which the child realizes that angry and destructive feelings are *directed towards the person whom he also needs and loves*, which in analysis constitutes a major point of growth. There does therefore seem reason to suppose that, however much of the concern was derived from a later period and was projected back into the past, some of it was actually felt at the time.

This is the point to introduce a formulation made by Michael Balint (1949), that in the earliest stages the human infant's attitude to his mother is that she must be there when she is needed, and there is hell to pay if she isn't, and when she has met his needs there is a state of quiet contentment in which she is more or less forgotten. Only later does she appear in his world as a separate person with needs of her own. Yet evidence from material like the present LSD experience suggests that embryonic feelings of love and concern arise very early in human development, and when they do arise can be of the utmost intensity.

Returning to the feelings of starvation that were so prominent in all this material, we may perhaps introduce the following speculation concerned with the quality of the feeding experience. It seems possible that some of the starvation was not so much physiological as emotional. Could it be that, ideally, breast feeding should have two qualities: it should be *strong* and *fierce* for the baby, and it should be *intensely enjoyable for both baby and mother*? It then becomes an example of the way in which the natural laws relating to material things do not apply in the area of emotions, in the sense that though something material passes *out of* one body and *into* the other, in emotional terms *both are enriched*. Correspondingly, if the fierceness cannot be expressed and enjoyed by both, then both are depleted. Could it be that it was some experience of this kind that the patient was symbolically recollecting? The parallel with an experience deriving from a much later stage of development, namely sex, is obvious, and is clearly hinted at in the association to the photograph of the girl and the mountain.

This leads to yet another observation of immense importance. The parallel between the interactions of breast feeding and those of sexuality is not superficial but profound; and time and again evidence will be found that feelings, fantasies and problems expressed in the later area have their derivation in the earlier.

The final point that I wish to make about this LSD experience is as follows: that I have chosen it because it illustrates so much about the nature of early human experience, but in particular it illustrates the intensity of non-selfish love that human beings are capable of. This is needed as a counterbalance to the theme of destructiveness and cruelty which play such a part in analysis and in writings about it. There will be plenty about these aspects of human nature in the rest of this chapter.

What then about such feelings in the present patient? There was no trace of them in the material presented. Well, as the reader may have guessed, this was the same patient as the Man of Sorrows described on p. 152 in Chapter 13 – here, fed upon his mother's tears – there, *vergiftet mit ihren Tränen*, poisoned by her tears; who once momentarily had the apocalyptic vision that his resentment about the loss of his relationship with his mother was leading to his *spoiling his whole life*. There was then no problem about identifying his solution to the problem of expressing his destructiveness.

This LSD experience, and its subsequent prolonged working through, had a powerful but at the same time limited therapeutic effect. Formerly he had always been troubled in many situations either by not knowing what he felt, or else by finding himself unable to feel. He now knew that what he felt included this profound sadness which always lay beneath what he felt on the surface, and which it was inappropriate to express except in his analysis or when he was by himself. At the same time, because the destructive anger mentioned above was never fully reached, the therapeutic effect was never completely fulfilled. Once more we meet the depressive defence of using genuine feelings of grief and compassion to hide the central conflict of *hating someone deeply loved*. Thus this was an example of failing to reach the central point of the analysis of most (all?) deeply disturbed patients, the depressive position – the point to which once more we return, and which must inevitably be the central theme of the present chapter.

The Cricketer: attacking the good

This patient has already been mentioned in Chapter 14 (pp. 158ff.), where some of his sessions were used to illustrate certain kinds of phenomenon that were only likely to be encountered in long-term therapy.

He was a married man in his mid-thirties, brought up in a professional home, with an older and a younger sister. Some years before he came to analysis he had had a breakdown containing marked depressive and mild paranoid features. His breakdown had left him with a large part of his creative potential stunted and untapped, and it was for this that he sought help. From his long and complex analysis (with a male analyst) I shall pick out a single theme, namely *attacking the good*.

This theme appeared in two different types of circumstance. One was when he was deeply frustrated by other people, when in his rage he would feel like destroying everything good *of his own*. The other was in the very opposite kind of situation: that is, that when he was offered satisfaction for his needs, he would feel like attacking the thing he was offered or the person who offered it.

The latter aspect of this theme clearly arose in the following passages from his analysis:

There had always been much criticism of the building in which he was being seen, and he was constantly on the look-out for evidence of neglect, as shown, for instance, by failure to clean the room properly.

When he arrived one day there was a new mat beside the couch, which he noted as possibly indicating that the authorities had taken some trouble for him. Two sessions later, after a preliminary interpretation that the air of gentleness and peace which he created might well be defensive, he said that the real question was whether his feelings were going to get out of hand. He then took hold of the mat, folded it up, and threw it across the room. To this his analyst said that although the mat represents our care of him, which is just what he wants, the only way he can express his anger about the over-all inadequacy of our care is by rejecting it when it is offered. Not long after this he gets up off the couch and kicks the mat, first into one corner, and then right across the room into the other corner. Having done so, he says that he agrees: only the fact that it's a new mat, and represents our care of him, makes it any good to him to behave in this way.

A second episode took place at a time when some Roman remains had been exposed by a bulldozer during the rebuilding of the City of London. After a long pause in the session he suddenly remarked, 'I wonder why so many people go to see those Roman remains. There are plenty of others to see – why those in particular?' To this his analyst said, 'Perhaps, since they are going to be cleared away and built over, their fascination is that they are a beautiful thing that is going to be destroyed.'

In the next session the patient said, 'I'm cross with you about yesterday, because you were right. I think the next thing I was going to say was that the Roman remains are a beautiful thing that is going to be *spoilt*. And I want to spoil a woman's bottom by beating it – I want it to change from white to red, and from red to black, and blue, and yellow'.

Thus there arose, in this highly dynamic fashion, a reference to his particular sexual deviation, which was that he wanted to be able to beat a woman – and, to a lesser extent, to be beaten by her – before he made love to her.

Obviously, sexual deviations of one kind or another are encountered fairly frequently in patients who ask for psychotherapy. A potential therapist should approach such a deviation with a combination of attitudes: first, the realization that there may well be present factors that are little understood, e.g. heredity and phenomena resembling conditioning and imprinting; second, the expectation that analysis will reveal that the deviation – at least in part – represents identifiable emotional conflicts expressed in the sexual sphere; third, he should retain an entirely open mind about what these conflicts may turn out to be; and fourth, nevertheless he need not be surprised if the conflicts turn out to be something entirely familiar and frequently encounted in other contexts.

This particular patient had spoken of these sexual impulses early in his analysis. Now, it appeared that they represented the sexual expression of a more general phenomenon, namely his above-mentioned need to attack the good.

It may seem a strange thing to say, but during the course of his long analysis evidence steadily accumulated that his impulses were not really sadistic. There was no preoccupation with torture, or with causing suffering for its own sake, nor did he create the impression that he wanted to take revenge on a woman or destroy the relationship with her. Rather, he gave evidence that this aggressive element represented an essential part of his love, without which it was shallow, and with which it was of the utmost depth and intensity. This was illustrated clearly by the following passage, taken from earlier in his analysis:

The passage started with a discussion of why, after the Second World War, 'good' Germans didn't want Germany to be re-armed. This was symbolized in the person of Pastor Niemöller, who had been a U-boat commander in the First World War, but who had suffered a revulsion against all destructiveness and didn't want it revived. The analyst now interpreted that he, the patient, had aggressiveness in him against which he had reacted and which he didn't want revived – he didn't want to be re-armed. The patient said, 'But you *are* re-arming me. Nowadays if someone pushes in front of me in a queue I protest.' He went on to say that another difficulty over Germany is that Germans are afraid that they will start demanding back Germany's Eastern possessions, which might lead to war.

In the next session this theme recurred, and the analyst interpreted that one of the fears was that, if Germany made war to recover her possessions, the possessions would be devastated. The parallel between this and the patient's revived ability to make demands, and the feared destructive effect on anyone on whom the demands were made, was obvious to both, and the analyst added that this destruction would give rise to a mixture of *satisfaction* and *guilt*.

At once the patient said, 'This links with the idea of your having a breakdown. With my previous therapist I used to have the fantasy – partly with *guilt* and partly with *satisfaction* – of his breaking down.' The analyst had then linked this with the patient's beating fantasies, saying that his demands for love got inextricably mixed up with aggression.

The analyst was quite unprepared for the effect of this comment – yet another example of the immense power of correct interpretation. Suddenly the patient was plunged into the depth of his feelings, and in a voice choked with guilt-laden passion started to quote the opening lines of Shelley's poem, *Night:*

Swiftly walk over the Western wave,
    Spirit of Night!
Out of the misty eastern cave –
Where, all the long and lone daylight,
Thou wovest dreams of *joy* and *fear*
Which make thee *terrible* and *dear* –
    Swift be thy flight.

He explained this totally unexpected and initially very obscure association by saying that the idea of his analyst's breakdown was both *terrible* and *dear* to him, arousing in him *joy* and *fear*; and he went on to say that the point about *being beaten* by a woman was that 'I let her do this to me to show her how much I'm willing to suffer because I want so much from her.'

Here one might add that presumably the converse was also true, namely that he wanted the woman to show how much she was willing to suffer in order to give to him what he so desperately needed.

As with the previous patient who had the experience under LSD, it is now high time that this theme of 'attacking the good' led to some elucidation. Why should anyone have such a paradoxical feeling?

This becomes clearer from the following:

On the face of it he came from a normal and caring middle-class home, but at the same time there was evidence from the beginning that his true needs and feelings had been met by unresponsiveness and lack of emotional understanding. In his own words, 'I had everything material, but inside it was absolutely barren.'

The result of this was a sense of emotional deprivation accompanied by a powerful underlying aggressiveness, which could only be expressed in fantasy, and which of course was met by conventionally-based condemnation if any hint of it ever appeared overtly. The whole situation was summed up for him, for instance, by his not being allowed to bang about on the piano, but made to practise properly such pieces as 'Down there in the valley, look, what a pretty farmhouse' – said with bitter contempt. This kind of thing was understandable enough on the part of the people in his environment, of course, yet it also accurately symbolized the gulf that existed between his inner feelings and their understanding.

The evidence therefore suggested the following hypothesis, which clearly links in part with the patient who had the LSD experience: that in his sexual impulses he was desperately trying to combine a number of different needs – first, the natural fierceness of instinctual expression, second the violent and destructive anger about frustration, third the need to have these aggressive impulses recognized and accepted, fourth the need to *produce a response* in the woman that matched the intensity of his own, and fifth, of course, the full depth of his love and need.

This is a satisfactory hypothesis as far as it goes, but, as so often throughout this book, there seems always to be yet another layer. This is suggested by the following piece of history:

When he was about 8, because some guests were staying in the house, he temporarily slept in the same room as his very much older sister. At this time he began to have fantasies of *carving up her breasts*. At the beginning of his analysis he was quite conscious that these fantasies had later been transformed into his impulse to *beat* a woman on her *buttocks*, which had first emerged in his teens.

Now the fact that the woman's *buttocks* appear to be a substitute for *breasts* does not in itself necessitate the hypothesis that the patient's impulses have anything to do with breast feeding. Here one can only say that the deeper one goes into such phenomena in any given patient, and the more often such patients are studied, the more clearly does the evidence point towards this hypothesis, as was illustrated in the present patient by such sessions as the following. (These sessions, incidentally, afford an example of the 'good enough analyst' – compare Winnicott's 'good enough mother' – who is struggling with his own difficulty in understanding the patient's material, but gets there to a reasonable approximation in the end.)

The sessions to be described are the first three after the patient's return from a holiday in some of the wilder parts of Northern Greece. There is an air of extreme constraint from the beginning, with long silences and the patient unable to find anything meaningful to say. Eventually he says that on holiday he met a Greek doctor who *refused to eat* unless his wife actually served his food to him – if she had to be out and left his food on the cooker and all he had to do was to light the gas to heat it, then he *went to bed in a huff*.

This communication needs a considerable amount of discussion. First of all, in deprived patients, breaks in treatment usually mean a feeling of neglect by the therapist, leading in turn to unexpressed anger and lack of communication, and the deadlock can only be broken if the anger is brought into the open, which often needs repeated interpretation over several sessions. Second, if the patient is well into his analysis and is in a potentially regressed state, both the neglect and the anger are likely to be seen in terms appropriate to a baby rather than to an adult – and themes related to *feeding*, the need to be *looked after*, and *early ways of expressing anger*, will be prominent. Seen in this light, the reason why the above communication appears at this point is not hard to discern.

The full interpretation must therefore presumably be that: (1) the patient is angry about being neglected during the holiday; (2) that he sees the analyst's care in terms of feeding; and (3) that the air of constraint is due to the fact that, like the Greek doctor, he wants to refuse what he is offered unless everything is done for him and he is in some way actively fed.

The patient was well aware of most of these issues himself, and the analyst tried to approach them by simply saying that in the present situation the patient felt he was asked to give something before getting anything back, and the analysis was no use to him on these terms. Either this interpretation, though basically correct, was insufficient, or else the patient was in no state to accept anything at all; in any case it didn't help.

The patient goes on to say, 'You won't tell me anything about your holiday, so why should I tell you anything about mine?' to which the analyst says, 'You need your analysis to be a two-way process and you feel it isn't.' The patient now says that, unlike most English people, *he* took the trouble to learn modern Greek so that he could communicate with the natives. Here the message that the analyst is failing to communicate is absolutely clear, but such accusations are not easy to bear, and the analyst didn't see it.

In the third session after the resumption the patient finally gets into a state of frustration, says 'for crying out loud', gets off the couch, sits on the table and starts rocking it, and makes as if to bang the wall. The analyst interprets that it's as if the patient is left in his pram, is full of frustrated anger, and will rock the pram and upset it if he isn't attended to.

At this he lies down and begins to say: 'Horrible, horrible, horrible. Terrible, terrible. Grim. The desert is in the heart of your brother.'

This communication also needs a good deal of elucidation. Words like 'terrible' probably include a reference both to the patient's present inner state and to his former breakdown – when he had *psychiatric* but no *psychotherapeutic* help and felt utterly abandoned and neglected. As he made clear later, the quotation about the 'desert' (from Eliot's *The Rock*) meant that he feels his analyst has nothing to offer him; and this must link with his feeling about his own home background in general, and the relation with his mother in particular, which he had said was 'absolutely barren'.

Now, from the patient's point of view, analysis is a situation with very special characteristics. On the one hand, he is offered what I have described before as very potent gifts – unconditional acceptance and understanding – and on the other hand he is offered nothing more than this, and undoubtedly he wants far more. Therefore the analysis can be seen either as deeply satisfying or utterly frustrating, according to the patient's state of mind at any given time. There is no question that at the present moment it is the frustration that is being emphasized, and yet it is the patient's own inner state that is responsible for this – the characteristics of the analytical situation haven't changed. Moreover, we know from previous material, first, that the Greek doctor *refused what he was offered*, and second, that the patient himself wanted to *attack and spoil the good*. Therefore this statement that 'the desert is in the heart of your brother' may well represent an angry depreciation of what the analyst has to offer. Moreover, if the patient depreciates what he is offered and refuses to accept it, then he himself will be left desolate, so that the desert will be in his own heart as well. And finally, we may ask, what has happened to everything he has received in the past? As was described in connection with the Personnel Manager in Chapter 15 (see pp. 177ff.), it is possible that there has been some *internal* spoiling as well, which has further contributed to the inner desolation.

The problem in this kind of analytical situation is to know which of all these aspects to emphasize at any given moment, and it is very easy to make an inappropriate choice. Here, the analyst chose to emphasize inner destruction, saying, 'You feel desolate, everything is destroyed in you, because I haven't fed you for so long, and what I have fed you with in the past is now destroyed by your anger.'

It is to be noted that this interpretation is probably correct, but is really inappropriate, because it is not sufficiently linked to what the patient has said. The patient himself makes this clear, saying that he said the desert was in the *brother*, and he feels it is not in himself but in the *analyst*, who has nothing to give him. Nevertheless, this is progress, because the patient now openly acknowledges that he is talking about giving-and-receiving in the analytical situation. The analyst then says, 'I think the desert in me is a reflection of the desert in you, and is concerned with your wanting to destroy what I offer you because I haven't fed you.'

This interpretation is sufficiently correct to produce a marked deepening of rapport, in which symbolic communications become transformed into direct feeling. The patient first says, 'But you *don't* feed me', and then suddenly, 'I have the feeling you don't want me as a patient. Your expression says so.'

This is another communication with profound and complex implications. First of all, it is a misperception on the patient's part – the analyst was deeply involved with this patient and it was not true to say that he didn't want him. But what was true was that the patient had been told openly by his *parents* that when he was conceived they had not yet been ready to have a second child, i.e. that he was to some degree unwanted. Thus the patient is imposing on the analytical situation something derived from the past.

Yet is this the whole story? The earlier communication about the Greek doctor makes clear that probably the patient is rejecting the analyst rather than the other way round, and if this is true it is this that needs to be dealt with, Moreover, this situation in which hostility is felt to be in the other person, when really it is in oneself, seems to lie at the heart of paranoid feelings, and one of the crucial tasks in the analysis of borderline patients is to undo this paranoid mechanism and enable the patient to acknowledge the hostility in himself. There was a preliminary discussion of this point under the heading of the Nurse in Mourning, p. 143.

Yet again, if the feeling of being unwanted results from 'paranoid projection', how can this be reconciled with the fact that there was objective evidence that the patient was in fact unwanted? The answer can only be that, although he was indeed unwanted, his angry and paranoid feelings have in some way exaggerated this, and it is this that needs to be brought out in the present situation.

This need not to be carried away by sympathy for our patients' deprivation is crucial to being an effective therapist – but it can also be taken too far, leading ultimately to the implication that all their deprivation is imaginary, which of course cannot be true either. It requires constant vigilance to strike a balance between these two extremes.

In the present session, therefore, the analyst said, 'I think that what you see as my hostility is really a reflection of your own. We're so close together that you don't know what's in me and what's in you.'

To this the patient at first continued his depreciation, but now with more open anger, and now also overtly in terms of food: 'English bread is foul, it's like tissue paper, there's no nourishment in it' (and, he might well have added, 'there's nothing to get your teeth into'); and then, without making any link, he suddenly launches into the following story: 'There was a cricket match between two teams who had challenged each other for a barrel of beer. Team A was winning hands down until someone came in to bat for team B and started beating the ball all over the place. There were several lost balls, and then finally all they could find was a very old and dilapidated one, and he beat this so hard that the cover came off, and one half went for six into a tree while the other half was caught! They didn't know which result to choose; and since there was now no ball anyhow, the game had to be abandoned.'

Here the reader will recognize all the hallmarks of an *unconscious communication* as described in Chapter 3 – a sudden change of subject accompanied by an increase in animation – but he may well be puzzled as to what it can possibly be about.

Let us take the elucidation stage by stage. First, this communication, together with the two previous ones, represents a very important shift: from the feeling that the *analyst* is hostile, through overt *depreciation*, to *overt aggressive impulses in the patient* – obviously the patient is identified with the batsman who beats the ball till it comes in two. Thus what has occurred here is an undoing of the paranoid projection – the patient has 'taken the aggression back into himself'. Second, the angry and destructive quality in the aggression has by now been considerably mitigated – the reference to cricket is to something 'good', and to a perfectly acceptable and non-sadistic form of aggression – as one West Indian cricketer said, 'Man, that ball's there to be *hit*' – though since the ball comes to bits in the end, the element of destructiveness is not entirely eliminated. Third, there must be a reference to the patient's beating fantasies, which – by displacement – can be traced back to feelings about *women's breasts*. Fourth, the themes of neglect and deprivation, food and feeding, run throughout the whole of the material. In other words, all the clues are there for a comprehensive interpretation.

The theoretical basis for such an interpretation, as I see it, leads on from what I said about the LSD patient:

Feeding at the breast should be fierce and highly 'instinctual'. If the mother is 'good enough' in the sense of meeting the infant's needs; and if she can accept the fierceness and enjoy it, all is well. On the other hand, if she fails badly in these two areas, the fierceness becomes not merely aggressive, but overwhelming, destructive, and terrifying. One of the primitive mechanisms that the infant uses to deal with this is 'paranoid projection' in which such impulses seem not to be in him but to be coming back at him from the outside world. In the analysis of paranoid patients one of the main tasks is to undo this mechanism and enable the patient to acknowledge the destructiveness in himself. When this is done at the right moment, and the patient realizes that the analyst/mother whom he wants to destroy is also the one whom he loves and needs, there occurs what may be called the 'miracle of the depressive position' – graphically illustrated by the present patient.

At this point the analyst said, 'I think you feel my food to be worthless because of your anger with me, and you want to beat and beat my breast, which I feed you with, till it's destroyed' (when one is operating at this level of fantasy, the fact that the male analyst is never likely to be able to breast feed a baby is neither here nor there).

In reply to this, suddenly the patient says, 'Glub's being resurrected. The cube of ice has been brought out for it to melt.'

Even without any inside knowledge this reference to *resurrection* should be enough for the reader to realize what has happened (compare 'the Arctic landscape transformed into grass', p. 144). Reaching the *attack upon the good* in the *transference relationship*, together with the *reason for the attack*, namely a *feeling of neglect*, and tracing it all back to the *earliest relation with the mother*, has led to the temporary resolution of the inability to make use of what the analyst offers, and therefore to the possibility of taking in something good and coming to life again.

The reference in fact is to a strip cartoon which was appearing at that time in the *News Chronicle*. Glub was a cave man who had been discovered frozen in a block of ice in Siberia. The ice had been melted and he had come out alive, and later had begun to undergo an analysis! At some point he had become dissatisfied and had decided to get frozen again, but now he was once more being resurrected. He had been mentioned many times in the analysis before, and it was always clear that, being a cave man, he represented primitive aspects of the patient.

The analyst makes use of this in his next comment: 'Yes, when I understand these things in you, you come to life; and what comes to life is the cave man, the primitive part of you.' The patient now says, 'They're very primitive in parts of Greece. I saw them threshing the corn with a flail.' Here again there is an overt reference to aggression and food, but the aggression is no longer destructive at all – threshing is an essentially constructive process, producing food for man and seed corn to perpetuate the plant. The analyst, who doesn't see these implications, says simply, 'Yes, they beat their food with a whip'. This is the end of the session.

The central theme of the present chapter is inevitably the *depressive position* in all its aspects. The Cricketer's original complaint was an inability to reach his creative potential. The reason for this was almost certainly an inability to reach the depressive position. His sexual impulses can now be seen clearly to represent an attempt to reach this position – to fuse love and aggression – which had been unsuccessful because the origin of the aggression remained unconscious. In the sessions just described the origin was revealed with considerable clarity.

The Refugee Musician and the treatment of near-psychotic patients

This patient came to therapy at the age of 23, complaining, amongst other things, of becoming distracted by sexual fantasies about small boys. In Chapter 19 he will be used as an example of inadequate initial assessment, because – although all the clues were there – the interviewing psychiatrist quite failed to see the severity of his disturbance (see pp. 249ff.).

Michael Balint used to say, 'Paranoid patients are my favourites', which seemed to me at the time absurd, since I was used to the chronic, deluded, litigious, hostile, rigid type of paranoid schizophrenic whom one encounters in mental hospitals – than whom few patients are less attractive. What he meant was patients like the one described here, whose psychotic unconscious is at their finger tips; who know all about psychodynamics without ever having read the books; and who then lead their – fortunately – less disturbed therapists into profound insight about the darkest areas of the human psyche.

The patient was Jewish, born in Germany. His father, who never married his mother, lived with her for perhaps the first year of the patient's life and then left and was not heard of again. The patient and his mother suffered considerably from Nazi persecution, but managed to escape to this country in 1939, when the patient was eight. Thereafter he was evacuated, without his mother, to a number of different English homes during the war. Not surprisingly, he had a profound sense of deprivation, both of maternal and paternal care; and underlying this was a basically psychotic disturbance.

He received a diagnosis of 'personality disorder' and was originally assigned, as a routine disposal, to a group. This was not as inappropriate a disposal as might be imagined – as, with his relative absence of neurotic defences, he certainly stirred the other patients out of their lethargy. But of course it was inadequate treatment, and when he later came back asking for further help he was taken on by his original therapist individually at once a week. What was intended as an essentially supportive type of treatment gradually transformed itself into an attempt – still at once a week – to help him radically, and thus became a sort of once-a-week, face-to-face, analysis.

This was a heroic task, and in the end a hopeless one. He finally met an event that threatened the whole basis of his life: after a particularly disturbed episode he was dismissed from his job, being offered as the only alternative a transfer 250 miles away from London and everything that kept him alive. The result was a psychotic depression and a second determined suicidal attempt, this time successful, leaving his therapist with a feeling akin to the words from the last scene of King Lear:

> Vex not his ghost; O, let him pass. He hates him
> That would upon the rack of this tough world
> Stretch him out longer

The technique with near-psychotic patients

This is an appropriate point to consider the technique of treating these near-psychotic patients in interpretative therapy, at any rate in anything short of five-times-a-week analysis. For neurotic patients the classical analytical technique of distant, free-floating attention, and refusal to give anything other than interpretations, which heightens anxiety and tends to intensify transference, may be appropriate; though in my view it needs to be tempered with everyday humanity. In patients such as the present, however, there is no need whatsoever to intensify anything, and indeed it is inappropriate and dangerous to do so; and in such patients the use of this kind of technique – certainly at once a week on an out-patient basis – will often rapidly lead to uncontrollable disturbance, destructive or self-destructive acting out, impossible transference situations, or premature withdrawal. The appropriate technique is not easy to learn or to describe, but it contains the following elements, of which the second is the most important:

(1) A friendly and flexible attitude, which needs to be free of any trace of falseness (which the patient will immediately detect).
(2) The establishment of a strong *therapeutic alliance*, within which the therapist *speaks to the sane part* of the patient *about the mad part*, trusting the sane part to hold the mad part under control. This is the most difficult aspect to learn.

(3) A very cautious attitude to interpreting defences, which will break down of their own accord and do not need any help to do so.

(4) When the patient becomes disturbed, then is the time for major interpretations, and then *nothing need be left unsaid* – no punches need be pulled – the patient is well aware of his most disturbing impulses, and it is only a relief to him to have them recognized and accepted, particularly in the transference relationship, and traced to their origin.

(5) At times of maximum disturbance, hospital admission may well be imperative; and when a really strong therapeutic alliance has been established the patient himself can often be trusted to say when this is necessary.

Finally, it needs to be emphasized that *no one should undertake the interpretative therapy of such patients without a good deal of experience, together with some personal analysis, and, if he is only moderately experienced, without experienced supervision.* The opportunities for catastrophe are too great – suicide is perhaps an acceptable risk, but homicide, which is often close beneath the surface, is not.

The Refugee Musician (contd)

From this very long therapy I shall pick out three related themes: the meaning of the patient's sexual fantasies, the meaning of paranoid phenomena, and the resolution of paranoid fantasies into the depressive position.

As I wrote in connection with the previous patient, one needs to adopt an open mind about the meaning of sexual fantasies – and indeed of any other neurotic manifestation – and yet one should not be surprised if they turn out to represent a variation on familiar themes.

Before the final catastrophe occurred, the patient showed some remarkable improvements. Prominent among these was a gradual move away from being sexually interested in young boys, first towards young girls, and then to grown-up women. 'I now realize', he said, 'that little boys are a defence against little girls, and little girls are a defence against women.' But why did he need to defend himself against women?

The answer seemed to be twofold:

First – as I mentioned in Chapter 8 (see p. 63), he was an example of a man suffering from the most intense Oedipal anxieties in spite of really never having known a father to act as a rival to him. He was the patient who used to have to carry a knife around in order to protect himself against rival men who would attack him in the street. It was noticeable that this fantasy became greatly intensified if he ever got close to heterosexual feelings. Here the fusion between Oedipal and paranoid anxieties is unmistakable.

But the little boys represented much more than a defence – they also represented the return-of-the-repressed, the impulse, with an extraordinary degree of over-determination. We may ask, what exactly did these paedophilic impulses consist of? The answer was, mainly, that he wanted to suck the little boy's penis, an act that would be accompanied by the most intense feelings of sexual love. During the course of his analysis the fantasy became more and more conscious that the boy had been filled up with all the good things that he himself had never had, and that by the act of sucking he could draw these things into himself, and thus give himself life.

Thus, once more, we come upon primitive and literal feelings concerned with 'drinking in' and enriching the inside of the body, which – it would seem – most probably have their origin in feeding at the breast.

Yet there was a further complication, for not only did he feel that the little boy had been enriched by his *mother* but also by his *father*. Not only would the patient drink to give himself *life*, but also to give himself *manhood*. Thus we meet another primitive kind of fantasy, that of literally drawing in manhood from a father.

When I entered the field of psychoanalysis and dynamic psychotherapy I used to read this kind of thing, often described by analysts as if it were self-evident, with irritation and disbelief. I have gradually come to realize that not all such fantasies are imposed on patients by some kind of psychoanalytical madness.

The reader by now will hardly be surprised if we go on to further complications. So far we have reached the point that the little boy represents a kind of intermediary between the patient and both a mother and a father. But why should the patient need an intermediary at all? All the evidence suggests that what he was trying to avoid was the fact that, side by side with his love, his impulses included hatred and violence of the most terrifying intensity – the little boy was sufficiently far removed from the original figures (it would be wrong to say 'people', since one cannot believe that these feelings concerned his real father) to keep such feelings at bay. For instance, a little boy cannot be regarded as much of a threat as a rival – or can he? One may well ask this question in view of the following: at one period of his analysis the patient used to stand in the street watching boys come out of school at the end of the day, carrying his knife, with the fantasy of following them and murdering them. The degree of love and concern in this patient, and his extraordinary capacity for impulse control, made quite clear that there was really no danger whatsoever of his putting these fantasies into effect; but once more we reach evidence about the intensity of love and hate that can exist together in human beings.

The depressive position in a paranoid patient

This leads straight into the next theme, *the conversion of paranoid fantasies into the depressive position*, which is illustrated by the following passage in his analysis:

As mentioned above, his homosexual, paedophilic impulses gradually gave way to feelings about adult women; and although he did not get as far as an actual sexual relation, he began to form friendships with girls. There was a particular girl who invited him to come to her home, and then – for what appeared to be no more than reality reasons – had to cancel her invitation. Wisdom after the event suggests that this rejection started a period of increasing disturbance in him. He would come up in a state of mounting psychotic tension, conveying the feeling that sooner or later some kind of volcano was going to erupt. This reached a climax in a session in which he reported that his mother had developed flu, and he spoke with suppressed rage of two GPs in partnership who had both left it to the last moment to visit her. Fairly obviously, he was identifying himself with a feeling of being neglected; but this was not what he mainly emphasized, which was either that his mother might become so ill as to be unable to do anything for herself and thus would put excessive demands on him, or that she might leave him to clear up single-handed all the practical and legal consequences of her death. If this happened, he said, it would have such a disturbing effect on him that he would need admission to a mental hospital.

Once again we meet the theme of *needs* and *demands*. One can see that he would intensely resent having to meet demands caused by the mother who he felt had not properly looked after him, but there seemed something deeper than this – he conveyed the feeling not only that these demands would make him angry, but that they contained some psychotically terrifying quality. Remembering, therefore, that this patient had much paranoia in his make-up, the therapist made an interpretation involving paranoid projection: that the demands directed towards him by his mother in some way represented his own demands, which had an *overwhelming* and *destructive* quality. For good measure, the therapist linked this with himself, since that week he had 'demanded' that the patient should change the time of the session. What he should have done also, was to add that the patient's demands took on this destructive quality as a consequences of his being rejected by the girl; but this 'strategic' interpretation was missed, since the rejection had occurred 2 months before and its effects had been insidious rather than immediate.

Once more we meet analysis as an experimental situation. The *hypothesis* is that his mother's demands are terrifying because they contain by paranoid projection, the patient's own destructiveness, which in turn is a consequence of his feeling of deprivation; the implied *prediction* is that the patient will in some way 'take the destructiveness back into himself'. If this does occur, it will represent a confirmation of the hypothesis in this particular case, and will provide confirmatory evidence about paranoia in general.

So what happened? Suddenly the patient launches into the following communication:

'I was recently reading an article about the massacre at My Lai in Vietnam. According to this article, what happened was that a group of American soldiers were approaching a village, when a woman suddenly stood up and looked out at them from a cornfield. Their response was frenzied machine-gunning, so that she was absolutely cut to pieces. *This is how people react when they see a woman, or a mother, as an enemy.*'

In this communication the destructiveness was unequivocally directed against the mother, and thus by implication was in the patient, and the above prediction was thus fulfilled.

In the next session he was still in a very disturbed, potentially explosive state, with suicidal fantasies. The therapist made an interpretation of the depressive position: that the intensity of his disturbance was the result of his having impulses like the machine-gunning of this woman towards anyone whom he loved and needed, particularly anyone in the position of mother to him, which included his therapist. The patient could not accept the transference aspects of this interpretation; but in the next session he said that he had been thinking about it, and he now realized that a reason for hating his therapist was that although he gave the patient a great deal, he didn't give nearly enough. The therapist did what is always necessary when there are suicidal feelings present of this quality, and interpreted that suicide was a way of protecting the therapist from the patient's wish to kill him. The patient remained in an extremely disturbed state, with horrifying, sadistic images forcing themselves on his involuntary attention; and the therapist finally succeeded in getting him admitted to hospital, from where, fortunately, he was allowed to continue coming to his sessions.

Here the patient met a schizophrenic girl, with whom he made contact with the help of his own profound insight, but who then said something rejecting to him; and in the next session he proudly announced that the television set in the ward wasn't working any more, as he had put a chair through it. The therapist continued with interpretations about rage against anyone who rejected him, including the therapist himself, and – although there is no record of this – perhaps in this session finally gave the 'strategic' interpretation about the previous girl's rejection, which had started this period of disturbance. He also promised to try and persuade the hospital consultant – to whom the patient had not endeared himself by his destructive acting out – to reverse his decision to discharge him; which promise he implemented, but without success.

After this session the patient wrote the therapist a most touching letter: 'I found our session of yesterday very satisfying. I can now think of the young schizophrenic girl with much less disturbance. I want her to get well because she is a lovely person and she would be of more benefit to other people healthy than sick.

'I enclose something which I had brought along to the meeting yesterday but forgot to give to you.'

The enclosure was a review from the *New Statesman* of Marion Milner's book, *The hands of the living God* (1969). One of the major themes of this book is how Mrs Milner 'held' her patient, symbolically, through all her disturbances; and the review reproduced a drawing made by the patient of a mother holding a baby, drawn in such a way that the two are fused and it is impossible to tell where the mother ends and the baby begins.

Before his admission to hospital a married woman, separated from her husband, had begun to show an interest in him. A few weeks after his discharge she invited him around to her flat and made clear to him that she would like him to make love to her. He coped with this the only way he could, by talking to her about all his doubts and fears – that his penis was too small, that she might not give him as much as he wanted and he might get violent, and so on. Eventually he said to her that if she would be willing to take her clothes off and go to to bed, he would join her there and he didn't know whether he would be able to do anything more than read her a bedtime story. In fact he was able to give her the most intense feelings and to satisfy her, though he himself was unable to ejaculate. He told his therapist that this did not matter, and that in fact it was the most powerful and beautiful experience of his life.

Thus, throughout this long series of sessions, we meet once again the miracle of the depressive position.

Discussion

I propose to leave the patient at this high point of his therapy and his adult life, and to discuss some of the psychopathology that he illustrates. As always, it must be remembered that, although the observations are clear and incontrovertible, the inferences made from them are about processes that it is impossible to observe directly.

Perhaps a good starting point is a comparison with the Cricketer. Examination of the process of the sessions described here will show: (1) that both patients suffered from a feeling of hostile forces in the outside world; (2) that both responded to interpretation of paranoid projection by producing an association that indicated aggression in themselves; and (3) that there was evidence in both patients that this aggression arose in, or at least was partly concerned with, the early relation with the mother.

There was, however, a major difference in the quality of the aggression, which in the second patient had a far more savage, terrifying and destructive quality. Correspondingly, there was a far greater need for disguise. In the first patient the situation seemed to be largely that sexual need and love were inseparable from aggression. In the second patient, (1) the aggression did not appear overtly at all, and only appeared in the form of powerful paranoid feelings if he was threatened with getting close to a woman; and (2) although the sexual feelings overtly contained the element of sucking or feeding, this was directed not towards an adult woman, not even to a young girl, not even to a breast at all, but to a young boy and his penis – in other words just about as far away from a mother and her breast as was practicable. All the evidence suggests that this was necessary because of the terrifying intensity of the mixed feelings aroused in him by the threat of a close relation with a woman. In therapy, the process of displacement had to be retraced in the opposite direction, stage by stage, and the origin of the aggression traced to his feeling of rejection, before such a relation could become feasible at all.

'Oral, anal, and genital'

I hope that enough has now been presented to illustrate three generalizations that are of course derived from clinical experience throughout the whole of the present century: First, that in certain adult patients both *needs* and *aggressive feelings* are seen in very early mother-child terms; second that, among the feelings involved, those to do with breast-feeding are prominent; and third, that such feelings may become incorporated into *adult sexuality*. (It should perhaps be added here that it doesn't seem to make much difference if the baby was in fact bottle-fed – presumably the bottle and its teat are felt to be part of the mother in the same way as the breast and its nipple.)

Freud made this observation about breast-feeding quite early in the history of psychoanalysis, and in the 'Three essays' (1905) he put forward the view that the child's 'sexuality' passes through three phases, being mediated first through the mouth, then the anus, and finally the genitals – the oral, anal, and genital phases. As far as the oral phase is concerned, the reader will see from the foregoing case histories the kinds of clinical observation on which Freud's theory was based.

It is, of course, not in question that feeding her baby is probably the most important of all a mother's functions – obviously the baby's life depends on this function more than any other – and the intensity of feeling associated with it has been sufficiently illustrated.

Nevertheless, the formulation put forward by Freud leads to all sorts of implications which seem to me to be over-simplifications or distortions, or at least need to be carefully scrutinized before being accepted. The danger is, for instance, that at this stage the infant is considered to be just a mouth, and the mother to be just a breast and nipple, and the over-all mother – child relation gets lost. This kind of approach then gets carried over into the 'genital' phase, and a boy or man gets considered as if he were little more than a penis, and you then get the absurd situation in which all fear of physical injury is seen as fear of genital injury, and all drive for achievement as a drive for 'potency' and so on. Returning to the 'oral' phase, I well remember, in my early days as an analyst, being firmly put in my place by a woman patient: 'After all,' I said, 'at this stage a mother is just a breast to her child.' '*And* arms, *and* a lap' was her reply. This clearly implies feelings about being *held*, emphasized by Winnicott and so touchingly illustrated by Marion Milner's patient mentioned above, and leads away from the narrow-minded concentration on the feeding relation.

Nor do I think that this narrow view is in accord with the findings of modern biology, as has clearly been formulated by Bowlby (1969, pp. 210–20). Here it is worth a digression to discuss one of the observations of the Harlows: that infant Rhesus monkeys, if offered a dummy mother made of wire from which they could feed, and another made of cloth from which they couldn't, in fact spent far more time clinging to the second rather than the first. If we assume that the clinging represented some form of 'attachment', then this means that the attachment developed not to something that provided food, but something that provided *soft physical contact*.

Now, of course, this tells us nothing about human beings – for instance infant monkeys are carried around clinging to their mother's fur, while human infants are not – but it permits us to question the widely held view that attachment develops in the human infant solely because of feeding. We all know that human beings have a need to be cuddled. When does this develop? Should we postulate a stage of 'cutaneous erotism' in between the 'oral' and the 'anal' stage?

As for the anal stage itself, it seems to me very questionable whether this should be elevated into a 'stage' at all. Michael Balint, who never succeeded in getting away from many psychoanalytic views which I regard as outdated, nevertheless used to say that he thought the anal stage was a purely cultural phenomenon – presumably over-emphasized and handed down from mother to child, especially as part of the legacy of Victorian times. *Of course* there are certain kinds of obsessional patients whose whole preoccupation is with lavatories, and certain homosexuals (and indeed heterosexuals) who use the anus as the main sexual orifice, but in my own practice I have found such problems to be of very little significance in the majority of ordinary neurotic patients. Psychotherapists should be aware of what Freud said on this subject, and be prepared to use it occasionally in their work with patients, but also should be prepared to treat it as a part of history. In my view, the whole concept of oral, anal, and genital stages is one of the *very* many examples of ways in which Freud drew attention to something of immense importance which no one had ever noticed before; and yet, by his particular emphasis and theoretical framework, somehow got the understanding of human beings off on the wrong foot. It is immensely important that clinicians from within psychoanalysis should have the courage to say this.

It is however unquestionably true – as I hope to have shown in the foregoing case histories – that in patients who have suffered severely from maternal deprivation in one form or another, feelings about breast-feeding and the inside of the body tend to emerge with unmistakable clarity and intensity. Moreover, such feelings often appear when the manifest deprivation has occurred long after infancy (both the Refugee Musician and the next patient, the Foster Son, are examples) and then the question arises of the extent to which later deprivation is merely *being seen in terms of,* or is actually *reviving memories of,* an earlier kind of deprivation – a question that is usually unanswerable.

Nevertheless, when due importance has been given to these feelings about feeding, the following needs to be said: surely the truth is that the mother – child relation is mediated in many different ways, not all of them concerned with bodily pleasure; and although the importance of each of them waxes and wanes during the course of development, so that it is correct to speak in terms of 'stages', they overlap in a highly complex way. And moreover, although physical expression and bodily pleasure are immensely important – and anyone who ignores this, at whatever stage of human development, does so at his peril – it is at least arguable that what really matters is whether the mother is *there* sufficiently often when needed, is responsive and accepting, and conveys the feeling that the infant is wanted and enjoyed. Correspondingly, what matters in the infant is not so much parts of the body, but – in more or less random order – love, hate, security, separation, loss, frustration, anger, grief, concern, guilt, need, demand, giving and receiving, and the ways in which these aspects of his relation to the mother develop and interact.

All this leads to another immensely important and unanswered question: what is the source of the truly horrifying aggressive impulses that we find in some of our patients – heredity or environment, or what combination of the two? This is best considered after the following patient has been presented.

The Foster Son: savagery and closeness

This was a married man of 24. He will be encountered again in Chapter 23 in connection with the problem of assessing a patient for psychotherapy. The issues relevant to this latter problem will be highlighted if the phenomena about to be described are borne in mind. Equally, if the reader wishes to hear the story from the beginning he should turn to p. 274.

The main traumatic event of the patient's childhood was that he arrived home from the pictures on a Saturday morning, at the age of 8, to find that his mother had gone; and although he continued to live with his father for a time, it soon became clear that this was an impossible situation, with the result that he spent most of the rest of his upbringing in institutions and foster homes.

It was difficult to know exactly what he considered as his main complaint. Let us say, simply, that he knew he was a very disturbed young man, and he wanted help. In contrast to the Refugee Musician, the extent of his disturbance and the kinds of danger likely to be encountered in psychotherapy were realized from the beginning – though not, perhaps, the severity of them – and this was reflected in the therapeutic organization provided for him (for details see p. 278). The therapist was a woman psychologist.

The patient showed very disturbed behaviour from the beginning. By the end of the first 6 months he had already been in and out of hospital four times, the cause of which was that at times of stress he had an uncontrollable urge to trace the veins on his forearms with a razor blade. This did not have the quality of a suicidal impulse, but rather of some act of self-mutilation connected in part with a fascination with blood.

The self-mutilation tended to occur especially in connection with long gaps in treatment such as holidays – not so much, as one might expect, during his therapist's absence, but usually after her return, and often after a delay of one or two weeks or more. This is unmistakable evidence that it represents *acting out* of transference impulses to do with reunion after separation. Obviously it was an extremely dangerous game that he was playing, and a potential threat to himself and to his therapy. Whenever such a phenomenon appears *it is essential to try to bring the underlying transference feelings into the open as soon as possible*. On the face of it these feelings seem to be of three kinds:

(1) A primary form of aggression, in which a wish to attack or injure his therapist is turned against himself;
(2) A secondary form of aggression, in which he takes his revenge on her for abandoning him by making her anxious – in which of course he unquestionably succeeded; and
(3) A cry for help and an attempt to prevent her from leaving him again.

Such feelings must be interpreted to him. It should also emphasized that this is one of the few situations in which interpretations should be persisted with *whether there is any direct confirmation of them or not* – it is the only way to hold the situation under control. This the therapist did, and in fact confirmation was meagre.

I shall now jump ahead to a series of sessions which followed a 6-week summer break, three years after he started treatment. Much of this is told in the therapist's words:

'The first sessions concentrated on his despair at making me understand his feeling – he can't say it right – he would like to "open up his mind and invite me in". He read about two snakes devouring each other – he'd like that sort of relationship. As an alternative to this wish for perfect unity he shuts down and denies wanting any relationship or having any feelings – and then he has an image of gas leaks which ultimately explode in your face. He pushes away any ideas of being responsible for such damaging feelings or forces, though he merrily indulges in fantasies of being a "hit man" – i.e. someone hired to carry out a murder. He thinks he could design the perfect crime.

'The tension increases because I have to change his times and he misses sessions because buses fail to run. Once he rings me at home to tell me that he is very frightened because a man bumped into him on the Underground – he was afraid he (the patient) would lose control and hit him because he was not recognizing the patient as a person.' Again, this kind of incident needs to be seen for what it is, namely one to which transference feelings have made a major contribution. The clear statement about fear of loss of control needs to be taken seriously – the therapist is only not in danger provided (1) she has established a good therapeutic alliance, and (2) she interprets and accepts the hostile feelings in the transference wherever there is evidence for them. This she did, linking his feeling of not being recognized as a person with the fact that the time of a number of sessions had to be changed.

The patient's intense dependence on his therapist, which of course is the source of his hostile feelings, becomes clear from the following passage:

'He complains that he wastes sessions: he can't start because he knows we have to stop; he needs half the time to get used to being there and my being still there. He can't bear the time between sessions, waiting to see if I am still there. He barrages me with questions about why I leave such a long gap between sessions, and about this crazy relationship. He gets terribly angry if I turn my head aside, and then is worried. An interpretation about his sadness over wanting to hurt me, who means so much to him, precipitates anxious feelings about not knowing what is fantasy and what is reality' – in other words, when he begins to be faced with the true intensity of his ambivalence, near-psychotic phenomena are intensified. 'Soon after this he appears wearing a painting of a woman's corpse, mounted on wood, around his neck.'

This is the beginning of openly sadistic treatment of his therapist. 'He rings and demands an extra session, to which he brings a letter opener in the form of a stiletto, exceedingly long and sharply pointed.' He is dressed in new brown clothes, which both patient and therapist know is a reference to the colour of dried blood, and behaves in an increasingly flirtatious way. The therapist makes a link between stabbing and sexual impulses towards her.

The patient now talks of how one of his principal fantasies is coming closer to reality. This is a fantasy about which he has spoken often before, which goes as follows:

He kills a woman by breaking her neck. Then, with the precision of a skilled leather maker, he skins her. He then covers the whole of his body with her blood. In his own words, 'As it dries out it pinches my skin and makes me feel like I am being cuddled tight.'

His therapist has a written version of this fantasy, which is so horrific, and is told in such loving detail, without a trace of concern for the woman, as to make it quite unsuitable for publication. It is only slightly mitigated by the fact that the woman is already dead before he does these things to her. If the Cricketer's fantasies were violent but not really sadistic; and those of the Refugee Musician were violent, savage, and destructive, but again only rarely sadistic, those of the present patient were all three of these, and in addition sadistic in the true sense of the word.

The reader may make of this fantasy what he chooses. For my part I see in it ambivalent feelings carried to the limit – a combination of the *ultimate savagery* with the *ultimate need for closeness*. On the other hand, it does *not* represent the depressive position, precisely because the element of concern is totally absent.

The terrible thing is that at that point in therapy the patient was making a habit of *actually* hiding in the bushes at night, and following women, in imagination putting these impulses into effect. If anybody wants tangible evidence for my previous statement that this kind of work should only be undertaken by experienced therapists, surely it is to be found here.

The patient blatantly uses this sadistic fantasy to be sadistic to his therapist. 'He gleefully talks about his wish to kill a woman, and wants to know if I would stop him. After his childhood history, prison would be no hardship. He goes on torturing me with sadistic pleasure and demonstrations with the "knife". Interpretations make him threaten to kill me because I maintain my professional attitude towards him.'

In retrospect, the therapist said that she had enough faith in her relation with this patient not to feel in any personal danger from him; but that what was unbearable was (1) her anxiety that he would really translate his fantasy into reality outside the sessions, and (2) the way in which he made macabre jokes about it all, breaking her control and making her laugh and collude with his own pleasure.

In such situations therapists have nothing but words and other intangibles with which to preserve themselves, their patients, and innocent victims from catastrophe. Chief among these intangibles are sincerity and the therapeutic alliance. At these moments of desperate psychotherapeutic emergency one of the cardinal rules is *objectivity but no pretence*. For instance, one can point out to patients the fundamental reality, in so many words: '*I* can't control you, only *you* can control yourself' (see p. 229). There is no point in concealing your anxiety, which is obvious, and which is deliberately aroused by the patient in any case. This therapist chose from among the many possibilities one that was certainly correct: she told him straight out that she *could not stand his pleasure in making her so unbearably anxious*.

Probably two important elements in this remark of hers were, first, bringing his pleasure out into the open; and, second, openly acknowledging how much he was affecting her, which may well have made it less necessary for him to go on doing so. Anyhow, what emerged immediately was the hidden therapeutic alliance, for the patient admitted his own anxiety about his impulses, and pleaded with her to share it with him. At this point, quite rightly, she implemented a decision already taken before this session started, namely to offer to increase his sessions to three times a week, which he accepted.

What does one do about the knife? It is certainly possible to persuade him to give it up; but the only trouble with this is that it leaves the patient with the feeling that he is being controlled from outside, and hence conceals how large a part of him wishes to control himself – and in any case he can always go and buy another. With immense courage this therapist said nothing about the knife – and on the way out of the building he left it for her with the receptionist.

I shall now jump forward to a crucial session lasting two hours, some six weeks later, from which I shall pick out only the elements important to the main theme. Here there were three main communications:

(1) He spoke of the state of deadlock within himself, saying it was as if he was his own amplifying system. 'Something goes into the microphone, through the amplifier, and out of the speaker, straight back into the microphone. He's his own echo chamber.'

(2) Soon after this, he mentioned once more an extraordinary incident that had occurred not long after his mother left, when he was about 9. His father had had a series of women in the house. One of these, in a touching but crazily misguided attempt to comfort him for the loss of his mother, had bared her breast and offered him her nipple to suck – thus showing deep insight into one aspect of human beings and rather less insight into others. He had of course refused to respond and later had pointed an (unloaded) gun of his father's at her. The transference aspects of this communication were made clear in his next remark: 'She wasn't my mother and there was no way she could be. You aren't my mother and never can be. Some things won't change.'

(3) He then went on to illustrate this immutability with a strange and graphic analogy: 'He used the example of dragging his nails down a hard and rough surface. If he drags them enough, gradually his nails get grooves in them, so that eventually his fingers go down smoothly. He changes, the wall doesn't.'

Before I describe what the therapist said, it is worthwhile to consider these three communications together. There is nothing difficult about the second, which is clear and direct, and contains the by now familiar reference to many of the themes of the present chapter: breast-feeding, deprivation, and aggression. The other two communications are much more obscure, wrapped up in the imaginative language typical of many of these near-psychotic patients. All one can do is to cut through the detail into what one does understand, namely that the state of deadlock is most probably about the inability to reach the depressive position, i.e. the realization that the ultimate savagery expressed in his murderous fantasies is directed towards the very person whom he needs and loves so much; that he cannot face the conflict between hate on the one hand, and love, guilt and grief on the other; and moreover, that he may well be afraid that his mother left him *because he was the sort of person who could have impulses like these*. In this connection the therapist remembered a crucial symbolic incident that had occurred not long before his mother left: they were playing together before his bed-time, and in play *he bit her nose*, but harder than he had consciously intended, and hard enough to put a stop to the play immediately. There is enough evidence in the material to suggest that this may be a reference to the impulse to bite her breast; and it probably links also with the reference to another primitive form of aggression, namely clawing with the finger-nails, which is contained in his third communication.

Perhaps these considerations will make clear what the therapist was trying to convey, which I now continue in her own words: 'In his amplifier system, he has missed out his anxiety that maybe he does something to make these women so hard and unjust to him – anxiety that keeps the system going. And he leaves out the initial woman, his mother. Perhaps his anxiety is that he wanted to, and did, claw and tear at this woman who was so hard and unrelenting, but he can't be sure whether this wish happened before or after she left him.'

Thus, with the greatest possible skill, she reached his grief – the *depressive position* expressed in an atmosphere of quiet, bewildered misery, with huge drops rolling down his cheeks: 'He couldn't believe that he was a bad child, that he could do that. And he couldn't hate his mother. She is that warm, cuddly little woman who made going to bed such fun. How can he hate her? She is only a mother because he is her son, and he is only a son because she is his mother. Should he go to see her to ask why? Why did she leave? Why did she leave *him*? Somewhere along the line he lost something; he'd like to have it back, but he doesn't know what it is. Something to do with soul – he'd do anything for it.'

The therapist now says, 'His good, cuddly mother has been lost. He can't make her link up with the cruel mother who had or has no space for him.' And later, when an atmosphere of peace and dreamy reflectiveness has been established, she says that, after being so sadistic to her, he can't believe that he can so much enjoy being with her in the session. She thus interprets the depressive position in relation to both his mother and herself.

Finally I shall describe a passage that occurred a few months later. He reported once more having followed a girl with his knife; and then, having felt his actions were 'like a blue-print', he cut himself instead – thus giving a sure pointer to the meaning of the self-mutilation as at least in part the displacement of his murderous fantasies onto himself. He asked for admission to hospital, saying he was tired of living a lie and wanted to sleep for a fortnight.

The therapist went downstairs to phone his GP, who wasn't there, and when she came back found the patient asleep on the floor. She woke him and said that the major lie is that she is good and caring; and that at present everything about her is so bad that he needs to get away from her until he can feel good about her again. At this point he sits up; and there follows a discussion of how much she can bear. He insists that she cannot bear what he imposes on her. She now uses another crucial therapeutic move, which every therapist should be familiar with. It contains two elements: (1) the absolute truth; and (2) the principle that 'everything is possible in fantasy': that indeed if he sets about murdering her she will be helpless; but it needn't be in reality – if he murders her in fantasy, *that* she can bear. Later she points out his conflicting views of her: 'when I am doing the hateful thing I am a hard, callous, insensitive bitch. But when he feels hate I am suddenly a delicate lady who is terribly fragile.'

This makes him laugh, and he says that he couldn't use such a word about her, it's not polite. Not long afterwards there is an amazing change of atmosphere: 'I could dream here and not be bothered. I'd like a cup of hot Horlick's in a cold cup. It makes a nice cup, cold outside, warm inside.' Thus the act of accepting the patient's truly terrible savagery against the therapist, whom he also loves, leads to a moment of the utmost warmth in which he can now take in something good. Once more we meet the miracle of the depressive position.

This therapy continued for a total of 6½ years, and we now have a follow-up of 2 years by interview and 10 years by letter. The patient got divorced and later re-married a divorcée with a teenage son. This second marriage contains much companionship and ordinary difficulties. The savagery has largely disappeared, and one of the most impressive features is the way in which he has been able to use his aggression constructively to resolve difficult situations. This has included effective handling of his troublesome stepson and also of the latter's father.

There are very few accounts in the literature of the successful psychotherapy of near-psychotic patients, with adequate follow-up; but this therapy shows what can be achieved with a combination of psychodynamic insight, flexibility, management, sensitiveness, and courage, together with experienced support and supervision. The inference is that if similar conditions are available, such patients can be taken on with some degree of realistic hope.

The origin of human aggression

This is an appropriate point to ask what the therapy of such patients can contribute to the understanding of this most crucial of all human problems. What has been presented in the present chapter is unsystematic, naturalistic, clinical observation, leading nevertheless towards some clear generalizations which form part of the science of psychodynamics.

These are that there are certain severely disturbed adult patients in whom one can observe the following combination of phenomena:

(1) A history of emotional deprivation, sometimes severe, often occurring relatively late in childhood.
(2) Impulses of almost unbelievable primitive savagery and destructiveness, side by side with love of equal intensity.
(3) Incontrovertible cumulative evidence that the deprivation is felt to be mainly maternal, and that both the savagery and the love are ultimately directed towards the mother.
(4) Prominent themes to do with breast-feeding.
(5) And finally the observation that integrating the love and hate leads to moments of extraordinary transformation, in which the world, both past and present, changes from 'bad' to 'good'.

These empirical observations lead to a basic theoretical question: what does all this mean in terms of cause and effect, and what light does it throw on basic human nature and human evolution? Above all, to what extent is the savagery and destructiveness of human aggression the result of 'nature' or 'nurture' – i.e. to what extent is it innate, or caused by the failure of the environment?

Now the trouble with unsystematic clinical evidence is that, from the very fact that it is unsystematic, it is almost always incomplete. In this particular case there are two important empirical questions that need to be answered before we are in any firm position to start building hypotheses. The first is, to what extent, if at all, do primitive destructive impulses occur in the absence of serious deprivation? And the second is, when primitive fantasies appear to be associated with *later* deprivation, does this mean that there was *in fact* earlier deprivation, or merely that later deprivation is *being seen in terms appropriate to* an earlier phase of development?

It has to be said at once that these empirical questions remain unanswered, and consequently no one is in any position to answer the basic theoretical question. Nevertheless the world is not short of dogmatic opinions on what can only be a subject for speculation. This is no place to develop the argument in detail, and all I shall do is to add to the speculation, as follows:

Let us start with four quotations, all from p. 186 of Lorenz's book *On aggression* (1966):

A personal bond, an individual friendship, is found only in animals with highly developed intra-specific aggression, in fact this bond is the firmer, the more aggressive the particular animal and species is.

Intra-specific aggression is millions of years older than personal friendship and love.

The personal bond is known only in teleost fishes, birds and mammals . . . Thus intra-specific aggression can certainly exist without its counterpart, love, but conversely there is no love without aggression.

A behaviour mechanism that must be sharply differentiated from intra-specific aggression is hate ...

To these quotations we can add a further statement of fact, namely that a close mother – child relation has appeared relatively late in evolution, being principally found in birds and mammals.

Now it has been known since Haeckel, who wrote his major work entitled *The natural history of creation* in 1868, that 'ontogeny recapitulates phylogeny'; and although Haeckel overstated his case, a basic principle remains: namely that during the early development of the individual certain features occur which can only be explained on phylogenetic grounds. This can be made clearer by analogy with an aircraft factory: when the designer produces a new form of aircraft, he is able to modify production with the new aircraft in mind *from the very beginning*. It seems that evolution cannot do this, but on the contrary must superimpose the new design on the production of the old, often going some way towards making the old design and then having to modify it or undo it to produce the new. The development and later disappearance of gill slits in a mammalian embryo is the best known example – a feature that has no function whatsoever in the adult and can only be explained as a residue left over from the evolution of mammals from amphibia and fishes.

Therefore, if we accept Lorenz's second statement above that aggression is millions of years older than love – and we cannot fail to accept it – then we would *predict* that the first relation formed between a baby and its mother would be an aggressive rather than a loving one. This is in many ways an appalling thought, but if it is true it has to be faced, and it makes sense of a number of the observations of psychoanalysis. Could it be, therefore, that the initial interchanges between a mother and her baby – besides, obviously, being necessary to the baby's survival – are in some way analogous to the courtship rituals in other species, namely an elaborate procedure by means of which the more fundamental aggressive relation can be first neutralized, and then converted into a bond of love?

But what about the *quality* of the aggression at this earliest stage? Is it like that in the Cricketer, which as I suggested was simply primitive and fierce, or is it like that in the Foster Son, which unquestionably was destructive, sadistic, and revengeful? Obviously no one knows, and if it has the latter qualities then this also has to be accepted. There is, however, an alternative, namely that these qualities only – or largely – enter *when the initial exchanges go wrong*. It is then that the baby becomes enraged because he feels deprived and inadequately cared for, a situation to which he may have contributed by what his mother sees as demanding, unresponsive and unreasonable behaviour. Here obviously, as in the breakdown of a marriage, we are dealing with a vicious circle situation involving both partners.

Nevertheless it seems to me that, because the baby is helpless, it is the mother who has the responsibility for preventing the relationship from going wrong. It is her duty, on the whole, to be there when she is really needed, and to be caring and responsive, without of course allowing herself to be dominated or exploited – which is no good for the child either.

In any case, in therapy, the patient's hatred is principally encountered in situations in which the therapist is felt to have failed in one way or another, either through mistakes, or through 'reality factors' such as absences, or simply through the intrinsic limitations of the therapeutic situation. And usually – perhaps not always – these failures will be found to link with real failures on the part of the mother in the past.

When this has been passed through in therapy, the primary, non-destructive aggression is reached – 'I love you so much I could eat you' – and then patient and therapist together can pass through what Michael Balint (1952) has called a new beginning.

This speculation, whether it is correct or not, fits the clinical facts, and offers the therapist both a framework in which to make sense of the phenomena that he observes and the principles by which to handle them. It also partly – though only partly – gets away from the hidden and bitter controversy, which in an unacknowledged way lies behind much of the disagreement between different schools of psychoanalytical thought: the question of *whose fault it all is*, the mother's or the child's?

Even if this speculation is not correct, it points the way to something that is badly needed, namely the collaboration between psychoanalysts on the one hand and biologists who take psychoanalytic observations seriously, on the other. This collaboration has been pioneered by Sydney Margolin and Lorenz (see Lorenz, 1966, pp. 209–11), and later by Bowlby and Hinde,* but so far as I know has not addressed itself to the kinds of phenomenon described in the present chapter. This is urgently needed if there is ever to be hope for that lonely and desperate species, *Homo*, arrogantly and blindly calling himself *sapiens*, who is busily occupied trying to prove himself to be evolution's greatest mistake.

---

*For a list of references to Hinde's studies of mother – infant separation in primates, which were inspired by Bowlby's work, see Bowlby (1973).

17

Termination and breaks in treatment

When Freud, and the early analysts in their turn, entered the field of psychotherapy, each had to learn the hard way that the work did not simply consist of enabling the patient to ventilate unexpressed emotion about incidents in the past. In those days most therapies were of female hysterical patients treated by male therapists. A pattern regularly encountered then and still encountered to this day is that such patients improve symptomatically very soon, but that if the therapist is deceived by this into suggesting termination, he is in for a shock, for the patient immediately relapses.

The reason for this sequence of events of course has to do with the phenomenon of transference, and is both simple and not so simple as it at first appears. In these early hysterical patients the problem was usually concerned with intense, sexualized, unfulfilled, and guilt-laden longings for love from the father. The mere fact of being listened to and taken seriously by the male therapist fulfilled these longings in a symbolic way, and hence there occurred, first, the disappearance of the symptoms, which was then quickly followed by relapse when termination threatened that the love would be withdrawn.

What therapists did not realize at this time, of course, was the degree to which unfulfilled love, and unexpressed grief – and above all *anger* – about loss and deprivation, play a part in neurotic illness of all kinds. Nor did they realize the degree of symbolic love contained in what the therapist offers, in terms of unconditional acceptance, determination to understand, and what Truax and his co-workers refer to as genuineness and non-possessive warmth – gifts which the patient is never likely to have been offered in his or her life before. The intermeshing of these two factors, the patient's intense need and the therapist's response, result in transference phenomena of extraordinary intensity.

Here we may once more return to the theme of Chapter 14 (see p. 163), summarized in Winnicott's phrase that the function of the therapist is not to succeed but to fail. Where a major part of the patient's problem consists of loss, deprivation, or unfulfilled love, it is the therapist's task not to try and make this up to the patient – which is impossible – but to enable him to experience his true feelings about it, and to pass through them and come out on the other side. In such patients, feelings about absences and termination will play a crucial part. This is quite independent of the sex of patient and therapist, as has already been exemplified in the present book by such patients as the Personnel Manager, the Mental Welfare Officer, the Foster Son, and the Cricketer.

Thus in the Personnel Manager the dramatic session quoted on p. 182 occurred as a consequence of working through the patient's reaction to a 3-week break in therapy, in which her childhood feeling of being left alone with all the responsibility had been experienced in relation to the therapist. This was followed by a prolonged period in which she worked through her grief and anger about her mother's failure to care for her, as re-experienced over the issue of termination. The Mental Welfare Officer quoted on p. 155 developed such a feeling of need for his therapist that he told her 'The ending I feel most is the ending of each session'. In the therapy of the Foster Son, one crisis after another occurred on his return from breaks in treatment, usually after a delay of one or more weeks, in which the main feeling expressed was primitive rage. The major crisis in this patient's therapy, and its resolution into the depressive position, (p. 211), and the similar temporary resolution in the Cricketer (p. 198) both followed a break in treatment caused by the summer holidays.

I have the impression that in many long-term therapies, feelings about such breaks are so fully worked through that the final termination itself does not become nearly so great an issue. This was certainly true in these last two cases. Consequently the termination issue may often be seen in its most concentrated form in the brief time-limited therapies, and it is from this type of therapy that most of the following examples are drawn.

Here it is worthwhile making the following point, which needs to be especially taken to heart by beginners in the field of psychotherapy. Patient and therapist together may get drawn into deep and fascinating material, e.g. about sexual and Oedipal anxieties, and the therapist may find himself very reluctant to drag himself away to deal with the apparently quite separate issue of termination. What needs to be emphasized is that in fact termination is usually not a separate issue at all, but a crucial aspect of the main theme of therapy, so that there is really no question of 'dragging himself away' at all. Thus as mentioned above, in Oedipal problems in women, termination will highlight feelings about the essentially unfulfilled and disappointing relation with the father; and, since boys need love from a father almost (quite?) as much as girls, exactly the same can be said of them. In fact it is one of the most surprising experiences for a psychotherapist to observe the intensity of hidden love that may be found in a man whose father appears to have been nothing but brutal and overbearing. Where the father has been weak and inadequate the intensity of frustrated love is less surprising, but can equally be of staggering intensity – for an example see the Man with School Phobia (pp. 225ff.).

Before we go into cases such as these, however, it is also important to emphasize that termination is not always an issue at all – for instance the patient may have received what he came for and may leave in gratitude, or may want to see the last of his therapist and lead his own life, as in the first two of the following examples respectively.

Simple gratitude as a response to termination – the Geologist (contd)

The shorter the therapy the more likely this is to occur, the limiting case being the type of one-session therapy represented by the Geologist in Chapter 4. Here the patient received an important piece of insight about the conflict over his mother, and his feelings at the end of the session are well illustrated by the following quotation from the therapist's account: 'I said that if he wanted to talk over this again, he could always make another appointment, to which he replied that he did not think he would, but held my hand quite firmly for a long time, telling me how grateful he was for the interview.' At follow-up 3 years later he had clearly made use of the insight that he had received to reach a compromise over the problem that had brought him to seek help.

This particular case illustrates another phenomenon, namely that the therapist sees all the problems that his brief therapy has not resolved, and – in ignorance of systematic follow-up evidence – has no faith in the patient's ability to mature further. This therapist wrote that his interview 'may well have helped him with the immediate situation, but I have very strong feelings that he has considerable neurotic problems', and he went on to speculate about the patient marrying a girl who was socially isolated like himself, and this eventually leading to some kind of breakdown. In fact, follow-up showed that the patient made a seemingly creative marriage, to a girl who was 'good at people', and in doing so was enabled to overcome his social problems to a very considerable degree.

The patient has received enough help – the Gibson Girl

An example of similar unjustified misgivings on the part of the therapist is given by the following example. The patient, aged 18, sought help for the recent onset of agoraphobia. During a therapy lasting 28 sessions (with a female therapist) she came to the realization that her symptoms had started when the man to whom she was engaged began pestering her for sexual intercourse. Her symptom dramatically improved, she immediately got a job, and she began mentioning the possibility of managing on her own. However, her feelings about this were apparently not whole-hearted, and the therapist interpreted that she felt abandoned now that she no longer obviously needed to come. The patient seemed relieved at this, and arrangements were made to continue for a few more sessions. In the discussion in Balint's Workshop the consensus was that the patient needed much further work on her fear of violent sexuality; and when in the next session she seemed to be denying her sexual anxieties by saying it would be all right when she was married, the therapist more or less persuaded her to go on for another 6 months. The final result of this was that the patient first failed two appointments, and then wrote saying that she felt so much better that she preferred not to come any more. At follow-up, 5½ years later, she was symptom-free and happily married to the same man, with two children and an apparently happy sex life. There was possibly some question about her having avoided rather than solved her problem over violent sexuality, but since this apparently caused her no trouble whatsoever, it is legitimate to ask, 'who cares?'. (For further details see Malan, 1976a.)

In a situation like this, the patient's wish to stop can be regarded from two different points of view. On the one hand it is defensive, in the sense that there are further problems which she does not wish to face. On the other hand it is a healthy move – she senses that she has received enough help and can manage on her own, and follow-up shows that she is right, and that in her case therapeutic perfectionism is misguided. It is usually almost impossible to estimate the relative importance of these two opposite factors, which clearly can lie on a continuum.

'Flight into health' – the Factory Inspector

This leads to a consideration of 'flight into health', a concept which at first sight may seem to contain an inherent paradox. The paradox can be resolved by making it clear that the flight is into *apparent* health – the patient believes he has recovered but the clinician believes that unsolved underlying conflicts will give rise to more or less serious difficulty in the future:

The patient was a married man of 41 who asked help because of the acute onset of impotence 8 months before. He was seen by a male therapist. From the beginning he showed highly ambivalent motivation for therapy, on the one hand withholding communication, and on the other suddenly beginning to communicate about the heart of his difficulties when it seemed the interview was about to come to an end. From this it became apparent that part of his problem concerned intense competition with other men. The acquisition of this piece of insight seems to have relieved the pressure, and in session 5 he began to say that his problem was merely 'petty jealousy', that he wasn't sure he was getting anywhere; and now that he realized that his attitude was 'silly' and 'wrong' he wondered if he might be able to manage on his own. The therapist made some cautious remarks, ending by saying that surely the test was whether the patient's potency had been restored. To this, much to the therapist's astonishment, he said, 'Oh yes, it has, for some time now' – a fact that hitherto he hadn't thought fit to mention.

The patient's extreme ambivalence towards the whole process of therapy should be evident. If he came in order to recover his potency: (1) why didn't he mention before that this had been attained; and (2) why did he say he wasn't getting anywhere? When this is coupled with his attempt to dismiss his basic conflict as 'silly', it looks as if he may be using the restoration of his potency – which may well be precarious – as a way of avoiding either further painful conflicts or anxiety-laden feelings about his therapist.

Nevertheless the improvement cannot be ignored, and an obvious way of handling the situation is to accept his wish to withdraw and thus put his potency to the test. This the therapist decided to do, suggesting that they should meet again in three weeks' time to see how he was getting on. At this point the patient suddenly started communicating again – saying that he wondered if his problem was that he had always wanted to be a leader, but he didn't feel he had all the qualities a leader should have. He was clearly unconsciously asking for further therapeutic work, and in spite of the fact that the session had already run 55 minutes, the therapist decided to plunge in with interpretations, with which the patient worked actively, ending a 2-hour session with the remark that to-day he felt he had got further than ever before. He came back in 3 weeks' time and continued therapy for a total of 18 sessions.

The evidence that this was a potential flight into health came from the fact that he made no further attempt to put his potency to the test during the whole of the next year. When he finally did so, he was successful, but his potency remained precarious and was never restored to its original level.

Premature withdrawal as a way of avoiding feelings about termination – the Neurasthenic's Husband

A frequently encountered situation is for the patient to come for the penultimate session fully intending to come again, and then suddenly to decide not to come for the last session. In this way, although it is impossible *in fact* to avoid having a last session, emotionally speaking he succeeds in doing exactly that.

Another pattern is that when the therapist starts talking about termination the patient announces that he doesn't want to come any more. Here the mechanism is somewhat similar to that in the Medical Student described in Chapter 2 (see p. 7): although the patient suffers by losing even more therapeutic time, he gains by retaining control of the situation and turning the tables on his therapist by *leaving* rather than *being left*. Because of the importance of making the patient work through his feelings about loss, this premature withdrawal should be interpreted and prevented if at all possible. The following is an example.

The patient was a man of 54, who was married to an exceedingly neurotic woman, and whose basic disturbance was a lifelong inability to function effectively in any sphere of life. The male therapist took as his main focus the hypothesis that the patient: (1) was angry about his father's ineffectiveness; (2) as a consequence of this anger depreciated his father even further, symbolically castrating him; and then (3) out of Oedipal guilt, became unable to be effective himself. With hindsight it can be seen that the element of hidden disappointment in his father might well be activated by the loss of the therapist at termination, and thus might highlight the whole of this pathology in the transference.

The therapy was clearly of the kind which, if not effective quickly, would become interminable; and therefore, when in the 8th session the patient began to show signs of greater assertiveness, the therapist began to speak in terms of termination. He suggested that they should continue to meet weekly for 4 more weeks, and then twice more, in August, on his return from an absence abroad. The patient's response was that 'he didn't want to be independent on anybody' – a slip of the tongue for 'dependent' – thus revealing very clearly the conflict between a need for his therapist and a defensive determination to manage on his own.

In the next few sessions he alternated between these two positions. In the 9th session he said, 'I just do not believe that you will stop, that you will leave me', to which the therapist made plain that he meant what he said. The patient's face fell, he closed up, and the rest of the session consisted of mere politeness.

In the 10th session he was sad-faced and gloomy, and said he didn't see the point in coming any more, since clearly nothing could be done in the time remaining. The therapist interpreted that underlying this lay his need for strength from a man. The patient responded by speaking of an employer for whom he had worked so hard and to whom he owed so much, but who in the end had got jealous of him and had transferred him to another town.

Of course in the context of the therapist's previous interpretation the meaning of this communication is obvious; but it can be used to emphasize the need to be on the look-out for communications of this kind as termination approaches – remarks containing themes such as loss, abandonment, parting, neglect, people being fed up with demands, poor service in shops, etc. etc. In the present session the therapist gave the obvious interpretation about reproaches towards himself, which the patient understood intellectually but did not really feel. Nevertheless he ended by being quite keen to come the next time.

When he did come, for the last session before the therapist's absence, he appeared doubtful about whether the therapist would see him in August – though the therapist had made absolutely clear that he would – and mentioned that he might be 'too busy' to come himself. He spoke of the position between him and his wife as hopeless and said that he was now leading a separate life from her. This was in fact a statement of a realistic position, but it also probably contained a transference communication, which the therapist interpreted: 'I tried to interpret his independence as his turning away from me in retaliation for my turning away from him.' To this his only response was to say 'Why should I be critical of you, you have done your best, it's me that's no good' etc.

He did in fact come back for his two sessions in August, opening by saying that he'd at first decided not to come but had then thought it would be impolite. The climax of the whole of therapy came with a major interpretation of the basic focus in terms of termination, as follows:

'The patient spoke of his father's return from the war with presents for the family. It was a tragi-comedy, for all these gifts were no good – a watch that fell to pieces for the daughter, some silver thing that almost broke in your hand for the son, etc. I interpreted this in the transference, how he appreciated my goodwill but thought little of what I had given him, and I pointed out how his father, impotent and unable to be anything but laughable, was his view of all men including himself and me. He went on to say that of course he hadn't known his father much – when he was near puberty his father had gone away to the war. The hint here was that his father had not helped him with his sexual problems as I had not, and I took this up. He repeated that he had been independent from an early age. I pointed out that he was now being independent, and that on three occasions when the prospect of ending the treatment had occurred he had become independent and threatened to leave – rather than to be deserted he was doing the deserting, to avoid having feelings of disappointment, longing, and dependency on a man. I pointed out his loneliness all his life, his need for men, and this really shook him. He paused, sat back in his chair and thought, and said, "I have always felt my independence to be virtuous and never allowed myself to be owned by anybody".' Using material from a dream, the therapist then interpreted that the patient symbolically castrated his father by his constant depreciation, with the aim of having his mother to himself. 'He again took this soberly and said, "Like Moses, like the Virgin Birth", and went on with a dawning realization that he had never allowed himself to have a father.'

This was an example of the termination issue being used first to highlight, and then to force the patient to experience, his nuclear problem in the transference, and to link it with the past in a way that had the maximum impact. The therapeutic result, in what appeared to be an impossibly chronic and intractable character problem, was spectacular (for further details see Malan, 1963, pp. 99–103).

Intense grief and anger – the Swiss Receptionist

All that needs to be known about this woman of 31 is that she was complaining that when depressed all her good feelings about anyone close to her disappeared;

and that when she was 14 her mother had died of the complications of asthma, by which she had been partly incapacitated for the previous 3 years. The reader will at once recognize in this the probable pathology represented by several previous cases – e.g. the Imaginary Therapy, the Nurse in Mourning, the Daughter with a Stroke – namely ambivalent feelings which have caused the normal process of mourning to remain incomplete and unresolved. This was confirmed when, in one of the cards of her projection test she saw a ghost looking in at a wedding and associated this with her mother. Because, although she had initial difficulty in making contact, she was clearly a responsive patient with plenty of inner resources, she was assigned to brief psychotherapy with a limit of about 30 sessions set from the beginning, in the full knowledge that therapy would be largely concerned with the issue of termination. The therapist, deliberately chosen from several possibilities, was an extremely mature and sensitive woman, capable of withstanding and sharing the intense feelings that were expected to be aroused.

This expectation was fulfilled. The patient felt very deeply but also found difficulty in expressing her feelings, with the result that there were long periods of brooding silence in which the therapist either had to press her to speak, or else had to use every fleeting expression that passed over her face in order to guess what was going on in her mind. The elements of profound sympathy and compassion, coupled with a relentless determination not to let her escape from angry feelings, with much non-verbal communication on both sides, were therefore prominent features of the whole process of therapy.

Because of circumstances that were partly but perhaps not entirely beyond the patient's control, her own summer visit to her home in Switzerland did not exactly coincide with her therapist's holiday, with the result that the summer break was 6 weeks long, with only four sessions left after the resumption. There was possibly in this the element, observed in the Neurasthenic's Husband, of 'leaving in retaliation for being left'. Another feature, also observed in this previous patient, was the denial that the therapist meant what she said in setting a time limit. This was mentioned in Session 18, and again where we take up the story in Session 21, the last but one before the break.

From the beginning the patient shows her ambivalence, on the one hand creating an atmosphere of disdain for her therapy, and on the other saying that she doesn't believe it is going to end and that the therapist *has just been saying this in order to provoke her.* Throughout the session the therapist, while remaining profoundly sympathetic, is determined to try and bring the underlying hostility into the open. Here she says that surely it is the patient who is angry and is wanting to be provocative. To this the patient says that in fact she will be *relieved to get away.* The therapist again interprets the patient's anger, now expressed by openly depreciating her therapy, and, in a further attempt to get in contact with strong feelings, makes the link with times when her mother left her and she felt abandoned, dissatisfied, and angry. Moreover, she is clinging to the idea that therapy will go on indefinitely because she equates the ending with her mother's dying and leaving her. The patient, who has been sitting quietly and rigidly, eventually says she feels guilty now. The therapist, sticking to her guns, says the patient feels guilty because she is so angry, and there the session ends.

At this point the therapist made a prediction – always a hazardous occupation in the field of psychotherapy – namely that the patient's underlying anger was so intense that it would spill over against her boy-friend, John, before the next session.

In this session, the last before the break, the patient begins very silent but at the same time seems willing to listen. The therapist once more links the ending with feelings about the patient's mother who didn't give enough, bringing in an interpretation of the anxiety as well as the impulse, that in her imagination her resentful feelings had contributed towards her mother's being damaged. The patient says helplessly, it's all so complicated – how can she sort it out by herself? At this the therapist emphasizes the element of hope in the situation, questioning the patient's assumption that, when she stops coming, all she has got from her sessions will be lost.

After a long silence the patient tells of how she and John got very angry with each other during the last week, ending by actually hitting each other, and how she didn't want to make it up – thus entirely confirming the above-mentioned prediction. She then adds that she thinks *this must have something to do with coming here.* This is of course an almost open acknowledgement of the mechanism of displacement, and the therapist says 'You wanted to go for me but took it out on John instead,' to which the patient nods and says again that she was terribly angry and didn't want to make it up. The therapist, carefully including the positive, says that the patient both did and didn't want to make it up with her before the coming break. The patient remains with her head down till the end of the session.

When she returned 6 weeks later, after her visit with John to her home in Switzerland, she opened by saying, 'It's weird, you were right,' and she went on to tell how she had missed her therapy, it was like a physical pain right inside her, she had felt as if she were leaving for ever, and there had been explosions of anger with John. She later agreed with the interpretation that during the break it had felt as if therapy was already over, and when this was linked with her feelings about being left when her mother died, she quietly dissolved into tears. The therapist sat with her, acknowledging and sharing her pain.

Later she went on to ask, in a helpless tone, a number of questions about how she will be able to manage her feelings after therapy ends, to which the therapist says she is denying the resources she has in herself, and thus perhaps she hopes to persuade her therapist not to leave her. She agrees that this may be what she secretly hopes, but in her heart she knows it won't work. At this acknowledgement of the reality of termination the therapist feels it is natural to soften it by mentioning her own wish for a follow-up interview 3 or 4 months after the last session.

At this the patient is silent for a time but then dissolves into tears once more, and begins to tell in more detail of her explosions of anger, which had happened not only with John but – for the first time – also at work, and had left her shaking all over. After this had been linked once more with the transference, she was enabled to speak of some more positive moments, particularly one in which she had been able to confide in her father – though not as much as she would have liked – and of his gesture of affectionate contact in response, something that she remembers from her childhood.

The next time she came she immediately said that she *felt much better after the last session,* but she then went into resistance and made little response to further attempts to reach her anger.

In the penultimate session (no. 25), however, she tells of bouts of anger and misery during the week, which the therapist links once more with termination; and now she suddenly says, 'I do feel better for coming here. I used to feel dead inside, but now, though I have bad feelings I also have some good ones. But will I go back to how I was?' The therapist says she now has some choice, to bottle up all her feelings, or to struggle with the pain of loss and the effort to hold onto the good things she has got. To this she says that she does now know that part of her is better, stronger, more alive inside, and sometimes she knows it but at other times it is gone.

With greater animation she goes on to speak of a couple whom she visited over the weekend, who seem to get on very well together – by comparison she herself feels dull and unhappy. Here the therapist brings in another important aspect of termination: not only the fact of being abandoned, which involves two people only, patient and therapist, but also the three-person situation of being abandoned *in favour of someone else*. The therapist therefore first suggests that the patient felt left out; and when she agrees, suggests that this was like her feelings about her parents both when she was small and after her mother died, when her father turned to another woman; and completes the interpretation by saying that she may well feel left out because the therapist will have another patient who will take her place. At this her face tenses and she says she feels *strange* inside. Shortly afterwards it was the end of the session. The therapist wrote: 'After she put on her coat and was going out she turned round and glanced first at her chair, and then round the room, before she closed the door. It was as if she was trying to take it all in to hold it in her mind.'

In the final session (no. 26) she again tells of having been angry and upset during the week, with rows with her boy-friend. However, she found herself getting calmer as she approached her session – she associates this to love-making, which she sometimes feels is messy and horrid. The therapist interprets how she begins by wanting to make love and then the bad feelings of anger and resentment get the upper hand, and how this is like what happens in therapy. She makes a clear response to this, launching into a detailed account of how *this has happened throughout her life* – thus reaching, through the transference, the basic interpretation of her original complaint, namely that all her good feelings for someone close to her tend to disappear. She elaborates, saying that she often starts by getting interested in something and then suddenly she gets fed up with it – this even happens with her own cooking.

There follows a long silence during which tears come and go in her eyes though she doesn't actually cry. The therapist says she must be feeling in turmoil inside and that it is hard to part like this. She says she knows she lets herself be worse, allowing herself to wallow in sadness or resentment. The therapist says, 'You let it get the upper hand and destroy the good experience?', to which she agrees and there is a further long silence.

She then begins to ask, what kind of therapy has she been having? The therapist, correctly, answers this question straightforwardly. 'It has been psychotherapy', she says, and she then goes on to interpret that the patient is trying to put a name to what she has received, in order to hold onto it.

In the last few minutes she sits mostly silent, and as she stands up and shakes hands her face flushes with emotion and her eyes flood again; and as she goes towards the door she twice turns back to look at her chair as if saying goodbye to it.

At follow-up a few months later, the patient seemed to be much less depressed and showed signs of facing the prospect of making a new life for herself.

The issue of termination carried to the limit – the Man with School Phobia

This was a young man of 24, whose main disturbance was anxiety of extreme severity at any attempt to break away from home. He had in the past been able to go out to work, but had had to phone his mother at least twice a day just in order to hear her voice. At the beginning of therapy he was making one more attempt to break away, by going back to University for further studies and trying to live in a student's hostel.

It seemed that the aim of therapy must be to try and resolve the pathological tie to his mother, which in other patients often arises out of intense unconscious ambivalence. What was not so clear was what part might be played by his feelings either directly about his father, or about the triangular relation between him and his father and his mother. Here the facts will not be given for reasons of discretion. Suffice it to say that the father had been a failure, was no longer at home, and had given the patient very little in the way of true contact or fatherly support.

In accordance with a policy of trying to explore the limits of brief psychotherapy, the patient was taken on at once a week (by a male therapist) with a time limit stated to the patient from the beginning. Therapy was due to end at Easter, after a total of about 30 sessions.

The early stages of therapy did indeed deal with mixed feelings about his mother and with the triangular relation between him and his parents; but though this work seemed highly meaningful, its therapeutic effect was negligible. The initial attempt to live away from home ended in severe anxiety and an ignominious return, followed eventually by his abandoning his studies altogether.

Later in therapy he began to speak of a new plan for leaving home. Some time ago he had used money that he had earned, supplemented by a legacy, to buy a house with a wine bar on the ground floor and a flat above; he had installed a friend as manager while he remained a sleeping partner; and he now intended to try and live in the flat and make it into a place of his own. The therapist offered to support him in every possible way while he made the attempt, giving the patient all his phone numbers and saying that he could ring at any time of the day or night.

This is of course something that can only be offered to the right sort of patient; but the therapist knew, from the strength and quality of the therapeutic alliance already developed, that the offer would not be abused.

We now take up the story in Session 20. Here the therapist, in talking about how the patient had displaced his father, emphasized not only *guilt*, but *love* and *sorrow*, at which the patient began to be in tears and remained so for most of the rest of the session. The next session was very resistant, culminating in a 5-minute silence, with the therapist in a state of despair about any possibility of making contact; when suddenly the patient broke the silence by saying, 'I think I've decided not to get upset to-day', and went on to say that he had been in tears all the evening after the last session, and again on many occasions throughout the week. (This determination to overcome his own resistance against facing painful feelings is, incidentally, an example of what is meant by true *motivation*, an aspect of the therapeutic alliance.)

There followed a passage in this and subsequent sessions in which he began to experience the deepest grief about what he had never had from his father, interspersed with periods of deadlock caused by resentment against his therapist because he was not his father. 'Why isn't it him? In a sense it's countless other people – it should only have been him. People I don't even bloody well know.' He spoke of his pattern of trying to build men up into father-figures, and of the inevitable disappointment, and the therapist very gently pointed out that what he wanted was really no longer available. To this the patient said, 'Yes, and I'm very bitter about it – so bitter I'm prepared to go on crucifying myself because of it.' During this period, however, he began to sleep in his flat, away from home.

This was the first time that his therapy gave the feeling that it was really beginning to move, but the trouble was that the original termination date allowed time for only six more sessions. This question was raised by the patient himself in Session 23, to which the therapist said only that they had 'better play it by ear'. Surprisingly, the patient answered that he didn't want it to last any longer than it had to, but he added that if he were to stop now he would feel that nothing had changed at all. The result was that in a later session the therapist decided to extend the termination date from early in April to the end of June, which would give him time for about 40 sessions in all.

The patient's flat held a tremendously powerful significance for him, and he began to have the impulse to invite his father to come to it and walk around it – 'every room, including the bathroom and the loo' – with the intense conviction that this would set the seal on his new-found independence. With the therapist's encouragement he tried to speak to his father about this; but his father, as always, hardly heard him – let alone appreciating the importance of what he was being asked – and immediately changed the subject to one of his own trivial preoccupations.

This changed the principal emotion felt by the patient from overwhelming *grief* to all-consuming *anger*, first in relation to his father, and then, as will be seen, to the therapist; and at first this was expressed in an utterly *self-destructive* way. In Session 30 he announced that he had been 'trying to destroy that house', and he no longer wanted to live in it. What this meant was that he had been behaving in such a way as to go far towards spoiling his relation both with his partner and with the other employees in the wine bar. He and his therapist together listed many other things in his life, all concerned with achievement and thus possibly representing his manhood, which he had destroyed because his father hadn't shared them with him.

The session continued relatively uneventfully until about 40 minutes after the beginning, when he said out of the blue that he had been 'having the fantasy of dying in that house'.

This is a kind of moment to which every therapist must be alert, and in which – whether he is medically qualified or not – he must immediately add the role of psychiatrist to his normal role. In my book, *The frontier of brief psychotherapy* (1976a, p. 345) a moment is described in which a patient remarks that 'she imagines herself deep in a grave'. The full meaning of this was not directly taken up with her, and the result was a successful suicide attempt a week later.

With the present patient, the therapist therefore immediately asked, did he mean suicide?, to which the answer was Yes. 'And I want you to sit with me while I'm in bed.' The therapist, now thoroughly alarmed, asked whether he meant alive or dead. The answer was, dead. 'I'll go round to the Clinic, late at night, and deposit the keys of the flat, with a note letting you know where to find me; and you'll go to the flat the next morning and find a chair by my bed, which you'll sit in for 5 minutes; and then you'll start making arrangements for my body to be removed.' His method of suicide would be by cutting his wrists. He had planned the whole thing in a most realistic way, and when the therapist asked if he thought he'd really do it, he gave the almost unbelievable answer, 'It would seem to me to be normal procedure.'

This is, further, an example of how the transference and the patient's real relation with the original people in his life become utterly entangled: although the rejection by his father is the primary situation, the rejection by the therapist who insists on ending therapy is felt almost – or quite – as deeply, and potentially leads to even more serious consequences. As always when suicide is in question, the therapist must consider it as a fusion of intense destructive anger expressed self-destructively on the one hand; and love, protectiveness, concern and guilt, on the other – the patient would rather kill himself than harm the other person – and it is usually the anger that needs to be brought into the open. Here, side by side with the love expressed by the chair beside the bed, the anger was hardly far to seek; and the therapist interpreted several times in different ways that 'this fantasy represented an extremely violent attack on me because, like his father, I had failed to be a proper father to him. I had been trying to help him and would have the shock of discovering his body and see all my efforts end in catastrophe. In addition, though, the chair was an expression of a need to be close to me, but only if he was dead, not if he was alive.' It is interesting to note that, although this interpretation was surely correct, the therapist missed interpreting the rejection embodied in *termination*.

By now the session had run for 55 minutes and the therapist had another patient waiting downstairs; but this was no time for half measures, and the therapist went down, asked her to wait, and came up again. Further enquiry now revealed that the patient intended to go back to his mother's house to spend the night, at which the therapist was greatly relieved. Eventually he sent the patient away with an appointment for next week, together with the further reassurance that he could phone at any time of the day or night in the intervening period.

Perhaps this demonstration of his genuine concern, together with his refusal to be panicked and controlled, was the right combination, as is shown by what happened the next day. The patient walked into the Clinic and was seen as soon as the therapist was free. The deeply touching purpose of the visit was to say that he wasn't going to put his suicidal plan into effect – it was what the thought *meant* that mattered, not something he was going to do. After delivering this reassuring message he was content to leave after about 20 minutes. Once more we see the power of the therapeutic alliance this time involving both partners, in the struggle to reach destructive feelings without bringing about catastrophe.

This was followed by a most encouraging session, in which the patient reported some forceful, effective, and seemingly extremely mature behaviour. At the end of the session he raised the question of future plans, saying that he would want to go on seeing the therapist after the end of June. The therapist took this to mean simply that he didn't want the relation to end completely at termination – which in fact had already been agreed in the original contract – and therefore said, 'Yes, that goes without saying. We'll stop regular sessions at the end of June but that doesn't mean you've lost me, and you can always come back if you need to from time to time.'

The next week's session was missed because the therapist was abroad. On the Monday of the following week (the normal session being due on a Wednesday) the therapist received a phone call in his private consulting room, saying that the patient was in the Clinic in a desperate state. Once more we meet an example of a *psychotherapeutic emergency* (for previous examples see the Refugee Musician and the Foster Son, pp. 204 and 209).

There are no set rules, and every situation has to be judged on its merits. It is not necessarily correct to respond, for certain types of patient may just be manipulating their therapist, and then need to be handled with the utmost firmness – something that they may deeply appreciate rather than resent. This present situation, however, was quite different. The therapist knew he must respond immediately – which in any case had been agreed as part of the current contract.

He asked to speak to the patient on the phone. The latter was almost incoherent with tears, but made plain that the cause of the emergency was twofold. First, he had tried once more to speak to his father, who instead of understanding had launched into a self-pitying account of the father-deprivation he himself had suffered in his own childhood. The patient almost shouted over the phone that he 'didn't want any more of this fucking crap from anyone'; and he then added the second cause of the emergency: 'and you dropped the bombshell about ending in June'.

Of course it shouldn't have been a bombshell, in the sense that he had known about it all along, and the therapist had merely said that the previously arranged termination date would stand; but the truth was that the patient's attachment had become so strong that he couldn't really believe that the relationship would end. This is one of many examples of the frequent observation that what the therapist says and what the patient hears or believes are not necessarily the same. In this kind of situation it is no good arguing about it – the patient's psychic reality must be considered as the only reality that matters.

The therapist interrupted one session with a private patient, made alternative arrangements for the next, and got to the Clinic as soon as he could. On the way to his room, his secretary showed him a weapon (a hammer) which the patient had brought into the Clinic and had then entrusted to her for safe keeping, which gave an inkling of the quality of the emergency. The patient said later that he hadn't intended to use it on anyone – which was by no means clear at the time – but that he might have either thrown it through a window-pane or used it on the fire alarm, just to make everyone understand how serious the situation was.

In the actual session he was again almost incoherent, giving more details, through his sobs, of the utterly hopeless encounter with his father. In addition he told of how he had been behaving in an extravagantly violent way ever since, going round his flat screaming, having rows with people, and – which was more alarming – driving dangerously, deliberately half-trying to run down pedestrians.

There was of course no need to say anything more about the patient's rage against his father; but the transference aspects needed to be brought out to the full. When the patient mentioned the ending in June the therapist said, 'You are as enraged with me for being a bad father as you are with your own father, and you want to kill me rather than be deserted by me.' To this the patient said, 'I just don't want to be alone.'

Towards the end of the session the patient became a little calmer, and smiling for the first time said, 'we talked about racing', referring of course to his conversation with his father. When asked, however, he denied that this had been of any value to him.

The therapist, in his role as psychiatrist, heard with some apprehension that the patient intended to sleep at his flat that night, but did not demur and sent him off with an appointment for the next day. On the way out he met the patient again, who apologized for the trouble he had caused, to which the therapist said 'not at all' and went away feeling reassured.

This was short-lived. His hope that the crisis was over was immediately dashed at the beginning of the next session, when the patient put his head in his hands and sobbed for about 10 minutes. Eventually he recovered enough to speak, saying, 'It's *all* anger', and adding something about being 'left to drift'. The therapist said, 'That's what you feel I'm doing to you in the present situation', to which the patient shouted at the top of his voice, 'YES LEFT TO FUCKING DRIFT', with an intensity of rage unparalleled in the therapist's previous experience. The therapist, when he got an opportunity, said, 'Surely you are trying to destroy everything around you because I've left you to drift; and you want to destroy everything I've given you, whether it's good or bad'; to which the patient said, 'Yes, because I've only got you on *these* terms. I'm angry with you before I start.'

Having got this into the open, the therapist decided it was right to give the patient something his father had never given him, namely firmness, and said: 'What I'm afraid of is that you're going to *succeed* in destroying everything, and you need to be stopped' – 'before it's too late', the patient added – 'and the trouble is that in this kind of situation *I* can't control you – only *you* can control yourself. But I don't like your taking out all this anger on innocent people, and still less do I like what you're doing with your car, and I'm afraid you really will kill someone, and I think it should stop.'

The patient made no obvious response to this, and they went on to discuss where he was going to spend the night, eventually coming to the conclusion that he had better go back to his mother's. In further discussion they agreed that another source of his recent behaviour was probably that he was trying to make everything so bad that the therapist would be forced to go on seeing him.

Towards the end he said three very positive things: 'I *can* be a nice person, you know', 'I don't want to lose the things I've got', and 'I want to make something of my life, at least to become an expert on *something*.'

This was in fact the end of that particular crisis, but it was by no means the last. I shall leave the story there. The ending in June was eventually revealed as quite unrealistic, and at the time of writing therapy continues in a much more relaxed and informal atmosphere. Of course I do not recommend this kind of messing about with termination dates as a regular procedure, but in this particular case it doesn't seem to have done any harm; and the existence of a termination date, even though it was not adhered to, almost certainly heightened the patient's feelings and shortened the therapeutic work.

During this later part of therapy the patient has reached the idea that one of the many factors tying him to home was the feeling that something existed there that he had never had from his father, for which he was turning to his *mother* as a substitute, and which he would give up for ever if he left. In any case, the tie to home appears to have been broken, and the patient is now in regular work, with the intention of going back to his studies later.

It is worth quoting a single moment from this period, when the patient said to his therapist, 'I suppose it's inevitable that you become for each of us the very thing that we've wanted all our lives. There must be a lot of disappointed patients around.' Thus, without having read the books, he showed a quite remarkable ability to stand back from his therapy, and grasp – no longer with bitterness – its central principle.

It is clear that he needs a long period of consolidation, and that he must be allowed to terminate in his own way and his own time. This is something that the therapist is very happy to grant.

There is one final comment. After events such as these, surely it is not possible for even the most hardened sceptic to go on disbelieving in transference and its origins in the past; and hence to go on disbelieving that psychodynamics deals in *observations* from which – even in a single case – inferences can be made that are virtually unassailable.

Postscript

It would be nice to report that this intense and dramatic therapy was a success, but unfortunately it is not so. Termination was eventually achieved, and at first things seemed to be going well, with gradual but steady improvement in his ability to handle his life constructively. However, it then began to become clear that this ability was fragile; and, particularly after the failure of a relation with a girl, the old self-destructive patterns began to reassert themselves. Moreover, it also became clear that his pathological tie to his mother, which seemed at first to have been considerably loosened, was largely unresolved. With hindsight this might have been predicted, since his therapy was almost entirely concerned with his relation with his father. The result was that he was referred for analysis to a highly experienced male colleague. The analysis was not a success, and the final follow-up showed very little evidence of improvement.

Coda

After the *Sturm und Drang* of this last therapy, it is fitting to end with something very different. The following are quotations from an account of the 17th and last session with a woman of 32 – a therapy which had contained its own crises, also to do with termination. No history is needed except that she had had a good deal of previous therapy and was living with a man called Arthur, who was in process of getting a divorce in order to marry her. The therapist was male.

'Miss D arrived looking slimmer and more attractive even than on the last occasion. She handed me a carrier bag containing a cake, which she had baked for me, and which of course I admired and accepted with thanks. She said we'd been talking last week about mourning, and she indeed had been mourning a great deal. On Friday, Arthur's mother, the 89-year-old lady who "ate like a gannet", had died in her sleep, and Miss D had not only wept for this potential mother-in-law whom she liked and whom she'd now lost, but she'd also wept for Arthur, who had been very moved by the loss of his mother. She told me in detail about the reactions of Arthur's family, none of whom had been able to hold him and cry with him. She was slightly surprised when I pointed out that their reaction had cheated her of the opportunity to mourn within the situation of family grief, and to bring together their mourning for their lost mother with her mourning for her father, and her mourning for the relationship with me. She was once again in the position of being the one who had to do it for the others, rather than being in a situation of mutual holding, sharing in a common experience. She agreed that this was so, and said that of course it had been different with Arthur, who by the way sent me his thanks and best wishes, because he was very grateful for the work which Miss D and I had done together. . . .

'She then went back to feeling that she'd also benefited from the relationship with me in terms of being able to speak up for herself. One of Arthur's relatives had been rather flirtatious with her, asking her to make a sweater for him like the ones she knits for Arthur. She'd replied that she does lots of things for Arthur she wouldn't dream of doing for him, which put him firmly in his place and made Arthur feel wanted and cared about – something that he had never received from his first wife.

'She went on to say that things were very different from how they had been before she started the therapy with me. She realized now that she had not been able to grieve about the end of her previous, group, therapy, whereas plainly she had been able to be sad about finishing the work with me. She was not depressed and she was struck by my remark of last week that there was a considerable difference between sadness and depression. She was quite sure that what she was feeling was sadness.

'At about this point Miss D sort of settled back in her chair, looked at her watch, and then said that it was odd that she felt she had nothing more to say, but that it was different – she could be quiet and didn't feel she had to rattle on. After a bit she said she thought it would be best if we ended the session now. I said of course it was her decision to do as she wished, but I'd be very happy if she'd come back in the summer and tell me how things had gone. "Oh", she said, "How nice. You've really made my day. I'd love to do that. Thank you very much." We agreed that she should get in touch with me after Easter, and we parted on very good terms.'

One could adapt a dictum of Winnicott's by saying that often our main function as therapists is to grit our teeth and survive; and that often all we can expect is for the patient to walk out and take all our forbearance and anxiety for granted; but sessions like this show that sometimes things are different and we are given our reward.

18
Assessment for psychotherapy: I. General principles

If a fault has developed in the smooth working of any system – whether this may be the mechanism of a car, human relations in a factory, the economic situation of a country, the ecology of some living population, a family, a marriage, or a medical or psychiatric patient – then any attempt to put it right must be based on the same fundamental principles. The first of these is that strenuous efforts must be made to identify the fault in terms of known defects or the interaction of known forces, so that any intervention can be *planned* and specifically based on undoing what has gone wrong. For this purpose the first step must always be the *preliminary enquiry*, the aims of which are to find out: (1) the exact nature of the fault; (2) how it developed; and (3) other features which may shed light on what has gone wrong and what should be done to correct it.

Now although we are often taught to view the 'medical model' of psychotherapy with contempt, the foregoing considerations will show that there is an obvious parallel between psychotherapy and medicine, the two being part of a much wider class of situations. It is true that psychotherapy shows certain features that distinguish it sharply from medicine, the main one of which is that the therapist does not so much *do something to* the patient as *interact with* him. Nevertheless the two have a very great deal in common: both involve a *system that is malfunctioning*, in which an expert carries out a *preliminary enquiry* in order to *identify what has gone wrong*, and then *prescribes an appropriate intervention* in order to try and set it right. Moreover, in psychotherapy exactly as in medicine, prescribing the wrong intervention on the basis of an inadequate initial assessment, or prematurely carrying out dangerous investigations, have potential consequences that vary from unnecessary pain at one end to catastrophe at the other (see pp. 237 and 245 for examples).

No matter what the system under consideration, the preliminary enquiry can only be carried out effectively by someone well grounded in the appropriate theoretical knowledge, and well experienced in the different kinds of defect that a given fault may indicate and the ways of distinguishing one from another. In the same way, the decision about what to do can only be taken by someone well experienced in the different possible kinds of intervention and the consequences of applying them in many different situations. This is the reason for the seemingly anomalous sequence of subjects in the present book: initial assessment, the *first* intervention that is made with any given patient, is considered *last of all*.

The truth is that the assessment of a patient for psychotherapy is probably the most complex, subtle, and highly skilled procedure in the whole field. It is very important to say that it is not the same as a psychiatric history, nor a social history, nor a psychotherapeutic session – it contains elements of all three, but is in fact more than all three put together.

The complexity arises because of the many different layers at which the interviewer has to operate, sometimes in sequence, sometimes simultaneously, and all of them overlapping with one another. A large part of the skill arises from the way in which he has to 'think on his feet', constantly switching roles and modifying his approach according to his changing view of the patient and the possible disposals that seem appropriate. Moreover, as will be seen, there is often no truly satisfactory order in which the various operations can be carried out.

The interviewer's basic aim has already been stated and is simple enough, namely to obtain sufficient evidence to enable him to *prescribe an appropriate intervention*. Since it is psychotherapy that is in question, he needs to be able to forecast the kinds of event that are likely to occur as the patient interacts with a therapist and begins to face his disturbing feelings. The conclusion may then be either that psychotherapy is an inappropriate or dangerous disposal, and/or that some other form of treatment is better, e.g. behaviour therapy, support, or medication. If the interviewer concludes that psychotherapy is appropriate, he must then decide on the type of psychotherapy – in-patient or out-patient, individual or group, conjoint marital or family, with how much of a supportive element, at how many times a week? As he thinks out these issues, he must pay attention to how he gets his information. He must make enough contact so that the information he is given is meaningful and reliable; and on the other hand he must not behave in such a way as to disturb the patient, to raise hopes that cannot be fulfilled, or to start a therapeutic process that cannot be continued.

Some of the ways in which the interviewer must think and behave can thus be summarized as follows:

(1) He must think *psychiatrically* – the psychiatric diagnosis has an important bearing on the prognosis, as will be explained in detail in the next chapter.
(2) He must think *psychodynamically*, that is he must try and identify the forces in conflict both within the patient, and between the patient and his environment, now and in the past – which, obviously, must form the main themes of any psychotherapy that may be undertaken.
(3) He must think *psychotherapeutically*, that is he must constantly use his experience to forecast not only the themes but also the probable *course of events* if this particular patient is taken into psychotherapy.
(4) He must think *practically* – although his first thought may be 'what is the ideal disposal?' his second thought must be 'what is there actually available that would be appropriate?'
(5) He must take care of the *interview*, that is he must create enough rapport to enable him to get the evidence that he needs in order to make a correct disposal.
(6) At the same time he must take care of the *patient*, if possible bringing into the open the expectations and apprehensions with which the patient approaches the interview, and constantly trying to be aware of the effect

of his own interventions, particularly in relation to what the patient is going to feel when he goes away.

Some of these issues can be further elaborated as follows:

A crucial aspect of *psychodynamic* thinking often consists of, first, identifying recent *precipitating factors* (see Chapter 5), and then seeing that these *repeat events or situations from the past*. This often leads to the identification of a theme that runs through much of the patient's history, which can be called his *life problem*.

Psychiatric, psychodynamic, and psychotherapeutic thinking come together in estimating the balance between the patient's *strength* on the one hand, and the *severity of his disturbance* on the other. With this balance in mind, the interviewer tries to forecast whether the patient will be able to interact with a therapist and face his hidden feelings without serious threats to himself (e.g. suicide), to others (e.g. violence), or to his therapy (severe dependence, uncontrollable acting out).

This kind of thinking also leads to an assessment of the amount of additional *support* that the patient will need, which will depend on the amount that his environment can provide, and which in turn will influence the recommended setting in which psychotherapy is to be carried out (e.g. out-patient or in-patient unit, day hospital).

Finally, the interviewer must *view the patient and his environment as a whole*, and assess whether or not other people in his life need to be seen either for diagnostic or therapeutic purposes, with such possibilities in mind as conjoint marital therapy or family therapy.

The use of interpretations in the initial interview: trial therapy

As already foreshadowed, all this leads to a fundamental question: how do you get your information? There is a saying that well illustrates the sterility of certain kinds of interview: 'All I asked was questions and all I got was answers.' What this means is that if the interviewer does no more than ask questions without taking pains to deepen rapport, then the answers he gets may well be defensive, cursory, and superficial, may leave out crucial information, and may lack the element of spontaneous and intimate communication that is so necessary to true understanding. And, as emphasized so often in previous chapters, the best way of deepening rapport is to *make interpretations*. Sometimes indeed this is absolutely essential to being able to continue the interview at all – see for instance the Mother of Four (p. 78) and the Foster Son (p. 275).

Moreover, so far we have left out one of the crucial functions of the initial interview, namely to get evidence about whether or not the patient can work in interpretative therapy. Once more, obviously the best way of doing this is to *make interpretations* – the best way of assessing the patient's capacity to use psychotherapy is to try it.

This leads to yet another extremely important function of interpretations, which is to get *direct* as opposed to *inferential* evidence about the patient's pathology. It is easy enough to make inferences from the history about what is going on beneath the surface, but the only way of being sure that these inferences are correct is to get an unequivocal positive response to interpretation.

The trouble is, as I hope to have illustrated incontrovertibly in previous pages, that interpretations are a very powerful tool, and – like powerful drugs – have major side-effects, not all of them desirable in an initial interview. They may cause increased disturbance, raise strong hopes that help will be available, or produce immediately a strong attachment to the interviewer. *The one thing we must not do is to produce these side-effects and then leave the patient high and dry.*

These considerations lead to two important and opposite statements: *You must not make interpretations until you have found out what kind of patient it is that you are talking to.*

And yet, as clearly implied above, *you may not be able to find out what kind of patient you are talking to without making interpretations.*

These two statements are clearly irreconcilable. Is there any way in which they can be reconciled? The simple answer is no, and an obsessional would conclude that the initial assessment interview is therefore impossible.

The realistic answer is of course that the situation is not as black and white as this. A parallel would be a young man who wishes to find out whether a girl will come out with him – there are many marginal ways in which he can test her out without actually asking her, and as he constantly watches for feedback he can become bolder as the signals become progressively more positive, or withdraw without loss of face as soon as they become unequivocally negative.

The approach to the patient in an initial interview can be described similarly in a series of steps, with a similar constant monitoring of the response. Some of the possibilities are as follows:

(1) The patient, or known facts in his history, may convey an impression of severe disturbance from the beginning.
(2) Alternatively, skilled questioning in the early stages of the interview may elicit crucial information – e.g. a history of repeated suicidal attempts, poor impulse control, or several previous admissions to hospital (see p. 236 for an example).
(3) Obviously, these features do not necessarily mean that the patient is unsuitable for psychotherapy; but they do mean that the interviewer must tread warily and immediately begin to tailor his interview according to the therapeutic resources available.
(4) Interpretations may be necessary in order to make contact at all, in which case the risk must be taken.
(5) But these interpretations must be no deeper than the moment-to-moment situation requires – they must be constantly regulated by the degree to which the required information has been obtained, the view of the patient that is emerging, the appropriate disposal for such a patient, and whether or not such a disposal is actually available.
(6) If all the signs are favourable, the interviewer can go ahead fearlessly, within reason; but he must always be aware of the possible effects of what he is saying, and what is going to happen to the patient after the interview.
(7) As already mentioned, there are three main types of effect that the interviewer must be aware of: increased hope, increased *disturbance*, and increased *attachment* (for a particularly striking example of these effects, see the Foster Son, Chapter 23).

(8) Obviously, these states in the patient must not be produced *inappropriately*, e.g. hopes of treatment that cannot be fulfilled, or disturbance which there is no opportunity to share and work through.

(9) Provided that the patient is going to be offered psychotherapy with *someone*, the risk of producing attachment to the interviewer, and to no one else, seems to be much less than one might imagine – the attachment is often easily transferred to another therapist with a similar approach.

(10) Once more, therefore, the interventions must be carefully regulated according to the purposes of the interview, and as soon as these purposes have been achieved the process should be gently halted (for an example see the Film Director's Secretary, p. 262).

(11) Finally, the interviewer must be prepared to take responsibility for whatever situation his interventions have created, and deal with it appropriately.

An example of the importance of avoiding deep contact in the initial interview

The following is an instructive story. A social worker referred herself for a 'training brief psychotherapy' with the stated aim of deepening her understanding of her patients' emotional problems. The interviewer, who knew nothing more about her than this, asked her for more details of what she was hoping to gain from her therapy. She answered that she wanted to come to life in her work – only on rare occasions had she felt properly alive. How had this happened? The answer was, when she had been in love and loved. The interviewer said he supposed it always went wrong, to which the answer was yes. How did this happen? She didn't know.

At this point the natural thing for a psychotherapist to do would be to enquire into the nature of the patient's close relationships, making interpretations where he could, in order first to deepen rapport and then lead towards understanding her life problem; which in turn would provide a focus for therapy and give an indication of what would be likely to develop in the transference relationship.

Instead, he abruptly changed the subject, saying that he would like to become a psychiatrist for a moment. He asked if the patient had ever been seriously depressed – on the above story this seemed to be the most probable psychiatric disturbance. The answer was yes. Gradually it emerged that the patient had had previous long-term psychotherapy from a male therapist; that this had begun to result in severe acting out – 'quite bizarre', 'parasuicidal gestures', 'it just didn't seem like me'. At one point she had smeared carbolic acid over her face. Therapy had had to be terminated because of her therapist's departure, and she had then threatened to commit suicide on his doorstep. She had finally had to be committed to a mental hospital.

Of course the crucial question was whether the patient had worked this out of her system, but the one thing that seemed most improbable was that she was suitable for brief psychotherapy. The interviewer then had to decide whether he wanted to consider accepting such a patient into long-term therapy, a decision which is largely a matter of personal choice. He decided he did not want to take the risk, and he closed up the interview as best he could. For the patient this was traumatic enough, but it was considerably less traumatic than two other situations would have been: either (1) that the previous history had only emerged after the interviewer had made deep contact and started a therapeutic process; or (2) that these phenomena had remained unknown and had suddenly erupted during the course of therapy.

The further consequences of this interview seem in fact to have been the preservation of a reasonably good relationship between interviewer and patient, as is shown by the fact that she has subsequently kept in touch with him. It should be added that she is now in therapy with someone else and so far nothing untoward has happened, so that the interviewer's caution may have been misapplied. Nevertheless the story illustrates a crucial point.

This was an example of an interviewer's decision to get information first, and on the basis of that information to refrain from any attempt to go further. In other words the step-by-step process described above stopped at stage (2). In Chapter 23 I shall give an example of the inexorable and dangerous chain of events set in motion by *responsibly* taking a calculated risk and going on to stage (4), that is making minimal interpretations in order to gain the patient's confidence and thus be enabled to make a psychiatric and psychodynamic diagnosis.

The irresponsible use of interpretations in the initial interview

Here I can give two stories illustrating the consequences of a clinician's *irresponsible* disregard of these principles by making disturbing interpretations without first finding out what sort of a patient he has before him: the first, I am afraid, from my own experience, and the second from that of a colleague.

Not long after I qualified I worked as a Casualty Officer in a London hospital. As a young doctor in psychoanalytic training I was full of enthusiasm for a psychodynamic approach to patients and trigger-happy with interpretations. One day a man in his forties came in complaining of the intrusive thought of killing his wife. I took his history and quickly discovered that during his absence at the War his wife had had an affair with another man, by whom she had had a child. Accordingly I said to him that, after such an event, surely he had good reason to have the idea of wanting to kill her. He made no particular response and went away. The next day he returned in a psychotically exalted state, demanding of every stranger whom he met, 'Do you believe in the Lord?', and the Mental Welfare Officer had to be called to go through the formalities of committing him to a mental hospital. The fact that this response on the patient's part was intelligible psychodynamically – his guilt having been intensified and now taking a religious form, and being projected – is neither here nor there.

At this time I was without the experience to know that intrusive thoughts may be a psychotic phenomenon; but even with a patient known to be neurotic and already in psychotherapy it would be irresponsible to plunge straight in with an interpretation of such a disturbing feeling. With a patient whom I did not know and might well not see again it was quite inexcusable.

I can only describe the second example in outline, since the patient has quite understandably withheld her permission for any details to be given. Let me say simply that she was extremely distressed by a deep and disturbing interpretation given in the initial interview, was unable to mention this in her subsequent individual therapy, and was preoccupied with the question of exactly what the interviewer meant by it for the next 6 years.

This kind of procedure can be justified like the use of lumbar puncture as a routine investigation for headache – undoubtedly sometimes informative, and after all only occasionally fatal.

Summary of the use of interpretations in the initial interview; motivation

Interpretations responsibly used are an essential part of most initial assessment interviews. Four of their main functions have already been discussed:

(1) To convey to the patient that he is understood, and thus to *deepen rapport* in order to obtain more meaningful information.
(2) To remove resistances.
(3) To obtain direct evidence about *psychopathology*.
(4) To test out the patient's *capacity* to work in interpretative therapy.

There remains a fifth function that has not yet been mentioned, namely *testing out motivation for insight*. The feelings that need to be faced in psychotherapy are almost invariably painful – after all, that is what unconscious conflict is about. Therefore a patient needs considerable determination to go through with the process of psychotherapy. There is overwhelming clinical evidence, and strong research evidence, for the importance of motivation (see Sifneos, 1972, and Malan, 1976b), and therefore the assessment of a patient's motivation is essential to making a prognosis. But until a patient knows what is involved in psychotherapy his motivation may well be unrealistic – for instance he may be very keen to *come* as long as he thinks that he can remain passive while something is *done to* him. His true motivation may only emerge after he – and his unconscious – have been given a taste of what to expect. This is yet another reason for making interpretations in the initial interview.

In fact the dynamic interaction between interpretation and motivation is often extremely striking. The interviewer aims to give the patient some degree of fresh insight, often summing up for him what his life problem appears to be. A good patient responds with increased motivation, and many unpromising or resistant patients have been brought into treatment in this way. At the extreme, the patient responds with a flood of unconscious communication, clearly wanting to start treatment then and there (see the Film Director's Secretary, p. 262; and the Foster Son, p. 276). Obviously this is a good prognostic sign, but it can be extremely double-edged – what happens if there is no therapeutic vacancy available? On the other hand the patient may respond by revealing ambivalent motivation, warning potential therapists that tactful handling will be necessary to keep the patient in treatment (see e.g. the Nurse in Mourning, p. 140); and at the other extreme the patient may respond by immediately withdrawing and revealing a total unwillingness to work in this kind of therapy at all, in which case therapists may well have been saved wasted effort, and some alternative disposal needs to be considered.

Conclusion

The issues involved are so complex that probably only someone who already possesses considerable experience will find the foregoing account properly intelligible. Perhaps these issues will become clearer from the following actual examples.

I have chosen six. The interviews are mostly described as they happened. None is perfect, and where the interviewer made mistakes this is freely admitted. They are weighted towards young people – only one is over 30 – but the principles are exactly the same whatever the patient's age. They are also weighted towards the more severe types of psychopathology, often with severe deprivation in the background, for the simple reason that it is with such patients that difficult problems of assessment and disposal tend to arise.

19

Assessment for psychotherapy (contd): II. The importance of the psychiatric enquiry and differential diagnosis

The Fostered Irish Girl

Let us consider the following application form, written by a young woman of 21:

'My main difficulty is a deep fear of cancer. Even seeing and writing the word makes me terrified. Despite all reassurance to the contrary I still feel I have the disease.

'As far as I can remember I have had this fear since I was 8, after I left my foster-parents in Ireland with whom I was left when I was only a few weeks old, to come to live with my parents in England, who were complete strangers to me, especially my mother who still is.

'I get pains in my stomach, various aches, and diarrhoea, which make me panic, rendering me incapable of thinking any other thoughts other than that my body is diseased.

'I went to my doctor for help because I was ruining my life.'

It also emerged from her written material that she had an illegitimate baby girl aged 20 months, whom she had kept, and that she was now engaged to be married to her baby's father.

It must be assumed, of course, that her General Practitioner, who referred her, has taken all reasonable steps to exclude organic illness. This being so, anyone trained in psychotherapy would have no difficulty in making a preliminary hypothesis: she has suffered a severe trauma, which has involved both the loss of people who have virtually been her parents since she was born, and a transfer to people who, though her real parents in fact, were total strangers with whom she clearly did not get on. We all know by now the kinds of unbearable feeling of loss, deprivation, and anger which such an event is likely to have aroused in her and might well be expressed in a symptom; and this interpretation is confirmed by the information that her symptom in fact dates from that time. We have thus already made a *psychodynamic formulation*. Obviously, the correct treatment is psychotherapy in depth, with the aim of bringing out the feelings and resolving them.

But this is going much too fast. We can ask several additional questions: Is she capable of responding to a psychotherapeutic approach? If the answer is positive, is she going to be able to bear the disturbance that is likely to be aroused in her? And what kind of disturbance is this likely to be? What in fact is the psychiatric diagnosis?

Did someone use that word, *diagnosis*? Does the author of this sophisticated book on dynamic psychotherapy still cling to using labels like 'anxiety state' or 'obsessive-compulsive neurosis' under the impression that he is furthering the cause of assessing and treating the patients under his care?

The answer is, yes, he does. Although it is true that psychiatric diagnosis has severe limitations – often it is purely descriptive and does no more than label the patient's most prominent symptom, and very rarely does it imply any generally agreed underlying pathology – nevertheless it sometimes describes a clear-cut syndrome, and even more frequently it implies a *prognosis* that is of crucial relevance to psychotherapy, and quite essential to therapeutic planning.

Once more, of course, it needs to be said that this planning must be undertaken in the real world, not in an ideal world – in other words it needs to take into account what kinds of treatment are actually available. With this particular patient, let us suppose that she has been referred to a purely out-patient clinic like the Tavistock Clinic, and that the only type of vacancy available is provided by a competent but relatively inexperienced trainee, who is looking for a case for intensive three-times-a-week therapy of a strictly psychoanalytic kind, under supervision.

What I propose to do is to go through the various possible psychiatric diagnoses, with the following questions in mind:

(1) What characteristics would lead towards this diagnosis?
(2) Where does the patient lie on the spectrum of possible degrees of severity?
(3) What dynamic psychopathology does the diagnosis imply?
(4) If the patient appears both motivated for and responsive to a dynamic approach, is dynamic psychotherapy necessarily the treatment of choice, even in an ideal situation? If not, what is?
(5) In the real situation postulated above, is the patient suitable for this particular kind of vacancy (i.e. three times a week with a trainee under supervision)?
(6) If the patient does *not* appear to be responsive to a dynamic approach, what are the appropriate alternatives?
(7) And finally, what is the prognosis with the form of treatment recommended?

Throughout the following I use the traditional terms, and not those that appear in the American Psychiatric Association's admirable attempt to codify psychiatric diagnosis, published in their *Diagnostic and statistical manual of mental disorders* ('DSM-IV') (American Psychiatric Association, 1994). For instance, the terms 'hysterical' and 'psychopathic' do not occur in the DSM-IV, but I explain carefully what I mean by them.

Phobic Anxiety

First of all, the prognosis would probably be best if we were able to make a simple diagnosis of *phobic anxiety*. This would imply that the patient's condition is largely *reactive*, in the sense that the anxiety only appears as a response to a stimulus, in this case either to reading or hearing the word cancer, or having some physical symptom which suggests the idea of cancer to her.

Hysteria

If we reached this conclusion we might also conclude that she was an example of phobic anxiety in a *hysterical personality*, in which case we would label her as a case of 'anxiety-hysteria'. This diagnosis might be made on the basis of a history of conversion symptoms, but it would be more likely to be made on the 'feel' of the patient. One of the characteristics of a hysterical patient is the subtle quality of appearing to *act* what are nevertheless *genuine emotions* – a kind of emotional 'lying the truth'.

Now clinical experience suggests that the pathology underlying phobic conditions or anxiety-hysteria often involves problems that are relatively responsive to a psychotherapeutic approach, such as sexual or Oedipal anxieties or fear of loss of control of aggressive impulses. This applies, for instance, to a number of the patients described in Chapters 5, 7, and 8, e.g. the Adopted Son, the Director's Daughter, and most of the patients used to illustrate the male Oedipus complex. If this were so, then the present patient might well be suitable for the vacancy available. But here an immediate word of caution is necessary: to psychotherapists, a fear of *cancer* has an 'internal' quality implying depth and severity of pathology; and when one takes into account the degree of deprivation implied in the history, then one would need a good deal of reassurance, for instance from evidence for basic strength and lack of other types of disturbance, before recommending this particular disposal.

On the other hand, if the anxiety is largely reactive, then *behaviour therapy* (in the form of either desensitization or 'flooding') must be considered as a possibility, the more so, obviously, the less responsive to a dynamic approach the patient appears to be. Here, however, the same kind of caution applies. It is almost certain that the 'internal' quality of the anxiety, which is most probably a reaction to the *idea* of cancer rather than to cancer as an external stimulus, would make a behaviour therapist very guarded in his prognosis. Nevertheless this form of treatment would need to be considered.

Obsessional anxiety

Let us continue. Might it be that her condition is essentially one not of *phobic* but *obsessional* anxiety? Here there is a spectrum that needs to be considered. At one end she might suffer from anxiety within the setting of an *obsessional personality*, e.g. being perfectionist, or preoccupied with tidiness and cleanliness. Here, as in some phobic states, the underlying pathology may involve *fear of loss of control* of forbidden impulses, psychotherapy may well be the treatment of choice, and the particular kind of vacancy that I have postulated may well be appropriate. At the other end of the spectrum, her symptom might be part of a severe *obsessive-compulsive neurosis*, involving the use of irrational acts or elaborate rituals in order to keep the threat of cancer at bay. The idea of cancer might then well represent some kind of punishment for the underlying impulses. Now, even though the psychopathology in such cases appears perfectly intelligible, accumulated practical experience suggests that often the symptom itself develops an autonomy, and no matter how extensively the pathology is interpreted and apparently worked through, the symptom remains untouched. It is apparently true, for instance, that there is no known authenticated case of an obsessional hand-washer being cured by psychoanalytic treatment. In my view, therefore, the treatment of choice may well become *behaviour therapy* – or, even more, perhaps the treatment of the future will be a combination of behaviour therapy with dynamic psychotherapy (see e.g. Segraves and Smith, 1976), but this combination is not at present available. In any case, placing the patient on this particular spectrum becomes a crucial part of the initial assessment procedure.

Hypochondriasis

Supposing we were to make a diagnosis of *hypochondriasis*? This is of course purely descriptive, and *theoretically* it is the least meaningful of all the possible diagnoses that I shall consider; but *practically* it may well have an important significance. There is a type of hypochondriacal personality in whom feelings have been entirely somatized and with whom the translation of physical symptoms into feelings is an almost impossible task. In such patients the prognosis with psychotherapy is very poor indeed, and for them there is nothing better to recommend than support, reassurance, and tranquillizers. This patient's written material does not suggest that she is such a person, but the possibility needs to be explored.

Psychopathy

Might she be *psychopathic* – or, an alternative term, *sociopathic*? These terms, though largely descriptive, have perhaps the most important prognostic significance of all. With her background we might well find a history of such features as truanting, shoplifting, teenage trouble with the police, poor impulse control, promiscuity, repeated unwanted pregnancies, or destroyed relationships. If these phenomena were severe, then the prognosis with purely interpretative, intensive psychotherapy becomes unquestionably poor. Probable events are an initial honeymoon period, followed by increasingly uncontrollable acting out, lack of response to interpretation, an inability to cope on the part of the therapist, and final complete breakdown of the therapeutic relationship. In my view such patients need a long-term relationship containing a very considerable element of support, and need to be referred either to specialists in this kind of work or to organizations like the probation service or social work agencies.

Anorexia nervosa

Does her main symptom involve problems to do with *eating*, the most probable of which would be under-eating – perhaps with the fantasy that eating increases the risk of cancer of the gastro-intestinal tract – leading at the extreme to severe *weight loss* and *amenorrhoea*, in other words to a diagnosis of *anorexia nervosa*? Now although this is a very mysterious condition, and although patients with these two cardinal symptoms are probably very heterogeneous, the diagnosis is one that needs to be taken very seriously, and almost always implies severe psychopathology. Again there is a spectrum. At one end, where under-eating is potentially controllable, the outlook for intensive psychotherapy is good; at the other end, where there has been severe weight loss and refusal to eat even though life was threatened, intensive psychotherapy is a difficult and heroic act, needs the support of an in-patient unit, and certainly should not be undertaken by a beginner.

The law of increased disturbance and its bearing on the choice of treatment

This is an appropriate point to introduce a fundamental law of psychotherapy and psychotherapeutic forecasting:

Under the impact of uncovering psychotherapy a patient always has the potential to become as disturbed as they have ever been in the past, or more so.

In the first edition of this book I wrote that this law has serious limitations: 'It is true of some patients and not of others; and in the present state of our knowledge there is no means of distinguishing the two categories.'

As I now realize, this statement completely leaves out a crucial factor, namely the form of treatment that the patient is given. In any particular patient, whether or not the potential for increased disturbance is fulfilled depends on the balance between the speed or intensity of uncovering, on the one hand, and the degree of support offered by the therapist, on the other. Therapy will be most anxiety-provoking or disturbing in two opposite kinds of situation: (1) the more the technique approximates to that of the unresponsive 'passive sounding board' used in standard psychoanalysis, which leaves the patient without support; or, on the other hand (2) the more actively the therapist tries to confront defences and reach anxiety-laden feelings and impulses. Variations in these two factors result in a complete spectrum. Therefore it is essential at initial assessment to get an idea of the potential for disturbance in the patient, and thus to be able to refer them (1) to a form of therapy in which the balance is likely to be correct, and (2) to a therapist who both knows how to find this balance and is flexible enough to put his knowledge into practice.

The factors relieving anxiety that can appropriately be used to mitigate the dangers of uncovering psychotherapy consist essentially of *being both flexible and human*, of which we may mention: explaining what is required of the patient and why, answering legitimate questions, offering support and encouragement, and (Truax' terms) genuineness and non-possessive warmth; and also the technique used with patients in which an alliance is formed with the patient's healthy part in an attempt to understand the neurotic or psychotic part.

In conducting an initial interview, therefore, you must always try to get an idea of the potential for disturbance in the patient, so that your referral can be tailored appropriately. In particular, if the choice is to be several-times-a-week on the couch, you must realize that this form of therapy definitely lies towards the anxiety-provoking end of the spectrum, and you must be fairly sure that the patient has the strength and motivation to withstand it and make use of it – or at least you must warn the prospective therapist that at times their technique may need to be modified. Group therapy of a strictly uncovering kind is also potentially highly disturbing, and moreover it has the disadvantage that the therapist is far less able to monitor its effects on any individual patient; so that it also is a referral that needs to be considered with caution.

An example of the potentially devastating effect of unmodified uncovering psychotherapy

A young woman of 26 was taken on at twice a week. Her problem was that all her life she had adopted a façade of what other people required her to be, and in consequence she felt she had entirely lost her own identity. Obviously, you might think, the main aim of therapy will be to enable her to get in touch with what she really feels, and this presumably is what the therapist attempted. However, within a few months of starting therapy she began behaving in an extraordinary way at work, telling everyone what she thought of them in the most offensive terms – she called a colleague 'a fucking pig'. The situation became quite out of hand, she was sent to a psychiatrist, and was committed to hospital, where she received a diagnosis of a manic state. Here she only stayed for a few days, but she felt it was the worst experience she had ever had, that everybody's attitude towards her changed from then on, and that now she was labelled a mental patient for life. If anyone asked her how she was, she felt they were implying that she was suffering from some incurable disease. This was still true when she was followed-up 6 years later.

It is clear that a serious miscalculation was made, and that the form of psychotherapy chosen was too intensive for the patient's fragile defences. Though with the best will in the world, we had violated the cardinal principle of *primum non nocere* – your first duty is not to do harm.

Could this have been foreseen? I do not know. There was nothing overt in the patient's history to indicate the dangers. But one thing is certain: if there is a history of previous breakdown or severe disturbance, then this must be taken seriously in therapeutic planning.

Assessing severity, strength, and support

Therefore, in practical terms, it is always very important to assess the following:

(1) The maximum severity of past disturbance, for which the questions 'have you ever had a breakdown?' and 'what were you like when you were at your worst?' are of great value. Here the non-specific and non-psychiatric term 'breakdown' is entirely appropriate, because it covers so many different possibilities. Some patients ask what is meant by this term, in which case the answer is 'a state in which you were unable to carry on a normal life'.

(2) The patient's strength, as shown by her inner resources and interests, the history of her relationships, and her capacity to bear stress and disturbing feelings in the past without breaking down.

(3) The degree of support available in her environment, and
(4) The capacity of any potential therapist to cope with the degree of disturbance that is likely to occur.

The above fundamental law, and these questions arising from it, are highly relevant to the next two possible diagnoses.

Depression and the question of suicide

First of all, with this patient's history, it seems hardly possible that her condition will not contain a major *depressive* component. This is true both *psychopathologically* and *psychotherapeutically* speaking, in the sense that problems of grief, loss, and anger, conflicting with love and guilt, are likely to figure prominently in any psychotherapy that may be undertaken. This depressive psychopathology may or may not be reflected in manifest clinical *depressive features*, and the nature of these, if present, will have a fundamental bearing on the treatment of choice and the prognosis. Once more, therefore, there is a spectrum of possibilities.

At one end we may find that there is no evidence of clinical depression, and in the absence of evidence for any other diagnosis, I think the most probable conclusion will be that her symptom is a *depressive equivalent*. In this case there will quite probably be no reason why intensive psychotherapy should not be undertaken – though the high probability that relatively severe depressive manifestations, including suicidal impulses, may develop under the influence of psychotherapy, would always need to be borne in mind.

At the other end, the fear of cancer could be part of a *depressive syndrome* accompanied by other depressive manifestations such as loss of interest and despair; and this could be a chronic condition always present, or a cyclical phenomenon; and moreover it could have *'reactive'* ('neurotic') qualities, or *'endogenous'* ('psychotic') qualities such as depressive delusions, early waking, and a family history of manic-depressive psychosis. In addition there could be a history of previous depressive breakdown with admission to hospital and ECT; or of hypomanic or manic episodes; and above all, there may be *suicidal* tendencies now or a history of suicidal attempts in the past. Such questions as, 'Have you felt like suicide?' and 'Have you ever actually made a suicidal attempt?' are mandatory. If the answer to the latter question is positive, it is essential to know the exact circumstances in which these attempts were made, and to assess both the *true suicidal intent* and the *actual risk to life* (which do not necessarily coincide), the degree of 'cry for help' or wish to take revenge on people or to manipulate them; and to try and assess the danger of another attempt. If the patient took an overdose, it is very important to enquire *how much* she took, of *what*, and her own knowledge of the likelihood of *being discovered*. There is a world of difference between someone who took a few tablets from a large bottle, knowing her husband was going to come in in half an hour; and someone who, like the Refugee Musician to be described below, took everything he could lay his hands on while living an isolated life in a bed-sitting-room. Finally, in all cases, it is essential to assess the severity of any depressive or manic attacks – whether, for instance, depressive attacks have made her take time off work or have been totally incapacitating; and whether manic attacks have led her to do things that cause harm to herself or others.

The information about the cyclical, or 'endogenous' quality of the condition is also crucial. The more these qualities are present the more probable it is – if psychotherapy should be contra-indicated – that she will respond to anti-depressants; and the more the manic-depressive element is present the more likely she is to respond to lithium. Here, also, the family history may be highly relevant. Obviously, an assessment of her probable response can be based on direct evidence if any drugs have been used in the past.

This brings us back once more to the fundamental law and the questions arising out of it that were formulated above. A history of severe, incapacitating depressive episodes, not precipitated by any identifiable external event, must be considered as a probable contra-indication to intensive psychotherapy, and an absolute contra-indication to the type of therapy by a trainee postulated here. I very well remember a patient with such a condition, a man in his fifties, who was finally referred to an experienced analyst. This analyst reportedly said to him at the beginning, 'now we will *really* get to the root of your depression and treat it'. The almost immediate result of taking him into analysis was yet one more totally incapacitating, potentially suicidal, depressive attack, making admission to hospital imperative and the analysis impossible. The patient responded quickly to anti-depressants and – in my view rightly – broke off his analysis. It would be nice if the analyst's reported remark corresponded to reality in the practical world, but I am afraid that with such a patient it is just not so.

The relation between 'neurotic' and 'endogenous' depression is a very obscure subject, still unresolved, and this is no place to become involved in it. Nevertheless, 'endogenous' qualities, though serving as a warning, do not mean that the condition is not basically psychogenic; and, provided they are not too severe, that it will not respond to a psychotherapeutic approach. Here is another instructive case history: A young woman in her early twenties was referred for a psychotherapeutic opinion. She was suffering from recurrent depressive attacks – not incapacitating, but still serious – with an apparently cyclical quality, for which no precipitating cause could be found. There were no obvious predisposing factors in her background, but there was a family history of depression. She was at University in a city away from London where psychotherapeutic resources were slender, and the immediate danger seemed to be that her depression would prevent her from studying and make her fail her Finals. The therapeutic plan was therefore based on the following considerations: that the characteristics of her depression indicated a favourable response to anti-depressants, and these would be tried in her final year; and after that she would be reassessed, and possibly move to London and consider undertaking an analysis. The outcome was, first, that her response to one of the tricyclic anti-depressants was dramatic, and she ended by getting a good degree; and second, that she then went into analysis, which rapidly revealed the psychogenic nature of her depression and the antecedent causes in her background, and which in the end was relatively successful.

Returning therefore to the original patient, the exploration of the depressive features in her history may well constitute a large and essential part of the initial assessment.

Paranoid and other psychotic conditions

The next part of the differential diagnosis is equally important, if not more so. Is her symptom not so much *depressive*, but essentially *paranoid*? For instance, has the idea of cancer a *sinister* quality allied to the paranoid fantasy of being poisoned, or are there other manifestations that would lead us towards the diagnosis of a paranoid condition? Here again there is a wide spectrum. At one end there might be evidence that she is a *paranoid personality*, a condition that is regarded as unlikely to lead to breakdown; while at the other end the idea of cancer may at times have had a truly *delusional* quality, and there may be a history of previous *overtly psychotic* episodes. This leads us into yet another utterly unresolved area, namely the meaning of the term 'borderline' and the prognosis in different categories of patient for whom this term is used.

Now the term 'borderline' is surrounded by confusion, and though I have used it freely in previous Chapters, in a discussion of *diagnosis* it is probably best avoided. Nevertheless, some term is needed to describe patients who contain psychotic features without actually being psychotic – there is no other term in general use, and I have none to suggest. The fundamental problem is a highly practical one both for psychiatrists and psychotherapists. For psychiatrists the problem is to distinguish between those patients who are basically stable and those in whom the psychotic features are pre-schizophrenic. The problem for psychotherapists is to distinguish between those patients who will react to an interpretative approach with relief and those who will react with increased disturbance.

During many years at the Tavistock Clinic, I have accumulated a long list of patients in whom this question arises; and, even being wise after the event, I have found myself quite unable to distinguish between these two possibilities. I am constantly being surprised by patients whom I would not expect to break down, who do break down, and those whom I would expect to break down, who don't. This remains an area where systematic research is badly needed.

It is also important to bear in mind the possibility that, whether or not the patient becomes overtly psychotic, suicidal feelings or other disturbed phenomena may at some time call for admission to an in-patient unit. This is not necessarily a disaster; and the process of holding the patient in this way, while she passes through her most disturbing feelings, may constitute an important stage in her therapy; but it *can* be a disaster if it results in the therapy being interrupted. At one time, mental hospitals around London passed through a phase of not being willing to accept the divided responsibility involved with patients who continued their therapy at another institution; but fortunately they seem to have become more flexible in recent years.

If anyone has doubts about the fundamental law of increased disturbance under psychotherapy, he should read again the stories of the Refugee Musician (pp. 199ff.), Foster Son (pp. 207ff. and also 274ff.), and Man with School Phobia (pp. 225ff.); and also the story of the girl described on p. 22, who made a clear unconscious communication foretelling her breakdown. Here, in order to emphasize the point, it is worth adding some further details from the Refugee Musician, where the initial assessment was quite inadequate and the consequences of taking him into uncovering psychotherapy were totally unforeseen.

The Refugee Musician (contd)

The patient, who was Jewish and aged 23, wrote on his application form as follows:

'I considered it necessary to suspend my study because my concentration was being distracted by fantasies which I was finding progressively more difficult to control. These fantasies were concerned with sexual feelings towards small boys; fear of anti-semitism; and suicide. During these periods when I was more depressed than usual I was aware that I was tending to think like a paranoiac.'

Like the application form of the Irish Girl, this written material offers clues that invite questions of differential diagnosis. Preoccupation with sexual fantasies is, after all, something that any frustrated young man is likely to suffer – and, on the other hand, intrusive fantasies can be a psychotic phenomenon; feelings about anti-semitism, in someone who is Jewish, are perfectly reasonable – and, on the other hand, may have a paranoid quality, and the patient himself uses the word 'paranoiac'. He also mentions suicidal feelings, and the whole question of depression and suicide must be gone into very carefully.

Now it is a frequent observation that when a psychiatrist becomes a psychotherapist, his knowledge of psychiatry tends to disappear out of the window, and he progressively forgets its extreme relevance to psychotherapy. Moreover, with any particular patient, this becomes more and more true the clearer he sees the psychodynamics. In fact, one can coin another saying: 'There is no greater enemy of a psychiatric diagnosis than a psychodynamic diagnosis.'

With the patient under consideration the interviewer was an extremely competent psychiatrist, and his description of the interview was warm and sympathetic. Nevertheless his account does not contain any detailed enquiry into the question of psychosis, nor into what the patient meant by the word 'paranoiac', nor into the exact nature of his depression. Of course it is quite possible that, at that stage of the patient's development, the psychiatrist would have found little overt to cause alarm; but he clearly did not have the combination of psychiatric and psychotherapeutic experience to realize he was seeing the tip of an iceberg, and to forecast (changing the metaphor) the kind of Pandora's Box that would be opened by taking this kind of patient into uncovering psychotherapy. He made the diagnosis of 'long-standing personality disorder', which was of course correct as far as it went, and put the patient routinely on the group waiting list without any special recommendations.

When the patient eventually came to individual psychotherapy after group treatment had, hardly surprisingly, proved inadequate – in one session of which, incidentally, he let off a gun – he showed the following phenomena:

(1) Intense paranoid feelings, not actually reaching the status of delusions, which were nevertheless literal enough to make him carry a knife around in order to defend himself against men who might attack him in the street.

(2) Destructive fantasies which his therapist was at times afraid he would translate into action, e.g. spreading oil over the streets in order to cause cars to crash. On one occasion, with the aim of demonstrating how destructive it was possible to be without tools or weapons, he stamped a clock to pieces in his therapist's presence (ending by saying, 'one shouldn't do that to something that's ticking'); on another he threw a heavy glass

ash-tray through a window-pane on the fourth floor of the Clinic, which might easily have severely injured someone in the courtyard below.
(3) Homicidal impulses, e.g. lying in wait with his knife for boys coming out of school.
(4) Depressive episodes with 'neurotic' characteristics, which were nevertheless severe and incapacitating enough to cause repeated admission to hospital. On one occasion he took a colossal overdose of tranquillizers – 2500 mg chlorpromazine, 2000 mg nembutal, and an unspecified amount of librium – under conditions in which he was unlikely to be discovered. He survived after lying unconscious for 3 days.
(5) Episodes of almost unbearable psychotic tension, in which he was hardly able to carry on an everyday existence at all.
(6) Manic episodes, in one of which he danced on the desk at his office and did target practice with an air pistol. Not surprisingly this resulted in his being dismissed by his employers, who hitherto had shown extraordinary tolerance in accepting his disturbed behaviour and repeated periods off work.
(7) This led to a final attack of depression with much more 'endogenous' qualities – quite severe retardation, and constipation to the extent of opening his bowels only once a month – failed ECT, and a further suicidal attempt, this time successful.

It should be obvious that a thorough enquiry into the nature of psychotic phenomena is absolutely essential with any patient in whom their presence is suspected; and that if they are found they must greatly influence the final decision about treatment. Uncovering psychotherapy in a patient such as this is a vast, dangerous, and long-term undertaking, not to be entrusted to anyone who does not possess a high degree of skill and dedication, and is not in a position to see the patient over a long period.

Hildebrand's excluding factors

It is now worthwhile to relate this long account of differential diagnosis to the 'excluding factors' devised by H. P. Hildebrand (unpublished). In 1963 he was appointed as Consultant Clinical Psychologist to the London Clinic of Psychoanalysis. The Clinic was at that time faced with a drop-out rate of about 60% of patients taken into analysis. He then devised a list of features which, if found, would mean that the patient would be automatically rejected. The following list is modified from his:

Serious suicidal attempts
Chronic alcoholism or drug addiction
Long-term hospitalization
More than one course of ECT
A confirmed homosexual asking to be made heterosexual
Chronically incapacitating phobic symptoms
Chronically incapacitating obsessional symptoms
Gross destructive or self-destructive acting out

It has to be remembered that this list is concerned with the selection of patients for full-scale analysis carried out by trainees. It does not necessarily mean that *no* patient showing any of these characteristics ever responds to a psychotherapeutic approach, particularly if there is a strong supportive element in it. But what it does mean is that *statistically speaking* such patients tend to be unsuitable, and that it is unfair on both patient and therapist to assign them to a trainee. Here the important observation was that once such patients had been excluded from the intake of the London Clinic, the drop-out rate fell from about 60% to about 10%.

The Fostered Irish Girl (contd): actual diagnosis

Once more we may return to the Irish Girl. I have completed my account of the differential diagnosis, which as the reader will see has covered a large part of non-organic psychiatry. The question is now, what was found in fact?

The answers are as follows:

The patient had two interviews, the first from a female psychologist and the second from a male psychiatrist, and I shall combine information obtained in the two, taking the headings somewhat out of order.

(1) As forecast, her fear is basically about the *idea* of cancer, and although it is exacerbated by reading or hearing the word, or by suffering from physical symptoms, it is present most of the time and cannot really be described as *phobic*. Moreover the air of quiet sincerity with which she approached the interview made a diagnosis of *hysteria* seem inappropriate.
(2) There are hardly any *obsessional* phenomena, although recently she suffered a period of mild checking after a row with her mother.
(3) She is not a '*hypochondriacal personality*' in the sense used above, is well able to talk about her feelings, and makes no attempt to run away into a description of physical symptoms.
(4) She has shown no behaviour that would cause her to be labelled as *sociopathic*.
(5) Surprisingly, manifest depression has never been a prominent feature. She does have attacks of feeling dejected, but these are hardly severe enough to be labelled as clinical depression. When she is feeling like this she suffers from insomnia to some extent, but not from early waking. She denies any suicidal feelings.

So far, then, the psychiatric enquiry has given largely negative results.

We now have to raise questions to do with the technique of interviewing. The patient started tense and anxious, but was willing to talk about the history of her life and the nature of her symptom. It is possible that if she had been asked direct questions about the other two headings, namely eating problems and psychotic phenomena, she would have given truthful answers, but it is by no means certain. What in fact happened was something quite different. The psychologist tried to ask her about sex, but found her extremely resistant to giving any information. The psychologist was therefore forced to try and ease the resistance, and she took the risk of making a number of 'defence' interpretations about the patient's unwillingness to look at this side of herself and her wish to pretend that it didn't exist.

The patient eventually responded to this and gave a full account of the development of her sexuality. When she came to recent events, the following emerged:

Three years ago her fiancé, John, had begun pressing her for sexual intercourse, and she had finally given in; but, in some irrational attempt to pretend it wasn't happening and to preserve the idea of virginity, she had not insisted on any contraceptive measures. As a result she had become pregnant at the age of 18. During her pregnancy she began to *refuse to eat*, became very ill, and had to be admitted to hospital. She was shocked out of this by her father, who pointed out the dangerous effects on her baby. In fact when born the baby weighed only 5½ lb. There was no history of under-eating before this, and her menstrual history was normal. Nevertheless, if she had not already been amenorrhoeic because of her pregnancy, an episode like this might well have led to a diagnosis of *anorexia nervosa*.

Finally, and even more important, the degree of contact that the psychologist had established with her enabled her spontaneously to reveal the following: during the first week after delivery of her baby, she had suffered from auditory hallucinations of voices telling her she was a bad mother (it is worth noting how this self-reproach fits in with Freud's formulation – see p. 149). She told no one about this symptom (the psychologist was the first person she had revealed it to) and after a week it went away. The symptom clearly has both *depressive* and *paranoid* overtones. To the psychiatrist she later added that at times she feels that the whole world is against her, and then everybody in the street looks hideous and she feels as if they are going to stab her. However, it was clear that this feeling did not have the force of a delusion. Nevertheless, we now know that the patient is not suffering from a simple phobic illness; and, taking this information together with the patient's starving herself during pregnancy, we can forecast with certainty that uncovering psychotherapy will have to deal with deep and primitive phenomena. It also clinches the final diagnosis, which is of an essentially *depressive* illness with *paranoid* features. The *anorexic* episode is almost certainly part of the depressive pathology.

This is an excellent illustration of the dilemma of initial assessment already described in the last chapter. If you do not try to establish deep contact with the patient you may miss vital information; if you do, you may establish a situation of trust and hope, and then be entrusted with information that raises questions about the patient's suitability for psychotherapy, or at least for whatever psychotherapeutic vacancies are available. Put succinctly: if you don't get the information, you may make a serious mistake in disposal; if you do, you may raise hopes that you cannot fulfil.

It is obvious, however, that the first of the two alternatives is worse than the second; and therefore the interviewer was entirely justified in doing what she did. Moreover, the situation was in fact retrievable.

The first question to ask is, what prognostic significance does a single episode like this have for psychotherapy – an acute, short-lived period of hallucinations under the impact of the major psychological and physiological stress of an unmarried pregnancy? The simple answer is that no one knows, and that each case must be considered on its merits. Therefore the next step must be to assess the patient's *inner strength* on the one hand, and the amount of potential *support* there is in her relationships and her environment on the other, both of which will help her to face her disturbance without breaking down.

Assessing inner strength and external support

Here the following information is relevant:

(1) Her early history is that she was illegitimate, born in Ireland, and because her mother felt unable to look after her, at the age of a few weeks she was given to a childless couple who lived nearby, where she remained till she was 8. Here we need to try and assess the degree to which these first 8 years gave her a good grounding for her emotional development – the more she was happy and secure during this time the more likely she is to have survived the later trauma without irreparable damage. In fact the information was encouraging. In her own words, 'As far as I can remember I was very happy with my foster-parents, especially my foster-mother, whom I loved very much.' However, the family was very poor, and she suffered from some degree of malnutrition.

(2) Not long after her birth, her mother left, with her father, to come to England, where they got married. They were not heard from for 7 years, until out of the blue her mother returned to Ireland and claimed her. Since the patient had not been legally adopted there was nothing that her foster-parents could do, and at the age of 8 she was taken back to live with her parents in England.

(3) Here there was constant marital strife and threats of divorce; and the mother seems to have never had a good word to say for her and blamed her for everything that went wrong. Thus the impression she created was that, after the age of 8, her home life had offered her nothing but unhappiness.

(4) In spite of this traumatic home background, and in spite of suffering from early bullying, *she did extremely well at school*, and eventually became head girl. She passed the necessary A levels and got a place at University, but was forced to give this up when she became pregnant. She is still looking after her child.

(5) The relation with the father of her child seems to be a relatively good one, and she and he are now intending to get married in 6 months' time.

(6) She is still living in her parents' home, with her fiancé. This is very unsatisfactory, and she complains that they are not really a family and there is hardly any privacy. Her fiancé, however, has saved enough money for a deposit on a house, where they will move when they get married.

(7) She appears to be a good mother and writes in a moving way about the satisfaction she gets from watching her child develop.

(8) She clearly is the kind of person whom people like. She writes of the pleasure she got at school from being *recognized* by the teachers and other girls; and she was in fact *voted* head girl. At her first, temporary, job, she was able to confide in her boss about her pregnancy, and both he and her work-mates gave her a good deal of support. It is clear that a similar good relation has developed with her present boss.

We wrote of her that, in spite of the traumatic background and the primitive disturbance in her, she seems to be a young woman with remarkable resources.

Two sets of questions now immediately arise. First, *can she use* an interpretative approach, and *has she the motivation* to do so if offered? And second, what is the *balance* in her between *disturbance* and *strength*, and is she likely to be able to respond to uncovering psychotherapy without breaking down?

As far as the first set of questions is concerned, she spoke throughout her contact with the Clinic with thoughtful insight and made plain that she wanted to understand herself. Moreover, there was a fact in her history that was of extreme significance – a rare situation in which the patient gave evidence about her response to psychotherapy without its ever having been tried: a few months ago her mother started telling her that she was incapable of looking after a home properly, and this had blown up into a major row in which the patient had got very angry. After this, she said, she had been almost free of her symptom for about two months and had felt as if she had been 'cleansed'. The significance of this incident was fourfold:

(1) It gave evidence that her symptom was at least partly concerned with buried anger against her mother.
(2) The word 'cleansed' even provided a more detailed tentative formulation of the fantasy underlying this particular symptom: anger felt to be 'bad', held inside, and threatening to contaminate and harm her.
(3) The incident showed that the buried feelings were accessible to conscious awareness.
(4) The improvement that followed showed that, on this particular occasion, getting in touch with buried feelings had resulted not in increased disturbance but relief.

The use of projective tests

This is a vast subject which I shall only touch on. At the Tavistock Clinic we use either the Object Relations Test (ORT, Phillipson, 1955), which is a psychoanalytically based version of the TAT, or the Rorschach. Both may tap areas that cannot be reached in an interview, and may give important additional information about psychopathology, strength, and severity of disturbance. The difficulty with both is that they need very skilled interpretation; and one of the troubles with the Rorschach is that the unstructured but highly evocative ink-blots are potentially very disturbing, particularly to a patient whose conflicts contain marked primitive features. The result may well be the impression that the patient is more disturbed than she really is.

This particular patient was given the Rorschach and saw a single percept on each card. The theme was monotonously repetitive – one creature attacking another creature. Also the 'form level' was not good, i.e. she tended to impose her own fantasy on the card without much regard for what it actually looked like. All this was far from reassuring, and was in marked contrast to the impression of strength conveyed by her history.

Referral and treatment

Here we may consider both the type of vacancy which I postulated, namely three times a week on the couch with a trainee, and the type that was actually available.

At the Tavistock Clinic the aim of the former kind of treatment is to train therapists in what is fundamentally psychoanalysis, the limitation to three times a week being caused by the need for trainees to use their vacancies as economically as possible. With this patient I would not have wanted to risk this kind of treatment, even under experienced supervision, since its anxiety-provoking qualities might well have led to breakdown. This would have been fair neither to the patient nor to the therapist.

In reality the only vacancy that was available was for obvious reasons even less suitable, namely once a week with the psychologist who tested her, who *was due to leave the Clinic in 6 months' time.*

In accordance with the principles described in this chapter, we concluded that the patient needed a long-term relationship with a therapist who knew when to make interpretations and when to refrain from doing so, and when to give support. We were very fortunate in finding such a vacancy with the Family Welfare Association, an organization that employs social workers highly trained in psychotherapy.

The patient was seen once a week. She rapidly showed that she could respond to fearless interpretation; and when one day she came complaining of a fear of cancer of the stomach, the therapist went straight in, relating it to her fantasies about the harmful effects of what she had taken in from her mother – and presumably also interpreting that this represented, by the mechanism of paranoid projection, her own hatred of her mother coming back at her. The result of work of this kind was that the cancer phobia soon receded into the background, and eventually the real-life situation with her mother considerably improved.

At the time of writing she had been treated by two separate therapists for a total of about 3 years, and she and her current therapist were beginning to talk about termination. Her therapist has now left this country and – apart from the fact that therapy has been terminated – we have been unable to obtain any further follow-up.

Conclusion

This story represented an important learning experience for me. At the time I was much preoccupied with a series of patients showing minimal signs of psychosis who had broken down under uncovering psychotherapy. I did not sufficiently realize that part of the reason for this was the rigid use of the 'passive sounding board' technique, without a strong element of support. Indeed the Fostered Irish Girl told her therapist that 'she felt we were dead scared of her' – an impression that it was unfortunate and inevitable that our over-caution would create. In the end, without my fully realizing it, the referral to the Family Welfare Association was exactly right; and it became clear that the combination of their flexible yet fearless form of therapy, together with the encouraging features in her story, far outweighed the danger signals.

20

Assessment for psychotherapy (contd): III. The psychodynamic assessment and psychotherapeutic forecasting

In the previous chapter the emphasis was on the relevance of the psychiatric history and diagnosis to psychotherapeutic assessment. In the present chapter I shall describe a somewhat similar patient, a young woman who developed symptoms in response to loss. The important differences, however, are first that the *psychiatric* diagnosis was not in doubt; and second that there was a much larger body of *psychodynamic* evidence on which psychotherapeutic forecasting could be based.

The Film Director's Secretary

This was a single young woman of 26. On her application form she wrote simply: 'Anorexia nervosa. Four weeks in hospital 15 months ago.' The (male) interviewer knew immediately that his interview would have to start with a prolonged period of assessing severity, strength, and weakness; that he might decide that it was quite wrong to try and make contact with the patient's unconscious; and that his final conclusion might well be that psychotherapy was contra-indicated.

The patient was petite, with a quite normal figure, attractive in a rather childlike way. She was very unsophisticated psychologically and had a somewhat artificial manner, but beneath this was an undercurrent of sincerity and good sense which commanded respect.

Invited to start where she liked, she opened with her worry and shame about her present condition. This is one of *over*-eating. If she is upset by something during the day she finds herself at home in a depressed state. At first she may just sit and stare at the wall, but often she then goes out and buys food, usually bread, and stuffs herself, and may eat a whole loaf at one sitting. She is then usually able to vomit spontaneously. She is horrified at herself for doing this,

256

and the physical act of vomiting disgusts her and may leave bruises on her cheeks. A binge of this kind may go on for as long as four days at a time. She has now got to the point at which she is totally obsessed by her weight. If she finds she has put on 2 lb when she weighs herself, her whole day is spoiled.

The main theme of these chapters is the way in which every piece of information needs to be assessed in terms of its implications for therapy. This craving to eat probably expresses an intense need in relation to human beings, and thus implies a severe dependence which would be likely to manifest itself in the transference; and therefore its severity did nothing to reassure the interviewer. In addition, her story implies that the eating is a cover for *depression*, which would be likely to manifest itself in response to any therapeutic approach, and the interviewer therefore sought information about another obvious danger of therapy, the intensification of suicidal feelings. Here she said that she had begun to feel that she could not go on like this and had got as far as counting her Mogadon tablets, wondering if there were enough to kill her. Of course this is not enough information, and the patient must be pressed. Had she ever actually made a suicidal attempt? The answer was that on one occasion, after over-eating, she had found herself unable to vomit, had taken an overdose of Mogadon and mandrax, and had gone round to the hospital to have her stomach washed out – after all, she said, one couldn't go round and ask for this simply on the grounds that one had been over-eating.

Again this information needs to be assessed in terms of its implications for therapy. There is clearly some tendency towards acting out, but neither the suicidal intent nor the risk to life appear to be serious. On the whole this information was therefore reassuring.

In fact the interviewer slipped up here, because in the referral data there was mention of a further suicidal gesture, in which the patient had taken 'all the sleeping tablets she had', but had simply slept this off and had carried on normally the next day. Here again, the *actual risk to life* was clearly small; and the *suicidal intent* was at least not serious enough for her to have made another attempt when she discovered that she was still alive. While this additional information therefore further emphasizes the risk of acting out during therapy, on the whole it does not change the over-all picture.

At this point there are many directions in which the patient could be taken, e.g. the interviewer could have asked about *under*-eating – which, surprisingly, has not yet been mentioned – or the current stresses that caused her to over-eat; but in fact he chose to ask her the standard question that is asked in all medical and psychiatric histories, namely how far back did she date these symptoms? This led her to go back to the beginning, and during the next phase of the interview her whole history, and that of her symptoms, was elicited.

She was born and brought up in the country in Suffolk, and she gave a picture of her parents getting on well together, of being amused by her father in the evenings, of friends and fights at school, in fact of a happy and normal childhood. The interviewer was relieved at the mention of fights, as otherwise the picture seemed somewhat idealized, and in order to get further information he asked if she remembered ever being naughty. The answer was that she didn't, thus confirming the impression of idealization. It was also notable that she did not specifically mention the relation with her mother. Nevertheless it was clear that at this time her childhood contained many good things, and from the point of view of prognosis this was reassuring.

Her conscious traumatic experience occurred at the age of 11, when the family moved into a small isolated village in Yorkshire and set up a General Store. Here she emphasized the change from warm and wooded countryside to bleak moors; and it seemed clear that this also symbolized the loss of warmth in the relation with her parents, who now were so occupied trying to build-up their business that they had little time for the children (she had two older brothers). She remembered coming back from school and finding no one at home, and it was at this time that she began to *over-eat to comfort herself*, and became considerably overweight. This caused her to be teased at school, but not in a way to make her life utterly miserable, and she had happy memories of school as well.

At 16 she left home and moved to a small Yorkshire town, where she started work. Here again she was lonely and unhappy, and the pattern of over-eating was intensified.

At 18 she came to London. She was very frightened of the big city and at first did not dare to take a job more than a few hundred yards away from where she lived. Later she got a job in the West End and for the first time began to realize that being overweight was caused by over-eating, and that it was possible to do something about it by dieting. She went to a doctor who prescribed a diet and who also put her on the Pill. From that point her menstrual periods, which had started at 13 and had always been irregular, often recurring as frequently as every fortnight, ceased altogether.

The history of her symptoms turned out to be intimately connected with her sexual history, and the interviewer asked her to go into this from the beginning. This is an essential part of every consultation. In our society man's basic and primitive instincts are mostly kept under cover, and though in many people aggressiveness may apparently disappear altogether, this does not happen nearly so easily to sexuality; and within sexual fantasies and sexual acts are often contained essential aspects of an individual's true close relationship to other human beings, which are revealed nowhere else.

This girl's actual sexual functioning appeared to be relatively normal, and she described a very convincing orgasm, but her relation to men showed an important recurrent pattern, which gradually became obvious. She had her first sexual experience at 16, and between then and 20 had only casual affairs. Then, having got her weight down from 10½ stone (say 150 lb, 68 kg) without clothes, to 8 stone (say 110 lb, 50 kg), she got a job as personal secretary to a film director, and eventually became one of his favoured mistresses. She accepted with apparent ease the fact that she had to share this much older man with several other women, and became quite attached to him. However, after 2 years she left both him and the job, when he wanted her to indulge in activities that went beyond her own tolerance.

She then became deeply involved with a Greek businessman, who was married and 20 years her senior. This man installed her in a flat, became intensely possessive and would not allow her to work; and they would meet whenever he left his own country on business. He would phone up and say 'take a plane and meet me in Madrid tomorrow', which she would do – but if she happened to be out when he phoned he would immediately suspect the worst and accuse her of being with another man, and there would be hell to pay.

The inference made above about the connection between her over-eating and *dependence* was amply confirmed by the story of her relation with this man.

She became increasingly attached to him; and it was in the early stages of their relation, during periods when she was apart from him, that she began her recent bout of over-eating, coupled with desperate attempts to control it. She read somewhere that if she kept to a diet containing *no carbohydrate at all* she could get into a state of ketosis, which would enable her to eat as much as she liked without gaining weight. She used to test her urine, and as long as it showed the presence of ketones she was happy. By this means she managed to get her weight down to 6 st 5 lb (89 lb, 40 kg). This naturally did nothing for her physical health, and she began to suffer from recurrent minor physical complaints for which she went to a physician. He got out of her the story of her diet and had her admitted to hospital. She made the important comment that if she got her weight down as low as this it made her feel so ill that she couldn't keep it up – thus reassuring the interviewer that her condition was not so malignant that, like some anorexics, she would bring herself to the point of death rather than give in to the impulse to eat.

Finally the situation with this man became such that she could not bear the feeling that if they met in some European capital it could only last a fortnight at most before they would be parted again; and the result was that when she was with him she got into a state of constant crying. It was a slight point in her favour as a candidate for psychotherapy that at least she finally had the strength – as once before – to break with a man with whom the situation had become intolerable. In addition, since then she has gone back to work and has managed to continue working; though as far as men are concerned she has returned to casual affairs. However, her very intense preoccupation with eating has continued. This is where we came in.

Identifying the life problem

At this point we may pause and take stock. The patient's story shows the following features, which represent part of the ideal situation for making a psychodynamic formulation:

(1) A *recent precipitating factor* can be identified, namely the tension involved in the hand-to-mouth relation with her much older lover.
(2) *Previous precipitating factors* can also be identified, namely situations involving *separation*.
(3) There is an obvious *parallel* between (1) and (2).
(4) An *antecedent event* can be identified, of which (1) and (2) can be seen to be a repetition, namely the loss of her parents' warmth consequent on the move from Suffolk to Yorkshire.
(5) The *hidden feelings* – clearly to do with dependence and loss – can be identified by inference.
(6) These feelings are clearly *expressed in her symptom*, which consists of an uncontrollable craving alternating with a defence against it.
(7) The *same feelings are expressed overtly in her human relations*, namely the desperate need for her lover, alternating with her defence, namely lack of involvement, which is expressed in her casual affairs.

These features can be summed up by the statement that the patient's *life problem* can be clearly identified.

There is a contrast from the previous patient, in whom although the precipitating event and its probable meaning were clear, there was no obvious repetition in the patient's close relationships, and the symbolism represented by the symptom itself was far more primitive and more obscure.

Psychotherapeutic forecasting

Once a life problem has been identified in this way, a *part* of psychotherapeutic forecasting becomes relatively easy. We can surely say without question that any form of uncovering psychotherapy with this young woman must come up against *dependence on the therapist* as a major issue; and that any radical attempt to deal with her problems must involve the working through of feelings of loss. It goes without saying that treatment must be long-term.

Severity, strength, and weakness

The above forecast is however only the beginning. How well is she likely to be able to stand up to the stresses of therapy?

Here the *evidence* is clear enough, though the final conclusion to be drawn from it is not.

First of all, her childhood up to the age of 11, though it may no doubt be somewhat idealized, seems to have been happy and free from trauma. In other words the evidence suggests that she has a basis of 'good experience', and that her early emotional development proceeded normally.

Her symptoms began in response to what seems to be a relatively mild, and certainly a relatively late, trauma. This is encouraging, but it also cuts the other way, because it suggests that she must be especially vulnerable to this particular kind of stress.

Moreover, her disturbance is of very considerable severity, as is shown by the intensity of the craving to eat, the all-pervading preoccupation with it, and the extreme measures that she has adopted to control it.

What about her *impulse control* and her *tendency towards breakdown*? Here again the evidence cuts both ways. She has made two suicidal gestures, but not a genuine attempt to kill herself. She has managed to carry on without actually breaking down, and she has managed to go back to work and to keep this up in spite of the severe stress of the break-up with her man-friend.

What about the quality of her human relationships? Here it can be said that in spite of the extreme dependence that her story reveals and her tendency to take up with unsuitable men, she has at least been capable of some degree of emotional closeness, and her sexual functioning appears to be unimpaired. She also has artistic interests which indicate the presence of inner resources.

Psychotherapeutic forecasting (contd): dangers

It seems we can say with some certainty that all the phenomena described so far will become intensified during psychotherapy. The most likely dangers are as follows:

(1) Extreme dependence on the therapist, with intolerance of strains in the relationship and particularly intolerance of absences and breaks in therapy.
(2) Intensification of both sides of her eating conflict, with binges and weight gain on the one hand, and efforts to starve herself, with gross weight loss, on the other.
(3) Acting out, especially in the form of suicidal gestures.

Against all this the following can be said:

(1) Her dependence on her man-friend never led her to reach the point of total breakdown, and in the end she had the strength to break with him and go back to work.
(2) Neither her weight gain nor her weight loss have ever been completely out of control.
(3) Her suicidal intent does not appear to have ever been serious.

Although all these dangers must be taken seriously, therefore, the evidence suggests the possibility that with careful handling they may be kept within bounds.

The question of support

There is little support in her current life. Her parents are in Yorkshire and she has no relatives near London. She has friends, but her eating difficulties make her tend to keep away from them. She has her job; but of course at some point she might easily find herself unable to maintain this. She is sharing a flat with a friend, so that at least she is not living alone.

Dynamic evidence

The patient has thus given a great deal of evidence about herself, which has enabled us to make quite firm predictions about many of the issues that are likely to arise in psychotherapy. On the other hand, the reader may have noticed a glaring omission – no information whatsoever has been obtained about the patient's reaction to a psychotherapeutic approach.

This has of course been quite deliberate, and it was equally deliberate that hitherto in the interview no attempt had been made to elicit this kind of information. The interviewer was not going to start any kind of dynamic process until he had mentally carried out all the operations so far described in the present chapter, the final verdict of which was that the patient – though difficult – might just be suitable for intensive psychotherapy.

Another piece of information fed into the mental computer was the fact that a *long-term vacancy could probably be found for her*. What then emerged at the output terminal, in a totally subconscious way, was a move towards testing her out, as follows:

He found himself *summing up for the patient an aspect of her life problem*. This is often a very useful procedure for both interviewer and patient, and it can be used, with discretion, to enable the patient to go away from an interview with the knowledge of having been *given something valuable in return* for all her self-revelation. What he said was: 'One of your difficulties that stands out is that you don't seem to be able to choose the kind of man with whom a relation could lead to anything permanent.'

The power of this intervention can be gauged from the fact that both interviewer and patient immediately got caught up in a process of psychodynamic dialogue, from which there was no drawing back, and which was clearly something that the patient had never experienced in her life before. She said first that she always had to k*eep people at bay* and not let them too close to her. She then immediately said that she had begun to feel she wanted to live by herself because her flatmate was *getting to know her too well*. The interviewer now found himself drawn into making an interpretation. Remembering the patient's extreme *shame* about her symptom, he said that there must be a part of her represented by her eating problem which *she felt other people could never accept*, and which she could therefore never allow to come into relation with anyone. She immediately confirmed this by saying that she had never allowed her Greek man-friend to know about her eating problem. The interviewer then went deeper by saying that her need for food must represent a *desperate need for something from another human being*, and that she could not bring this into relation with anybody. With obvious understanding she said, no, it would be '*too dangerous.*' The interviewer said that it looked as if it represented a *desperate kind of dependence*, like what she developed with this man, and indeed like what he developed with her. To this she said that recently she had found herself *wondering where her flatmate was going and getting angry if she didn't know*. The interviewer then summed up, saying that it seemed as if her eating problem was only the surface manifestation of a deep problem concerned with her needs from other human beings. In response she spontaneously said, '*and I have to keep everything tidy as well*', thus unconsciously inviting an interpretation of the probable meaning of this obsessional symptom in terms of feeling that everything must be kept under control. This invitation the interviewer, having obtained quite enough information and not wishing to be drawn into a therapeutic session, gently but firmly ignored.

The patient had thus shown abundant evidence of her ability to look beneath the surface, to make unconscious communication, and to respond to interpretation, but this is only half the story. We know that she *can* but does she *want to* enter a kind of therapy of which this is the basis – once more, the crucial question of *motivation*. The interviewer, whose whole attitude to this patient had been reversed by the above passage, therefore began to think aloud to her about therapeutic possibilities. He said he thought she needed long-term treatment, 'possibly more than once a week'. As already mentioned, she was very unsophisticated psychologically, and she began to ask details of what would happen. He explained to her that it would mean talking to a therapist about her feelings, that almost certainly one of the things that would happen would be that she would start by trying to keep him at a distance, but that later she might become very dependent on him, and they would have to try to work this through to a point at which she could let people close to her but wouldn't need to be so dependent. She clearly took all this in, and he therefore said (referring to the London Clinic of Psychoanalysis) that he knew of an organization that might be able to treat her, but that they insisted on seeing patients five times a week, and what did she think of that? Her reply was to say that the nature of her work would allow her to make arrangements so that this was possible. Thus, though we may question the extent to which she really understood the implications of undertaking an analysis – and who does before they have had the experience – she appeared to be highly motivated to give it a trial.

The patient's capacity and motivation for insight

Here the questions that need to be asked with any patient can be summarized as follows:

(1) Is she aware that her problems are emotional?
(2) Can she speak about feelings?
(3) Can she express feelings?
(4) Can she look beneath the surface?
(5) Does she give evidence of being able to widen her sphere of awareness by responding to interpretations?
(6) Does she appear to have the motivation to work in interpretative therapy?

With this particular patient the answers to all these questions are clearly positive.

Choice of treatment

There are of course many different ways of approaching the treatment of a patient of this kind. If she had been less responsive and more disturbed, she could have been referred to the Professorial Unit at St George's Hospital, which specializes in the in-patient treatment of anorexia nervosa; but this would probably cause the loss of her job, and in any case the Unit was known to be over-burdened at the time. Equally, behaviour therapy might have been considered, but experience suggests that this tends not to be very successful with eating problems of such severity. A long-term supportive/interpretative relationship, like that given to the Irish Girl described in the last chapter, would have been another alternative.

In the event, her extreme responsiveness and high motivation tipped the balance in favour of an attempt at a radical solution to her difficulties. If there had been a vacancy at the Tavistock Clinic, which there was not, she would have been assigned to three-times-a-week by a trainee under supervision. As it was, she was accepted for five-times-a-week by the London Clinic of Psycho-analysis.

21

Assessment for psychotherapy (contd): IV. The indications for brief psychotherapy

The Man from Singapore

This was a man of 47 complaining of impotence.

The complaint of impotence presents an immediate problem in differential diagnosis. In the vast majority of patients it is the result of neurotic anxieties which can often be quite deep-seated. On the other hand, in a man of 47 it can obviously be no more than the result of a natural falling off in potency, which has set up a vicious circle of failure and fear of failure. It can also be a manifestation of psychosis; and finally in a very small proportion of patients its origin is organic. The first step therefore is to take a history of the impotence itself, while at the same time getting a 'feel' of what the patient is like.

The problem of differential psychodynamic diagnosis

The patient was a large man with a frank and open manner, able to talk freely and spontaneously about any subject, and indeed clearly with a need to unburden himself. It very quickly emerged that the impotence: (1) was only partial, which implied a better prognosis than if it had been absolute; (2) had been present on and off for a number of years; and (3) that it had been thoroughly medically investigated. The whole feel of the patient was of a substantially normal man suffering from sexual anxieties, and from early in the interview no other psychiatric diagnosis was considered. The question was then entirely whether these anxieties could be identified.

We now enter the realm of *differential psychodynamic diagnosis*. Three common possibilities are: (1) guilt about sex; (2) problems of competition, with feelings of inferiority as a man; and (3) unconscious hostility against the woman. The history was taken with these possibilities in mind.

The male interviewer knew that the patient had been married (at 30), had separated from his wife 3 years ago, and was now divorced. Since then the patient had had a number of relations with women. He made it clear that his potency depended on the woman's attitude – 'I am not really impotent, you know'. One recurrent pattern had occurred when the woman was sexually forward and wanted him to make love to her early in their relationship; he would then become frightened and lose his erection, and she would then be contemptuous and make him quite unable to perform. On the other hand if the woman was not too forward and was 'very understanding' he could function normally.

He went on to say that though he had always led a sheltered life, at 14 he had had the same feelings about girls as other boys did, with sexual dreams and fantasies, normal erections and masturbation. Yet he had been extremely shy in the presence of girls, and by the age of 26 had not yet seen a woman naked. The interviewer asked him why this might be, to which he said that of course he had lost three years out of his life – he had spent his childhood in Malaya, his family had been caught by the Japanese in Singapore, and between the ages of 14 and 17 he had been in a Japanese prison camp. All four members of the family had survived.

The interviewer left this on one side for the time being and continued with the history of the patient's relations with women. When, at 26, he had been sent to Africa in connection with his job, he had managed to function sexually with an Asian prostitute who had been understanding and a bit motherly.

At 30 he was sent back to England on leave. Here he met his future wife and although he was not really in love with her both of them wanted to get married, which they did. She was half French and, like him, Roman Catholic. On their honeymoon they went to France and she was extremely contemptuous of him when he made a muddle in a shop over the currency. He said that already he should have seen the writing on the wall.

Nevertheless their sexual relation went well. After a few days of marriage, he said, sex was perfect, there were no problems and they climaxed at the same time.

To cut a long story short, the periods of harmony became fewer and the quarrels more frequent, and this affected his wish to make love to her, though it did not really affect his sexual functioning. In order to get an idea about aggressive feelings the interviewer asked what happened when they quarrelled. The patient described moments of passionate anger – 'I could almost kill her', 'I smashed her purse against a wall', 'I was afraid of myself ... I could have smashed her in blind rage ... with superhuman power I managed to control myself' – only on a few occasions had he actually hit her and then it was only to slap her.

This was very important negative evidence. The patient was entirely in touch with his anger, and moreover during this period his sexual functioning was little affected. This narrowed the *differential diagnosis*, making it very unlikely that his impotence was caused by hidden aggressive feelings against women.

The interviewer asked him what the quarrels were about. The impression he conveyed was that his wife was very competitive and had made him feel inferior in all sorts of ways *other than sexually*. This theme was continued in the next passage, as the patient told how his relation with a woman had ended within the past two years. He had concealed from her his true occupation and his very limited earnings – she had expected a big shot, which he had implied to her he was, and she found out he was only a salesman.

This was now important *positive evidence* – he was earning below his capacity and was sensitive enough about it to have allowed it to come between himself and a woman. The interviewer therefore made an interpretative comment: that the problem all seemed to come down to *lack of confidence as a man*, and asked him if he could elaborate on this. In reply the patient said that he was always 'pressed' by people *who were doing better than he was*, who had big jobs and titles. He always dreamed of doing the same but never took steps to better himself – 'I think I can't make it'. He thus confirmed both a sense of inferiority and intense feelings of competitiveness.

The interviewer then said that the patient obviously had the potential to do well – for instance he had lost three years of schooling and yet had graduated at University – what went wrong? In view of later material the patient's answer to this was highly significant. He said that his graduation was in order to please his father, 'whom he'd hurt for many years by not doing well at school'.

Why had he not done well? The answer he gave was 'just plain laziness'. He described his father's patient, firm, but ultimately unsuccessful attempts to get him to work. Only once had his father spanked him in his childhood for being naughty – on all other occasions his tone of voice and the look in his eyes had been enough. On the other hand his *mother* used to punish him quite severely with a stick she kept for the purpose. Here he described intense rebellion against her, his airily whistling while she hit him, and raging fantasies of what he'd like to do to her in retaliation. Yet at other times he was immensely close to both his parents – he described a feeling of togetherness, and a passionate physical relation with his mother 'I loved to kiss her and bite the lobe of her ear'. This evidence weakens the first of the three possibilities in the differential psychodynamic diagnosis, namely unconscious sexual guilt, though it may be that the Oedipal aspects of this relation still remain hidden.

One of the climaxes of the interview came later when he described events in the prison camp. His mother and sister had been in one camp and he and his father in another. He described his father's defiant refusal to be obsequious to the Japanese guards, and the terrible consequences. The interviewer braced himself for a story of atrocity, but found instead a supreme story of the human spirit – how the father had been beaten up in the patient's presence, yet had walked back into the hut almost laughing; and how he had later said that, throughout the whole experience, the only thing that had kept him from trying to kill one of the guards had been the thought of his wife and children – he knew if he had retaliated he would have been killed himself. The patient went on to say that under the pretence of not being hungry, the father had often given half of such food as there was to his son – and the patient said with shame that he had accepted it without realizing at the time what his father was doing.

The interviewer was lost in admiration. On a hunch he asked about the father's history after the war. The hunch was abundantly confirmed – the father had worked himself up to a very responsible position, and the patient added that as a boy his father had done very well at school and was top of his class.

Suddenly it seemed that the story made sense. In the following passage the interviewer emphasized several times that surely the patient's sense of inferiority must be due to the impossibility of matching up to this incredibly admirable man. 'Yes', said the patient, 'he was strict yet loving, a father and friend at the same time, good at his work, a loving husband, he spoke French, German, and Italian fluently. He was a wonderful man, perfect. Yet he died at the crucial point in my life, when I was 26 and just about to go to Africa. . . . You would have thought I would have made more of an effort ... I still think, "if only Daddy had been here I could have discussed things with him". I don't think I would have married that woman – he would have had no time for her.'

For reasons of space I shall omit most details of the rest of the interview. The father had later been killed in a motor accident. The mother had collapsed, but son and daughter had found 'an inner strength' to cope with all that the father's death entailed. Whether or not the son had really mourned his father properly was uncertain.

In answer to the question of what he felt about coming for treatment he said that 'he realized he must speak about intimate things, the more open one is the better, or one can't be helped. I feel it's going to help in the end. I have great confidence in it.' Thus his motivation seemed realistic and high.

Yet at the end the interviewer was left with the uneasy feeling that he had in some way missed the crucial point. As he later realized, perhaps the correct interpretation was more complicated: that the father's personality was such that the son's need for defiance, rebellion and competitiveness had never been allowed to emerge, *except in the relation with the mother*; and that the only way in which the son could rebel against the father was by failure. This inability to understand completely during the interview does not really matter. One does not have to reach an exactly correct interpretation – one only need find out basically what is wrong.

There is a postscript to the story. A few days later the interviewer phoned the patient to get some further factual details. During this conversation the patient said that he had been thinking a great deal about 'that discovery of yours'. The interviewer asked him, what discovery? 'That it all has to do with my relation with my father.' He went on to say that he would be *ashamed to meet his father again in the after life* because his own life had been such a failure – he hadn't even a penny in the bank. He went on to eulogize his father's life and his marriage once more, and then suddenly revealed that his father had been overworked after the war and had had a nervous breakdown. The interviewer did not go into this but simply said that perhaps it was not too late to retrieve the situation.

Thus the interpretative work in the interview about *comparing himself with his father* has brought out something beyond this, namely *guilt about failure in relation to his father*. If he felt so guilty, why did he not try harder? The answer strongly suggested by the evidence is that there must have been an *impulse to fail*. Thus the interpretation elaborated above about expressing rebellion by failure is confirmed. This is an example of the phenomenon described in Chapter 8 (see pp. 62ff.), namely the devastatingly malignant feelings underlying the quite genuine love and admiration for a good father.

Finally, the clear impact of the interview suggests very strongly that the patient is highly suitable for an interpretative approach.

Choice of treatment: the criteria for planned brief psychotherapy

We may now consider the exact form of treatment. This patient offers a very interesting comparison with the Film Director's Secretary described in the last chapter. In both cases the following three conditions are fulfilled:

(1) The patient's *life problem* can be clearly identified, and this offers a clear-cut theme or *focus* for therapy.
(2) The patient has *responded to interpretations* concerned with this focus.
(3) The patient clearly has the *motivation* to work with this focus.

These are the first three indications for *planned brief psychotherapy*.

With the previous patient, however, it is really inconceivable that therapy could be brief – it is possible to predict with virtual certainty that the patient will rapidly become dependent on her therapist, and that any attempt to terminate will result in a severe intensification of her eating difficulties. In other words it is possible to identify a clear-cut *danger* to brief therapy, which seems unavoidable. With the present patient *no such dangers can be identified*, and there seems no reason why he should not work through the focus within a relatively brief time. He thus fulfils a fourth criterion, which reads as follows:

(4) Possible dangers to brief psychotherapy have been considered, and either none can be seen, or else it seems reasonable to suppose that they can be overcome or avoided.

These four criteria for planned brief psychotherapy have been worked out from extensive clinical and research experience (see Malan, 1976a). The patient fulfils them all, and this is the treatment of choice.

Experience has also indicated that it is best to work within a time limit set from the beginning. For this patient, whose problem is of long standing and appears to be deep-seated, a total of 30 sessions at once a week would probably be appropriate. Finally, since his main problem appears to lie in the relation with his father, it would probably be best if the therapist was male. It also seems reasonable to predict that after an initial honeymoon period the wish to fail in therapy, as a way of defeating the therapist, will become a major transference issue.

22

Assessment for psychotherapy (contd): V. Contra-indications to uncovering psychotherapy

As I hope to have made clear in previous chapters, the decision about whether or not a patient is given psychotherapy usually depends on the situation as a whole – the patient, his environment, and the forms of treatment actually available. Though there are plenty of patients who may be considered unsuitable, there are few contra-indications that can be regarded as absolute. Even Hildebrand's excluding factors (see p. 250) are presumably only valid statistically. Here are two patients with whom, for entirely different reasons, intensive uncovering psychotherapy was regarded as quite inappropriate. In both cases this was seen very quickly, and consequently the interviewer rigorously avoided making interpretations or even asking the kind of question that might bring the patient's unconscious nearer to the surface.

The Man from Borstal*

This was a man of 30. Extracts from the GP's referral letter are as follows:
'I should be most grateful if you can help this man in any way, as his life so far appears to have been an uninterrupted series of disasters.

'His mother sounds as if she suffered from a depressive illness during his childhood, as he says she often took to her bed and left the management of the household to him for long periods. His father is described as being too tired to do more than watch television or doze in his chair after work.

'In his late teens he was committed to Borstal for two years after being charged with attempted murder. He describes this period in Borstal as about the best years of his life. He seems to have appreciated the regulated life with sports and recreational facilities to the full. He obtained full remission and during the ten months that he served he was able to pass three O levels in Art, though he states that at fifteen he had hardly been able to read and write'.

The GP also writes that the patient has had two marriages, both of which have broken up.

---

* A resident rehabilitation centre for young offenders.

269

The patient's responses to the initial questionnaire were laconic in the extreme:

Do you experience any difficulties in your married life? 'Could not cope.'
In what way do your difficulties affect your life? 'Just cannot get things together.'
In what way do you expect treatment to help you? 'Do not know.'
What aspects of life give you satisfaction? 'Do not know apart from painting.'

It is almost possible to give a full assessment of this patient before ever he is seen. He can be compared with all the other people whom one has known, whose background contains severe emotional deprivation, and who have really not been given a chance to develop their potential or their capacity to deal with close relationships or the stresses of everyday existence. Important clues are also given by (1) the fact that he was able to flourish in the structured environment of Borstal, and (2) his evident artistic potential. Uncovering psychotherapy is one thing this man can do without. What he needs is a warm, long-term relationship, with the aim of developing his inner resources and supporting him through the stresses that he will inevitably encounter. But where is that likely to be found?

The (male) interviewer was quite clear in his own mind that a dynamic type of interview was entirely contra-indicated, and that what was needed was no more than an over-all assessment of the patient's strength and weakness, and in particular his frustration tolerance and impulse control. In this connection the history of attempted murder does not sound encouraging.

The interviewer deliberately adopted a friendly, sympathetic, natural manner towards him. No interpretations were made throughout the whole interview. The patient turned out to be an extremely pleasant young man. In place of the expected history of moving from job to job, he told of having kept jobs of the same kind throughout his working life; though it was also true that something always went wrong and he got the feeling he couldn't cope. His present position is that he just wants to sit in his room and drink. He had the insight to say that he knew the trouble was something in himself.

He said that he came from a background in the East End of London where one lived by violence, and anyone who wanted to be recognized had to come out on top. He said he used to be violent, but he 'had given up all that nonsense now'. The attempted murder had not been in a fit of rage but a deliberate act after extreme provocation – as he told it, it seemed almost like attempted justifiable homicide.

The two marriages had clearly been to feckless women with whom it was unlikely that any permanent relation would be possible.

Later in the interview he asked what was wrong with him. The interviewer said, 'Some people with bad backgrounds just don't develop certain qualities that enable them to cope with life.' In reply the patient said, 'Oh yes, my mother tried to kill me once or twice.' The interviewer did not ask for details and made no attempt to go into the background further.

All this information essentially confirmed the impression given by the doctor's referring letter. The interviewer ended by saying that there was no suitable treatment available at the Tavistock Clinic but he would make enquiries.

In the end the patient was referred to the Portman Clinic, which specializes in the treatment of patients who have been in trouble with the law, where he was offered a long-term group. The Consultant there said, 'It's a drop in the ocean, but it's better than nothing.'

The Man with Psychic Pain

A word like 'anguish' would probably be more appropriate but seems too dramatic.

The patient was 20. Extracts from his application form read as follows:

'First symptoms occurred at the age of 15: a sense of complete alienation from myself, as if I was inhabited by an entirely strange *persona*. For the first two years rather childish behaviour, after which a tendency to strike a solitary pose in company, and an inability to form any emotional relations. A sense of a very shallow existence ... I have attempted during recent months to penetrate into the obscured aspects of myself. This has only resulted in violent mental confusion and chaos, accompanied by obsessional thought.'

As with the Refugee Musician, this written material invites questions that have a crucial bearing on the kind of a person that he is, and hence on the prognosis with psychotherapy. The main questions are:

What is the quality 'being inhabited by a strange persona', how isolated is he, what does he mean by mental chaos, and what is the severity of obsessional phenomena?

In the account of the initial interview, with a male trainee psychiatrist, there is no record that any of these questions were investigated. The interviewer behaved in an unresponsive way, deliberately provoking transference phenomena, and eventually produced a good response to an interpretation that the patient wanted to humiliate the interviewer and feared humiliation in response.

He was given projection tests, both the ORT and Rorschach, which seemed to indicate Oedipal problems. The diagnosis and prognosis read, 'Adolescent character disorder. Should do well in a group.' He was put on the group waiting list.

About a year later, no group vacancy having become available, he asked to be seen to discuss the situation because he didn't want to go into a group. He was seen by a much more experienced psychiatrist, who at once recognized him as a type of patient not described in the books, and for whom there is no diagnostic label: someone disturbed at a very deep level, not psychotic, whose profound insight about himself must be taken as the absolute truth. In other settings this insight tends to make psychiatrists feel inferior and resentful, and that their job is being usurped; and they then tend to use labels like 'hysterical' or 'manipulating', with results that are not in the patient's best interest.

With quiet seriousness and total lack of histrionics, the patient told of his present position: that he is studying and has managed to keep going the whole time, but that he feels in danger of total breakdown; that he has managed to keep this at bay by developing a rigid routine – something that would arouse his contempt if he saw it in others – doing exactly the same things in exactly the same order day after day; that he feels the breakdown would occur if this routine were interrupted – e.g., since one of his solaces is music, if his record player broke down – or if his mother, the one person left in his life, should die. There was no difficulty in asking him what form he felt this breakdown would take. He said that he would not have the courage to kill himself or starve himself to death, but would just feel that life was no longer worth living and there was no point in getting out of bed. The interviewer accepted this as the truth and made absolutely no attempt to go deeper or to discover why the patient felt he had got like this.

Towards the end of the interview the patient began to ask questions about himself. With such a patient there is no point in anything but total honesty, and the interviewer answered straightforwardly to the best of his ability. What had gone wrong? The interviewer said he didn't know, but he knew the patient was in danger of a breakdown. Was he going crazy? The interviewer said he could see no evidence of this at all. If he had a breakdown, might it be for life? The interviewer, imagining the course of mental hospital treatment under medication, said he thought probably not, but that he would be likely to recover to the same kind of state as he was in at present.

The question was now what should be done. It seemed to the interviewer that with such a patient therapy should be *total* or *nil*. *Total* would almost certainly mean taking him into hospital and allowing him to regress and pass through whatever it was that lay underneath his defences, with daily psychotherapy. The Cassel Hospital might possibly provide this, but they quite rightly have a policy of short-term admissions; and it seemed only too probable that the patient, having lost his place at College and failed to qualify, would end up by being transferred to the only type of alternative institution, namely a mental hospital. As it seemed to the interviewer, any kind of half measures would just result in bringing on the breakdown and then mental hospital admission anyhow.

The patient himself had no wish to give up his studies, and the interviewer offered him the one thing that seemed appropriate, namely that he could get in touch at any time if he felt the need.

This is a kind of disposal that may be more valuable than it seems. At least the patient does not feel that he is entirely alone, and if he comes back in time, perhaps something can be done to prevent a breakdown that otherwise might seem inevitable. Again, just as this kind of patient can be entrusted with the absolute truth, he can also be trusted to tell the absolute truth; and the interviewer said that if the patient stated clearly how urgent it was, he would respond appropriately. The patient seemed grateful for this and went away.

The outcome of this is that he has asked to be seen just three times during the next 7 years (so much for any possible accusations of 'hysterical' or 'manipulating'). He has qualified and has held down a job throughout this period. Two brief extracts will give something of the quality of his experience.

Five years after the above interview he spoke of having begun to face his real self for the first time – he has found unfamiliar 'other personalities' within himself, sometimes as many as four or five. This is accompanied by the most intense psychic pain, sometimes bad enough for him to cry out in anguish when he is by himself. He spoke of himself in a way that conveyed the utmost profundity, but was largely beyond the interviewer's understanding. At 7 years, he spoke of physical symptoms accompanied by loss of weight, which he felt had been inadequately investigated by a physician. One day he weighed himself and found he had lost a stone, and this precipitated a state in which he couldn't stop shaking and was convulsed by what he called 'dry sobbing'. The interviewer could do no more than help find a second opinion for his physical condition, share his pain and despair, and reiterate that he was available for the patient to see at any time in the future.

Postscript

Many years later the interviewer was camping in a wild part of the Hebrides, and this patient himself walked past – few unlikelier settings for a follow-up interview can be imagined. The interviewer invited him to supper and used the opportunity to find out what had happened since he was last seen. The essence of this was that he had survived. He had not broken down, he was still working effectively in the same job, and he now appeared considerably less disturbed. It was also true that his mother had not died, so that he had not been put to the ultimate test. Nevertheless it does seem that the original action taken had been realistic and correct.

23

Assessment for psychotherapy (contd): VI. The consequences of making contact

In Chapter 18 I wrote of two incompatible statements: that you should not make interpretations until you know what kind of patient you are speaking to; and on the other hand, that you may not be able to find this out without making interpretations. Similarly, in Chapter 20, with the Film Director's Secretary I illustrated the flood of unconscious communication set in motion by a simple understanding comment. Finally, in Chapter 18 I also wrote that, whatever the consequences of your interview, you must take full responsibility for them. The present patient, who has been encountered before in Chapter 16 (see pp. 207ff.), gives point to all these themes.

The Foster Son (contd)

Anyone who recollects the material of Chapter 16 will perhaps have an inkling of what the present chapter is about.

The patient was a married man of 24 who wrote on his application form: 'Miserable, short tempered, insomnia, nightmares, no sex life, indifference. At least two years.'

The very helpful letter from the GP mentions that he had been studying at a college for further education in Liverpool and had been separated from his wife who was training as a nurse in London. On one occasion he had been picked up by the police in a fugal state at Crewe on his way home. His wife at this time had suggested that he had become *depressed at their separation*.

In his contacts with the medical profession he had shown difficult behaviour and a resistance to talking. He had once walked out of an interview with his GP, and when seen by a psychiatrist he had shown 'a selective refusal to discuss himself'. He had been on massive doses of tricyclic anti-depressants.

On his questionnaire he wrote about his childhood as follows:

'Never really knew father till he was home. I was 3 or 4. Mother left, I was 8. Went into Home [i.e. a children's home]. Went back to father for a while. Chose to go back to Home.'

The above statement, as laconic as that of the Man from Borstal, referred to the fact that he had arrived home from the pictures one Saturday morning to find that his mother had gone; and that the situation at home alone with his father had been so impossible that in the end he had preferred an institution. Later he had been fostered.

When he arrived for his consultation, the interviewer said 'I know you have difficulty in talking. How can I best help you to talk to me?' This sympathetic approach was ineffective. There was a passage that lasted about 25 minutes in which the patient could say little more than that he did not know what to say, even when asked questions. The most helpful communications that the interviewer was allowed were that 'sometimes things were bad and sometimes they were all right, and things were all right at the moment'; and when the interviewer said something about 'unhappiness' the patient said yes, sometimes he was unhappy but when this happened he 'didn't notice it'. The interviewer adopted the policy of breaking the silence from time to time with some comment that came to him, and conveying as far as he could an atmosphere of sympathetic acceptance. The best he could do for an interpretation was that the patient's silence must be due to his difficulty in trusting people, but this didn't seem to help any more than anything else.

The thought crossed the interviewer's mind that the patient was a simple schizophrenic, and he was beginning to despair, when the patient suddenly asked if he could smoke and began talking. When he did so it was clear that he was intelligent and insightful, and moreover there was a clear dynamic sequence to what he said.

From a long interview containing a great deal of information I shall pick out only a few moments. The patient described the situation of being in Liverpool and being visited by his wife for as much as a fortnight at a time. He said that when this happened they tended to be irritable with each other for a long period and when they began to recover from this it was getting near the time for her to go back. The interviewer felt it right to take the calculated risk of deepening rapport by the following interpretation: that surely what was happening was that at every separation each of them was feeling abandoned and angry with the other, and at each reunion it was necessary to go through these feelings before they could really feel together again. This seemed to mean something to him, the rapport did deepen, and he began to describe what it was like studying in Liverpool, ending by saying that he eventually got into a state in which he could hardly bear to leave home to go to College, and then to leave College to come home. To this the interviewer said that he could understand the first half easily enough, and surely the second half must mean that he had to put his armour on to face College and it was difficult to take it off again when he came home. The patient confirmed this by saying that home had become for him a place of absolute safety, and that once he got there he never wanted to leave again.

What had then happened was that he could neither face going in to College nor face telling his wife about this, so that he would leave in the morning, wander around Liverpool, and come back at his usual time. On one occasion, on impulse, he had gone to a chemist with a prescription for librium and had gradually taken the whole bottle during the course of the day.

This was not the kind of interview in which one could tie up ends, and the interviewer never heard the rest of the story. Instead the patient spontaneously associated to *violence* and *murder* – thus, as was shown clearly by subsequent events, unconsciously making the link between violence and suicide. He spoke of a TV thriller in which the villain had hit someone over the head and dropped him off a bridge into the traffic on a motorway. He said that his wife had been quite worried when he had begun to wonder if it might be possible to get away with something like this. The interviewer made a very carefully calculated comment, which was designed to help the patient to elaborate on his own violent feelings if he wanted to, and thus give evidence about the strength of his impulses and his capacity to control them: 'So first *she's* worried about your suicide and then about your violence.' In response the patient said that he had only been violent on a few occasions, and once he had grabbed his wife and had hurt her more than he intended.

This information was of course impossible to assess, but one thing that did seem certain was that he and his wife might well need help over their relation with each other. The patient said he was sure she would come for an assessment.

The interviewer felt that he had got about as far as he could in a single interview; and, as an attempt at forestalling potential resistance in the next interview, made an interpretation about the patient's silence at the beginning: 'surely just as you didn't want to take off your armour in Liverpool, you didn't want to do so with me.' The patient smiled and said, 'Well, it makes sense anyhow.' At the end he added, 'I'm glad I decided to start talking after all.'

To make interpretations of this kind, inviting trust, without knowing more about the patient, was a calculated risk to which the interviewer felt he had no alternative. The consequences of doing so will appear shortly.

The patient's wife was seen a week later. For brevity I shall leave out any details about her, and say only that the final result was that she herself was taken into individual therapy.

A few days after this the interviewer received a letter from the patient, from which the following are condensed extracts:

'I can write things down easier than I can talk so I'm doing just that.

'The doctor at out-patients in Liverpool said he thought he could help me better if I went to hospital [this was presumably after the overdose of librium mentioned above]. After a while his assistant in the hospital said that he could find nothing abnormal about my behaviour, goodbye . . .

'I cut myself with a razor not so long ago. Not to kill myself but out of anger and a curiosity to know if I could do it anyway. I was pleased I could do it but I would never cut my wrists – too slow. I wanted to watch blood mix with water till it was quite red.

'Once I killed one of the chickens in the yard but now we are the best of pals. I wanted to see if I could do it I suppose unless I'm just plain cruel.'

This statement is of course incomprehensible as it stands. As emerged later, what he had actually done was to half-kill a chicken and then bring it back to life by mouth-to-mouth respiration. This was made the more terrible as the chickens were known individually and each one had a name. It is now generally recognized – which the interviewer did not know at the time – that such acts are often found in the previous history of convicted murderers.

With this letter was enclosed a poem that he had written about 6 months before, the first and last verse of which are reproduced below (with the patient's permission, for which I would like to express my grateful thanks):

Stars and Time and Space and Life

Stars of shimmering violet, waning in their hues,
Changing into mellow golds and iridescent blues;
Shifting their positions round the Universe until
They come full circle, and they find that really they are still.

Life from Stars was born within the frame of Time and Space,
Changing ever is its form, the features of its face.
But Stars and Time and Space and Life are Universal toys,
That play with creatures such as me – and other little boys.

The trust implied in the letter and the poem, conveying the two sides of his true nature, were the first consequence of the contact established in the initial interview.

In a second interview he was much freer from the beginning. His wife had mentioned that he had been suffering from disturbing dreams, and as a way into his fantasy world the interviewer asked him about these. One was as follows:

'There was a sort of refrigerator in a room. He got into telepathic communication with it and realized it had more power than he had. There were two other men in the room and a pair of arms appeared out of the refrigerator and squashed one of the men till he was like a roll of beef done up in string. Then a knife appeared and cut him in half. The other man went on as if nothing had happened.'

Although this is only a dream, it possesses features which should alert any interviewer – telepathic communication with a machine, primitive violence with hints of cannibalism, total lack of concern – where has one met such things before? With sinking heart the interviewer went into the routine 'psychotic' questions, in response to which the patient freely admitted to ideas of reference – while walking down the street he would answer people back who he imagined were passing remarks about him – and visual and auditory hallucinations.

Towards the end he agreed to come and see a psychologist as the next step; and the interviewer said that he was not sure that the Clinic could help, though they would try. The patient said very warmly, 'It's the trying that matters.'

This warm reaction, though of course genuine, was not all that it seemed. His wife now reported that he had been exceedingly upset after this second interview: that he could see intellectually that it was reasonable for the Clinic not to promise anything, but emotionally it seemed like the rejection at Liverpool all over again; he had had the impulse to cut himself with a razor; he had had a nightmare in which something terrible was pulling him out of his own body, from which he had woken screaming; he had remained in their room for three days and refused to go out; and he had started a daydream one day which had lasted into the next.

These were the consequences of having made contact, invited trust, raised hopes, and then made no promises. One may ask, what on the other hand would have been the consequences of never having got this far, and having referred him back to his GP, or given him to an inexperienced trainee for individual psychotherapy without supervision, or made the judgement 'should do well in a group'?

With the situation as it was, we may pause to consider the possibilities. The patient has given abundant evidence of ability to work in interpretative therapy, very high motivation, and creative potential, on the one hand; and evidence of being on the edge of psychotic breakdown, suicidal and other self-destructive behaviour, homicidal fantasies, and an act which could indeed be the prelude to murder, on the other. Do we send him elsewhere – to a mental hospital where he will get drugs, or a day hospital where he will get a therapeutic community but little individual attention, or a psychiatric teaching hospital where at best he will get a series of psychotherapists who change every six or nine months? After this depth of contact, what will be the consequences of sending him anywhere other than to the Clinic to which he has become attached?

What, on the other hand, will be the consequence of taking him on for uncovering psychotherapy, and who is likely to want to take the risk? It would be an act of total irresponsibility to offer him to a trainee, and experienced therapists no longer have either the time or the inclination for this kind of heroic task. For most therapists, one such patient in a lifetime is enough, and the interviewer had fulfilled his quota.

With a certain amount of hindsight, it is possible to forecast some of the phenomena that will be encountered with this patient in uncovering psychotherapy. The trauma of his life was his mother's sudden betrayal and abandonment – and there seems little doubt that dependence on the therapist will become a major issue, and that the main dangers will occur around breaks in treatment. Similarly, there is little difficulty in forecasting that the kinds of impulse likely to appear will involve: (1) suicide; (2) self-mutilation; and (3) homicide; and that the central aim of therapy will be to reach the *depressive position* – destructive feelings directed towards the very person whom he loves and needs. This will of course be the therapist, representing his mother. Therapy will constitute the ultimate test of any therapist's sincerity, sensitivity, courage, and skill; and it will hover on the knife edge of arousing all these feelings uncontrollably on the one hand, and failing to arouse them and hence to resolve them, on the other. Absolutely essential will be the establishment of a strong therapeutic alliance, without which some catastrophe will inevitably ensue. Shall we call for volunteers?

Yet the strength of patients of this kind is their mute appeal. Quite unconsciously, and with total honesty, he had played his cards just right. He had told us the worst and the best about himself at the same time. It was the poem that tipped the scales: one sensed that he was not going to be a merciless killer – though as events turned out, and as implied by the dream, he was nearer to this than might be imagined. In the end it was possible to find not merely a volunteer, but someone who *wanted* to treat him.

This was the psychologist who gave him a projection test, a woman of moderate experience and exceptional sensitivity. The arrangements were carefully planned within the resources of a purely out-patient clinic. The therapist was given the constant support of a highly experienced analytically trained psychiatrist. The frequency of therapy was chosen as twice a week – once a week being felt to be insufficient, and three times a week to invite too much regression. Finally, there was careful liaison with a tough-minded but caring General Practitioner, who continued to treat him with major tranquillizers and anti-depressants throughout much of the course of therapy.

The patient showed exceedingly disturbed behaviour from the beginning. Suicide was less of an issue than one might suppose, though he did arrive for one session with 625 mg of Tryptizol inside him. Self-mutilation was a constant issue. At times of stress, particularly around breaks in treatment, he had an uncontrollable urge to follow the veins on his forearm with a razor blade. This did not have the quality of a suicidal impulse, but rather an act of self-directed aggression. On one occasion he brought the therapist a jar of his own blood, obtained in this way. He later explained in a letter that this was 'a sexual advance of a strange kind. You will see similarities of blood/life/closeness/ pain/pleasure, to semen/new life/sexual intimacy, etc. You may be interested to know that my fantasy was that my therapist would drink that blood.' In the later stages of therapy, as described in Chapter 19, homicide did become a serious danger. Finally, the climax of therapy did indeed involve the depressive position.

Although it cannot be claimed that these events were forecast in detail, they were sufficiently foreseen to make possible a realistic therapeutic setting. The patient therefore brings together some of the themes that have run throughout many chapters of this book: the therapist's need for sympathy and ruthlessness at the same time; the power of interpretation; the appalling load of conflicting impulses with which human beings have been burdened; and the fact that careful assessment can sometimes lead to accurate prediction, and the realistic planning of an effective intervention.

24

The future of psychotherapy and psychodynamics

The science of psychodynamics

One of the aims of the present book, obviously, has been to explain the principles of dynamic psychotherapy; but another, which is really much more important, has been to abstract from the principles of psychoanalysis the core of scientific truth, which we may call the science of psychodynamics. I do not believe that anyone truly impartial can fail to accept certain psychodynamic phenomena as scientific facts. This applies, for instance, to 'defence, anxiety, and hidden feeling', and hence the existence of 'the unconscious'; the 'return of the repressed'; transference; and the validation of these concepts through direct observation of the response to interpretation. It does not apply to such concepts as 'oral, anal, and genital', or the libido theory, both of which are in my opinion over-simplifications based on a narrow and unsatisfactory view of human instinct. The slavish adherence to them has held up the proper understanding of human beings for generations.

Dynamic theory and learning theory

It follows from all the above that any theory of the human psyche, and any form of psychotherapy, *must* be incomplete unless it incorporates the psychodynamic point of view. This applies particularly, of course, to learning theory and behaviour therapy. But the converse is also true: dynamic psychotherapy itself is incomplete unless it incorporates the theory and techniques of other forms of therapy, of which behaviour therapy is probably the most important. It seems to me undeniable, for instance, that the success of behaviour therapy in dealing with certain symptoms, without dealing with unconscious conflict, means that there is something missing in psychodynamic theory in this area; and that some process such as self-reinforcement must be operating to maintain symptoms and give them autonomy. On the other hand, honest behaviour therapists will readily admit that their own explanations of the *origin* of symptoms – a question to which the psychodynamic approach has a fairly complete answer – is hopelessly insufficient.

The incomplete effectiveness of both dynamic psychotherapy and behaviour therapy

Something very similar applies to technique. During the course of many years of following up the results of dynamic psychotherapy, I have repeatedly observed patients who have recovered from almost all their personality problems and yet still suffer from residual symptoms, which are often phobic in nature. Such patients are crying out for the addition of behaviour therapy to their dynamic psychotherapy.

Clearly – once more – the converse is also true. Pure behaviour therapy deals well with symptoms but leaves many kinds of personality problems untouched. Patients with such problems are crying out for dynamic psychotherapy to be added to their behaviour therapy.

The integration of dynamic psychotherapy and behaviour therapy

A number of therapists have experimented with this combination and have obtained encouraging results. Examples are Birk (1970), Birk and Brinkley-Birk (1974), Feather and Rhoads (1972), Segraves and Smith (1976), and Fensterheim (1993). In particular, Segraves and Smith have presented strong evidence that the introduction of behaviour therapy activates the unconscious of patients who have got stuck in their dynamic psychotherapy, thus bringing into effective therapy patients who might otherwise never come out of their state of resistance. Nevertheless this type of approach has apparently not been used *routinely* by dynamic psychotherapists in patients for whom it might be thought appropriate.

The 'passive sounding board' technique

Let us now consider the pure technique of psychoanalysis itself, in which the therapist acts as a passive sounding board and confines his interventions to interpretations and nothing else. During a follow-up study of 114 patients who had been given individual dynamic psychotherapy, we accumulated much evidence of the bitter resentment left in patients by this technique, which had either been taken too literally by the therapist and/or had been inappropriately transferred from psychoanalysis to less intensive treatment. Below is a quotation from the follow-up interview with a male patient who had been seen by an experienced therapist for 700 sessions at twice a week:

'When he congratulated me on my son's birth and shook my hand, I thought, "Christ, it's the first time he's made any gesture of human contact towards me".'

How can patients who feel like this, and above all who cannot bring themselves to speak of it, be expected to open their hearts to their therapists?

Remarks of this kind were reported considerably more frequently by patients who had done badly, which suggests that in many therapies the passive sounding board technique is not only *inhuman* but *ineffective*.

As the other side of the coin to this observation, we found that a number of patients remembered above all, not interpretations from their therapist, but moments of straightforward humanity. The following is an example:

The patient had had an argument with her tutor at College. She described this to her (woman) therapist, expecting to receive comments that she would have interpreted as criticism. Instead, she got the answer, 'Oh yes, these situations can be so trying, can't they?' At follow-up the patient said, 'Here was someone who was fond of me as a person and prepared to be sympathetic. This was the most positive experience in therapy that I can remember. It was a turning point. Up till then I had found it very difficult to trust her.'

Remarks of this kind were reported more frequently by patients who had done well, which implies that therapists who behave humanly towards their patients tend to get better therapeutic results.

These two complementary observations need to be taken to heart by therapists of all persuasions – including psychoanalysts – but above all by those practising less intensive methods, in which the passive sounding board technique is in my view totally inappropriate and should be summarily abandoned.

(Aspects of this study are reported in Clementel-Jones and Malan, 1988, and Clementel-Jones, Malan and Trauer, 1990.)

The need to integrate further the techniques of different forms of psychotherapy

Here I can only scratch the surface of developments in psychotherapy in the past decade.

The present book has concentrated on the principles of working with patients of a special kind, namely those with whom a psychodynamic dialogue may be readily set up. Obviously, such patients are the best to use for an exposition of psychodynamics and dynamic psychotherapy. There are enough of them to occupy psychotherapists thousands of times over, but they may still represent only a small proportion of the total psychiatric population. In particular, there are two classes of patient with whom purely dynamic psychotherapy tends to be ineffective: (1) those who are very fragile or badly damaged emotionally; and (2) those who either start with massive resistance or else develop subtle forms of impenetrable resistance during their therapy.

Fragile patients

'Cognitive analytic therapy', as developed by Ryle (1990; Ryle and Low, 1993) seems particularly suitable for this kind of patient. Here the technique is essentially psychodynamic, but it also incorporates powerful collaborative and directive elements, within an atmosphere of warmth and support: e.g. writing in collaboration with the patient an essay summarizing the patient's problems, together with ideas about their origin, and setting tasks for homework. Clinical evidence suggests that for fragile patients this may be both more effective and safer than purely interpretative therapy.

Resistance

We may now turn to the problem of intractable resistance. Here there are two different kinds of patient, both of which are encountered only too often. The first consists of certain patients suffering from chronic character problems, who are not in the least motivated to give up their ingrained defences, are quite unsuitable for behavioural methods, and are utterly resistant to purely interpretative work. The second kind consists of those who show a much more subtle kind of resistance: with them, therapy reaches a stage in which there are clear responses to interpretation in every session, so that the therapist is kept happy feeling he is doing excellent work, the only trouble being that the patient doesn't change. How we could wish that there were a technique of dynamic psychotherapy which could be used with both these types of patient, and could produce major therapeutic effects!

Davanloo

Well, perhaps there is. In the first edition of the present book I wrote of the work of Davanloo, as follows:

> Even within the framework of pure dynamic psychotherapy, it has been shown incontrovertibly that a highly active, confronting technique can reach and *cure* certain phobic and obsessional patients within a few months who have been quite unresponsive to both behaviour therapy and psychoanalytic therapy for many years ... Some of this work, most of which remains unpublished, has been presented on videotape at three International Symposia on Short-term Dynamic Psychotherapy, and has already had considerable impact on psychotherapy throughout the world [see Davanloo, 1978, 1980, and 1990]. I am convinced, as a sober judgement made from intimate knowledge, that Davanloo's work is destined to go much further than this, and to revolutionize both the practice and the scientific status of dynamic psychotherapy within the next ten years – anyone who has seen these tapes cannot fail to be convinced both of the effectiveness of dynamic psychotherapy and of the truth of basic psychodynamic theory.

What of the situation now, as I write some 15 years later? I stand by most of what I wrote then, but there is one exception. This is the statement that Davanloo's work will revolutionize dynamic psychotherapy within the next ten years, which clearly hasn't happened. The obstacle has been the difficulty of transferring Davanloo's highly idiosyncratic style to other therapists.

Developments from Davanloo's technique

Some of Davanloo's supervisees have reacted against his technique, finding that they cannot use it effectively, and are developing a technique diametrically opposite to his. Thus Alpert and his collaborators at the St Clare's Riverside Center in New York are experimenting with an approach which they call 'Accelerated Empathic Therapy' (see Alpert, 1992 and articles by other authors in the same issue of the *International Journal of Short-term Psychotherapy*). In this approach the emphasis is on therapists' expression of overt sympathy for the patient's suffering, even to the point of openly acknowledging their own distress about it. They have elevated *grief* to the principal place in therapy, at the expense of anger, which in my view is going much too far. Nevertheless I have seen videotapes in which this approach achieved a breakthrough in patients unresponsive to a more confronting technique.

McCullough (1993a), also one of Davanloo's former trainees, has adopted a more eclectic approach to his teaching. Like him, she starts by concentrating on the defences, but in a more overtly sympathetic way. She gives as a typical example an intervention dealing with secondary gain: not the confronting, 'What are you getting out of this?', but the more sympathetic, 'It must be terribly hard to give this up. Let's see if we can discover what it gives you.' There is little doubt that many therapists feel much more comfortable with an approach of this kind.

In conformity with the tendency towards integration, McCullough has also introduced a number of techniques and aspects of theory derived from other forms of psychotherapy. The following quotations are from an unpublished application for a research grant (McCullough, 1993b). The italics are mine.

(1) 'Difficult' patients need more than mere insight regarding their feeling life. They need to be literally *desensitized* to their internal affective state until their underlying feelings no longer terrify or shame them.'
(2) 'The interventions used to achieve the relinquishing of defenses are drawn in part from *cognitive therapy*. The therapist must identify the anxieties which maintain the defensive behaviors and assist the patient in coming to see the lack of logic in their fears.'
(3) 'The techniques used to help the patient to experience conflicted feelings are drawn from *gestalt therapy*. Guided imagery to elicit affects, and close attention to the physiological concomitants of emotion heighten the experience.'

Thus one of the most hopeful developments in the whole field is the growing tendency to break away from rigid and compartmentalized systems, practised with religious fervour, to the adoption and integration of what seem to be the most effective elements in each.

A look into the future

It does appear that Davanloo has developed a method of brief, purely psychodynamic, psychotherapy applicable to a far wider range of *patients* than can be treated by conventional methods. What is needed now is a technique incorporating some of his discoveries which is applicable to a wider range of *therapists*. As described above, this is what some of Davanloo's ex-trainees are trying to explore. In fact it may well be that two of his major contributions do not consist so much of his particular style of confrontation, but: (1) the need to begin therapy by actively concentrating on the defences to the exclusion of all else; and (2) the emphasis not merely on *response to interpretation* but on the *direct experience* of the formerly buried feelings.

In the field of commercial invention, one of the dangers of patenting a discovery (and thus of necessity publishing it), is that other scientists – encouraged by knowing that such an invention is *possible* – may start searching for their own version which the patent does not cover. In our field, fortunately, this would be regarded not as a danger but as a welcome development. It might therefore be that Davanloo's *most* important contribution is simply the demonstration that widely applicable brief dynamic psychotherapy is possible, so that other therapists are encouraged to use some of his ideas in order to find equally effective methods that suit their own personalities. This may be the crucial development of the next decade.

References

Alexander, F. and French, T. M. (1946) *Psychoanalytic therapy*, Ronald Press, New York.

Alpert, M. C. (1992) Accelerated emphatic therapy: a new short-term dynamic psychotherapy. *Int. J. Short-term Psychother.*, **7**, 133.

American Psychiatric Association (1994) *Diagnostic and statistical manual of mental disorders, 4th edn*, Americal Psychiatric Association, Washington, DC.

Balint, M. (1949) Early developmental states of the ego. Primary object-love. *Int. J. Psychoanal.*, **30**, 265. Reprinted in *Primary love and psycho-analytic technique*, Tavistock, London (1964): Liveright, New York (1965).

Balint, M. (1952) New beginning and the paranoid and depressive syndromes. *Int. J. Psychoanal.*, **33**, 214.

Birk, L. (1970) Behavior therapy – integration with dynamic psychiatry. *Behavior therapy*, **1**, 522.

Birk, L. and Brinkley-Birk, A. W. (1974) Psychoanalysis and behavior therapy. *Am. J. Psychiat.*, **131**, 499.

Bowlby, J. (1953) Some pathological processes set in motion by early mother–child separation. *J. Ment. Sci.*, **99**, 265.

Bowlby, J. (1969) *Attachment and loss.*, vol. I: *Attachment*, Hogarth, London.

Bowlby, J. (1973) *Attachment and loss*, vol. II: *Separation: Anxiety and anger*, Hogarth, London.

Browne, S. E. (1964) Short psychotherapy with passive patients. *Br. J. Psychiat.*, **110**, 233.

Clementel-Jones, C. and Malan, D. H. (1988) Outcome of dynamic psychotherapy. *Br. J. Psychother.*, **5**, 29.

Clementel-Jones, C., Malan, D.H. and Trauer, T. (1990) A retrospective follow-up study of 84 patients treated with individual psychoanaytic psychotherapy. *Br. J. Psychother.*, **6**, 363.

Davanloo, H. (1978) *Basic principles and techniques in short-term dynamic psychotherapy*, Spectrum, New York.

Davanloo, H. (1980) *Short-term dynamic psychotherapy*, Jason Aronson, New York.

Davanloo, H. (1990) *Unlocking the unconscious*, Wiley, Chichester.

Feather, B. W. and Rhoads, J. M. (1972) Psychodynamic behavior therapy. II. Clinical Aspects. *Psychiat.*, **26**, 503.

Fensterheim, H. (1993). Behavioral psychotherapy. In Stricker and Gold (1993), pp. 73–85.

Freud, S. (1905) *Three essays on the theory of sexuality*, Standard edn. Vol. VII, Hogarth, London, pp. 125–245.

Freud, S. (1913) *Totem and taboo*, Standard edn, vol. XIII, Hogarth, London, pp. 1–62.

Freud, S. (1914) *Remembering, repeating* and *working-through*, Standard edn, vol. XII, Hogarth, London, pp. 145–56.

Freud, S. (1915) *Observations on transference-love*, Standard edn, vol. XII, Hogarth, London, pp. 157–73.

Freud, S. (1917) *Mourning and melancholia*, Standard edn, vol. XIV, Hogarth, London, pp. 243–58.

Freud, S. (1920) *Beyond the pleasure principle*, Standard edn, vol. XVIII, Hogarth, London, pp. 7–64.

Graves, R. (1955) *The Greek myths*, vols. I and II, Penguin, Harmondsworth.

Handford (ed) (1954) *Aesop's Fables*, Penguin, Harmondsworth.

Horowitz, M. J. (1976) *Stress response syndromes*, Jason Aronson, New York.
Jones, E. (1953) *Sigmund Freud: Life and work*, vol. I, Hogarth, London.
Klein, M. (1975) *Love, guilt and reparation.* Hogarth, London.
Lorenz, K. (1966) *On aggression*, Methuen, London.
Malan, D. H. (1963) *A study of brief psychotherapy*, Tavistock, London. Reprinted by Plenum, New York (1975).
Malan, D. H. (1976a) *The frontier of brief psychotherapy*, Plenum, New York.
Malan, D. H. (1976b) *Toward the validation of dynamic psychotherapy*, Plenum, New York.
Malan and Osimo, F. (1992) *Psychodynamics, training, and outcome in brief psychotherapy*, Butterworth-Heinemann, Oxford.
Malan, D. H., Balfour, F. H. G., Hood, V. G. and Shooter, A. M. N. (1976) Group psychotherapy: a long-term follow-up study. *Arch. Gen. Psychiat.*, **33**, 1303.
Malan, D. H., Heath, E. S., Bacal, H. A. and Balfour, F. H. G. (1975) Psychodyamic changes in untreated neurotic patients. II Apparently genuine improvements. *Arch. Gen. Psychiat.*, **32**, 110.
McCullough, L. (1993a) An anxiety-reduction modification of short-term dynamic psychotherapy (STDP): a theoretical 'melting pot' of treatment techniques. In Stricker, G. and Gold, J. R. (1993), pp. 139–49.
McCullough, L. (1993b) STDP objectives – a process study. Unpublished application for a research grant.
Menninger, K. (1958) *Theory of psychoanalytic technique*, Basic Books, New York.
Milner, M. (1969) *The hands of the living God: an account of a psychoanalytic treatment*, Hogarth, London.
Phillipson, H. (1955) *The object relations technique*, Tavistock, London; The Free Press, Glencoe, Ill.
Robertson, J. (1952) Film: *A two-year-old goes to hospital*, Tavistock Child Development Research Unit, London; New York University Film Library, New York.
Robertson, J. (1953) Some responses of young children to the loss of maternal care. *Nurs. Times*, **49**, 382.
Ryle, A. (1990) *Cognitive-analytic therapy: active participation in change*, Wiley, Chichester.
Ryle, A. and Low, J. (1993) Cognitive analytic therapy. In Stricker, G. and Gold, J. R. (1993), pp. 87–100.
Sechehaye, M. A. (1951) *Symbolic realization*, International Universities Press, New York.
Segraves, R. T. and Smith, R. C. (1976) Concurrent psychotherapy and behavior therapy. *Arch. gen. Psychiat.*, **33**, 756.
Sifneos, P. E. (1972) *Short-term psychotherapy and emotional crisis*, Harvard University Press, Cambridge, Mass.
Stricker, G. and Gold, J. R. (1993) *Comprehensive handbook of psychotherapy integration*, Plenum, New York.
Truax, C. B. and Carkhuff, R. R. (1967) *Toward effective counseling and psychotherapy*, Aldine, Chicago.
Winnicott, D. W. (1958) Collected papers: *Through paediatrics to psycho-analysis*, Karnac, London.

Index

Note: In order to minimize the number of sub-headings, main entries will often be found under the adjective, e.g. 'obsessional anxiety', not 'anxiety, obsessional', and there may be several main entries beginning with the same adjective, e.g. in addition 'obsessional personality', 'obsessional rituals'.